BESTMEDICINE

Osteoporosis

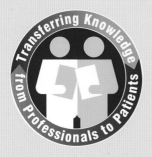

Dr George Kassianos
Professor Juliet Compston
Dr Pam Brown

Foreword by Claire Rayner
President of the Patients Association

Managing Editor: Dr Scott Chambers
Medical Writers: Dr Eleanor Bull, Dr Anna Palmer, Dr Rebecca Fox-Spencer
Editorial Controller: Emma Catherall
Operations Manager: Julia Potterton
Designer: Chris Matthews
Typesetter: Julie Smith
Glossary: Dr Susan Chambers
Indexer: Laurence Errington
Director – Online Business: Peter Llewellyn
Publishing Director: Julian Grover
Publisher: Stephen I'Anson

1 Bankside
Lodge Road
Long Hanborough
Oxfordshire
OX29 8LJ, UK
Tel: +44 (0)1993 885370
Fax: +44 (0)1993 881868
Email: *enquiries@bestmedicine.com*

www.bestmedicine.com
www.csfmedical.com

The content of *BESTMEDICINE* is the work of a number of authors and has been produced in line with our standard editorial procedures, including the peer review of the disease overview and the drug reviews, and the passing of the final manuscript for publication by the Managing Editor and the Editor-in-Chief or the Medical Editor. Whilst every effort has been made to ensure the accuracy of the information at the date of approval for publication, the Authors, the Publisher, the Editors and the Editorial Board accept no responsibility whatsoever for any errors or omissions or for any consequences arising from anything included in or excluded from *BESTMEDICINE*.

All reasonable effort is made to avoid infringement of copyright law, including the redrawing of figures adapted from other sources. Where copyright permission has been deemed necessary, attempts are made to gain appropriate permission from the copyright holder. However, the Authors, the Publisher, the Editors and the Editorial Board accept no personal responsibility for any infringement of copyright law howsoever made. Any queries regarding copyright approvals or permissions should be addressed to the Managing Editor.

You are strongly urged to consult your doctor before taking, stopping or changing any of the products reviewed or referred to in *BESTMEDICINE* or any other medication that has been prescribed or recommended by your doctor.

A catalogue record for this book is available from the British Library.

ISBN: 1-905064-81-0

Typeset by Creative, Langbank, Scotland.
Printed and bound by KHL Printing Co PTE Ltd, Singapore.
Distributed by NBN International, Plymouth, Devon.

Contents

Foreword

Claire Rayner
President of The Patients Association

Patients and their families are rightly entitled to have access to good-quality, independent and reliable information concerning a diverse range of conditions and a wide variety of medications that are available to treat them. Indeed, there is a growing recognition amongst the majority of healthcare professionals that well-informed patients are more likely to adopt a more active role in the management of their illness and will therefore feel more satisfied with the care that they receive. Such an effect has the potential not only to directly benefit the patient and their families, but can also maximise limited healthcare resources within an already over-stretched NHS. However, at present access to this kind of information is limited, despite the fact that as many as one-in-four adults (12 million people in the UK alone) want ready access to this knowledge prior to visiting their doctor.

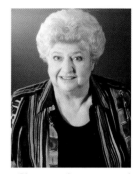

Photograph courtesy of
Amanda Rayner

    The importance of patient self-management is a key component of current NHS strategy. Indeed, this has been widely acknowledged in an NHS-led campaign called the Expert Patient Programme (*www.expertpatient.nhs.uk*). This is a self-management course which aims to give people the confidence, skills and knowledge to manage their condition better and take greater control of their lives. The Expert Patient Programme defines an Expert Patient as one who has had the condition for long enough to have learnt the language doctors use.

    BESTMEDICINE aims to meet the information and educational needs of both patients and healthcare professionals alike. The information found in the *BESTMEDICINE* series will assist patients and their families to obtain the level of information they now need to understand and manage their medical condition in partnership with their doctor. As *BESTMEDICINE* draws much of its content from medical publications written by doctors for doctors, some readers may find these books rather challenging when they first approach them. Despite this, I strongly believe that the effort that you invest in reading this book will be fully repaid by the increased knowledge that you will gain about this condition. Indeed, the extensive glossary of terms that can be found within each book certainly makes understanding the text a great deal easier, and the Patient Notes section is also very informative and reassuringly written by a doctor for the less scientifically minded reader. *BESTMEDICINE* represents the world's first source of independent, unabridged medical information that will appeal to patients and their families as well as healthcare professionals. This development should be welcomed and applauded, and I would commend these books to you.

Claire Rayner

Claire Rayner has been involved with the Patients Association for many years and has considerable expertise and experience from a professional background in nursing and journalism and her personal experience both as a patient and as a carer. She is well known as a leading 'Agony Aunt' and as a medical correspondent for many popular magazines. Claire has also published articles in a number of professional journals, as well as over forty medical, nursing and patient advice books.

An introduction to *BESTMEDICINE*

The source: information for healthcare professionals

Over the years, it has become increasingly apparent that there is a dearth of drug-related information that is independently compiled and robustly reviewed, and which also acknowledges the challenges faced by healthcare professionals when applying evidence-based medicine whilst practising at the 'front line' of patient care. As such, many healthcare professionals feel a certain ambivalence towards the numerous drug review publications that are currently on offer and, indeed, many do not have confidence in the information that can be found within their pages. In response to the need for a more impartial information resource – one that is independent of the pharmaceutical industry and the health service – we developed a novel publication, which was launched to meet this perceived lack of independent information. This peer-reviewed publication is called *Drugs in Context* and was launched in May 2003 and is the source of much of what you will find in this edition of *BESTMEDICINE*.

Uniquely independent

Drugs in Context is unique in that it reviews the significant clinical and pharmacological evidence underpinning the use of a single drug, in the disease area(s) where it is used and the practice setting where it is most commonly prescribed. Over 50 issues are published each year covering numerous diseases and conditions. The principal goal of *Drugs in Context* is to become the definitive drug and disease management resource for all healthcare professionals. As such, over the coming years, the publication plans to review all of the significant drugs that are currently used in clinical practice.

Reliable and impartial information for patients too

In addition to the lack of impartial information for the healthcare professional, we also firmly believe that there is a significant and growing number of patients who are not served well in this regard either. Indeed, it is becoming apparent to us that many patients would welcome access to the same sources of information on drugs and diseases that their doctors and other healthcare professionals have access to.

There are numerous sources of information currently available to patients – ranging from leaflets and books to websites and other electronic media. However, despite their best intentions, the rigour and accuracy of many of these resources cannot always be relied upon due to significant variation in the quality of the material. Perhaps the major problem facing a patient or a loved one who is hunting for specific information relating to a disease or the drug that has been prescribed by their doctor is that there is simply too much material available, making sifting through it to find a relevant fact akin to looking for a needle in a haystack! More importantly, many of these resources can often (albeit unintentionally) patronise the reader who has made every effort to actively seek out information that can serve to reassure themselves about the relevant illness and the medication(s) prescribed for it.

Can knowledge be the 'BESTMEDICINE'?

We firmly believe as healthcare professionals, that an informed patient is more likely to take an active role in the management of their disease or condition and, therefore, will be more likely to benefit from any course of treatment. This means that everyone will benefit – the patient, their family and friends, the healthcare professionals involved in their care, and the NHS and the country as a whole! Indeed, such is the importance of patient education, that the NHS has launched an initiative emphasising the need for patients to assume a more active role in the management of their condition via the acquisition of knowledge and skills related specifically to their disease. This initiative is called the Expert Patients Programme (*www.expertpatients.nhs.uk*).

Filling the need for quality information

Many of our observations about the lack of quality education have underpinned the principles behind the launch of *BESTMEDICINE*, much of the content of which is drawn directly from the pages of *Drugs in Context*, as written by and for healthcare professionals. *BESTMEDICINE* aims to appeal primarily to the patient, loved-one or carer who wants to improve their knowledge of the disease in question, the evidence for and against the drugs available to treat the disease and the practical challenges faced by healthcare professionals in managing it.

A whole new language!

We fully acknowledge that a lot of medical terminology used in order to expedite communication amongst the medical community will be new to many of you, some terms may be difficult to pronounce and sometimes surplus to requirements. However, rather than significantly abridge the content and risk excluding something of importance to the reader, we have instead provided you with a comprehensive glossary of terms and what we hope will be helpful additional GP discussion pieces at the end of each section to aid understanding further. We have also provided you with an introduction to the processes underlying drug development and the key concepts in disease management which we hope you will also find informative and which we strongly recommend that you read before tackling the rest of this edition of *BESTMEDICINE*.

No secrets

By providing the same information to patients and their families as healthcare professionals we believe that *BESTMEDICINE* will help to foster better relationships between patients, their families and doctors and other healthcare professionals, and ultimately may even improve treatment outcomes.

This edition is one of a number of unique collections of disease summaries and drug reviews that we will be making widely available over the coming months. You will find details about each issue as it is published at *www.bestmedicine.com*.

We do hope that you find this edition of *BESTMEDICINE* illuminating.

Dr George Kassianos, GP, Bracknell; Editor-in-Chief – *Drugs in Context*;
    Editor – *BESTMEDICINE*
Dr Jonathan Morrell, GP, Hastings; Medical Editor (Primary Care) –
    Drugs in Context
Dr Michael Schachter, Consultant Physician, St Mary's Hospital
    Paddington; Clinical Pharmacology Editor – *Drugs in Context*

Reader's guide

We acknowledge that some of the medical and scientific terminology used throughout *BESTMEDICINE* will be new to you and will address sometimes challenging concepts. However, rather than abridge the content and risk excluding important information, we have included this Reader's Guide to dissect and explain the contents of *BESTMEDICINE* in order to make it more digestible to the less scientifically minded reader. We recommend that you familiarise yourself with the drug development process, summarised below, before embarking on the Drug Reviews. This brief synopsis clarifies and contextualises many of the specialist terms encountered in the Drug Reviews.

Following this Reader's Guide, you will find that *BESTMEDICINE* is made up of three main sections – a Disease Overview, an overview of Management Options and Drug Reviews – each of which are evidence-based and as such have been highly referenced. All references are listed at the end of each section. Importantly, the manuscript has been 'peer-reviewed', which means that it has undergone rigorous checks for accuracy both by a practising doctor and a specialist in drug pharmacology. These sections are sandwiched between two opinion pieces, an Editorial, written by a recognised expert in the field, and an Improving Practice article, written by a practising GP with a specialist interest in the disease area. It is important to bear in mind that these authors are addressing their professional colleagues, rather than a 'lay' reader, providing you with a fascinating and unique insight into many of the challenges faced by doctors in the day-to-day practice of medicine.

The Disease Overview, Drug Reviews and Improving Practice sections are all followed by a short commentary by Dr Pam Brown entitled Patient Notes. In these sections, Dr Brown reiterates some of the key issues raised in rather more 'patient-friendly' language.

As mentioned previously, much of the content of *BESTMEDICINE* has been taken directly from *Drugs in Context*, which is written by and for healthcare professionals. Consequently, some of the language used may be difficult for the less scientifically minded reader. To help with this, in addition to the Patient Notes, we have included a comprehensive glossary of terms found throughout the text.

Disease overview

The disease overview provides a brief synopsis of the disease, its symptoms, diagnosis and a critique of the currently available treatment options.

- The epidemiology, or incidence and distribution of the disease within a population, is discussed, with particular emphasis on UK-specific data.
- The aetiology section describes the specific causes or origins of the disease, which are usually a result of both genetic and environmental

factors. Multifactorial diseases result from more than one causative element. If an individual has a genetic predisposition, they are more susceptible to developing the disease as a result of their genetic make-up.

- The functional changes that accompany a particular syndrome or disease constitute its pathophysiology.
- The management of a disease may be influenced by treatment guidelines, specific directives published by government agencies, professional societies, or by the convening of expert panels. The National Institute for Health and Clinical Excellence (NICE), an independent sector of the NHS comprised of experts in the field of treatment, is one such body.
- The social and economic factors that characterise the influence of the disease, describe its socioeconomic impact. Such factors include the cost to the healthcare provider to treat the disease – in terms of GP consultations, drug costs and the subsequent burden on hospital resources – or the cost to the patient or employer with respect to the number of work days lost as a consequence of ill health.

Drug reviews

☛ The pharmacokinetics of a drug are of interest to healthcare professionals because it is important for them to understand the action of a drug on the body over a period of time.

The drug reviews are not intended to address every available treatment for a particular disease. Rather, we focus on the major drugs currently available in the UK for the treatment of the featured disease and evaluate their performance in clinical trials and their safety in clinical practice. The basic pharmacology of the drug – the branch of science that deals with the origin, nature, chemistry, effects and uses of drugs – is discussed initially. This includes a description of the mechanism of action of the drug, the manner in which it exerts its therapeutic effects, and its pharmacokinetics (or the activity of the drug within the body over a period of time). Pharmacokinetics encompasses the absorption of the drug into or across the tissues of the body, its distribution to specific functional areas, its metabolism – the process by which it is broken down within the body into by-products (metabolites) – and ultimately, its removal or excretion from the body. The most frequently used pharmacokinetic terms that are used in the drug review sections of *BESTMEDICINE* are explained in Table 1.

Whilst the basic pharmacology of a drug is clearly important, the main focus of each drug review is to summarise the drug's performance in controlled clinical trials. Clinical trials examine the effectiveness, or clinical efficacy, of the drug against the disease or condition it was to treat, as well as its safety and tolerability – the side-effects associated with the drug and the likelihood that the patient will tolerate treatment. Adherence to drug treatment, or patient compliance, reflects the tendency of patients to comply with the terms of their treatment regimen. Compliance may be affected by treatment-related side-effects or the convenience of drug treatment. The safety of the drug also encompasses its contra-indications – conditions under which the drug should never be prescribed. This may mean avoiding use in special

Table 1. Key pharmacokinetic terms.

Term	Definition
Agonist	A drug/substance that has affinity for specific cell receptors triggering a biological response.
Antagonist	A drug/substance that blocks the action of another by binding to a specific cell receptor without eliciting a biological response.
AUC (area under curve)	A plot of the concentration of a drug against the time since initial administration. It is a means of describing the bioavailability of a drug.
Binding affinity	An attractive force between substances that causes them to enter into and remain in chemical contact.
Bioavailability	The degree and rate at which a drug is absorbed into a living system or is made available at the site of physiological activity.
Clearance	The rate at which the drug is removed from the blood by excretion into the urine through the kidneys.
C_{max}	The maximum concentration of the drug recorded in the blood plasma.
Cytochrome P450 (CYP) system	A group of enzymes responsible for the metabolism of a number of different drugs and substances within the body.
Dose dependency	In which the effect of the drug is proportional to the concentration of drug administered.
Enzyme	A protein produced in the body that catalyses chemical reactions without itself being destroyed or altered. The suffix 'ase' is used when designating an enzyme.
Excretion	The elimination of a waste product (in faeces or urine) from the body.
Half-life ($t_{1/2}$)	The time required for half the original amount of a drug to be eliminated from the body by natural processes.
Inhibitor	A substance that reduces the activity of another substance.
Ligand	Any substance that binds to another and brings about a biological response.
Potency	A measure of the power of a drug to produce the desired effects.
Protein binding	The extent to which a drug attaches to proteins, peptides or enzymes within the body.
Receptor	A molecular structure, usually (but not always) situated on the cell membrane, which mediates the biological response that is associated with a particular drug/substance.
Synergism	A phenomenon in which the combined effects of two drugs are more powerful than when either drug is administered alone.
t_{max}	The time taken to reach the maximum concentration of the drug in plasma.
Volume of distribution (V_D)	The total amount of drug in the body divided by its concentration in the blood plasma. Used as a measure of the dispersal of the drug within the body once it has been absorbed.

patient populations (e.g. young or elderly patients, or those with co-existing or comorbid conditions, such as liver or kidney disease) or avoiding co-administration with certain other medications.

A brief synopsis of the drug development process is outlined below, in order to clarify and put into context many of the specialist terms encountered throughout the drug reviews.

The drug development process

Launching a new drug is an extremely costly and time-consuming venture. The entire process can cost an estimated £500 million and can take between 10 and 15 years from the initial identification of a potentially useful therapeutic compound in the laboratory to launching the finished product as a treatment for a particular disease (Figure 1). Much of this time is spent fulfilling strict guidelines set out by regulatory authorities, in order to ensure the safety and quality of the end product. As a consequence of this, a drug can fail at any stage of the development process and its development abandoned. Once identified and registered, the new drug can be protected by a patent for 20 years, after which time other companies are free to manufacture and market identical drugs, called generics. Thus, the pharmaceutical company has a finite period of time before patent expiry to recoup the cost of drug development (of both successful drugs and those drugs that do not make it to the marketplace) and return a profit to their shareholders.

Potential new drugs are identified by the research and development (R&D) department of the pharmaceutical company. After a candidate drug has been selected for development, it enters a rigorous testing procedure with five distinct phases – preclinical, which takes place in the

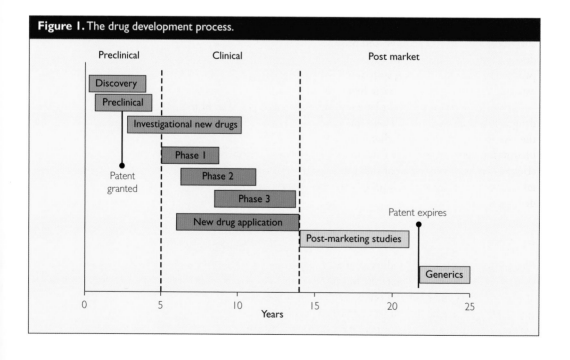

Figure 1. The drug development process.

laboratory, and phases 1, 2, 3 and 4, which involve testing in humans (Figure 1). Approval from the regulatory body is essential before the drug can be marketed and is dependent on the satisfactory completion of all phases of testing. In the UK, the Medicines and Healthcare products Regulatory Agency (MHRA) and the European Medicines Agency (EMEA) regulate the development process and companies must apply to these organisations for marketing authorisation. Within Europe, the Mutual Recognition Procedure means that the approval of a drug in one country (the Reference Member State), forms the basis for its subsequent approval in other European Union member states. This can make the approval process more efficient and may lead to approval being granted in several European countries at once. Once approval has been granted, the drug will be given a licence detailing the specific disease or conditions it is indicated to treat and the patient groups it may be used in. The drug will be assigned either prescription-only medicine (POM) or over-the-counter (OTC) status. POMs can only be obtained following consultation with a doctor, who will actively supervise their use.

Preclinical testing

Preclinical testing is essential before a drug can progress to human clinical trials. It is estimated that only one of every 1000 compounds that enter the preclinical stage continue into human testing (phases 1–4). Preclinical testing, or screening, is for the main-part performed in animals, and every effort is made to use as few animals as possible and to ensure their humane and proper care. Generally, two or more species (one rodent, one non-rodent) are tested, since a drug may affect one species differently from another.

Although a drug will never act in exactly the same way in animals as in humans, animal models are designed to mimic a human disease condition as closely as possible and provide information essential to drug development. *In vitro* experiments – literally meaning 'in glass' – are performed outside the living system in a laboratory setting. *In vivo* experiments are performed in the living cell or organism.

It is during the preclinical phase that the pharmacodynamics of the drug will first be examined. These include its mechanism of action, or the way in which it exerts its therapeutic effects. The drug's pharmacokinetics, toxicology (potentially hazardous or poisonous effects) and the formulation of the drug – the manner in which it is taken (e.g. tablet, injection, liquid) – are also assessed at this point in development.

Phase 1

Phase 1 trials are usually conducted in a small group of 10–80 healthy volunteers and further evaluate the biochemical and physiological effects of the drug – its chemical and biological impact within the body. An appropriate dosage range will be established at this point – the maximum and minimum therapeutic concentrations of the drug which are associated with a tolerable number of side-effects (secondary and usually adverse events unrelated to the beneficial effects of the drug). The mechanism of action and pharmacokinetic effects of the drugs are also further explored in this, the first group of human subjects to receive the drug.

Phase 2

If no major problems are revealed during phase 1 development, the drug can progress to phase 2 trials which take place in 100–300 patients diagnosed with the disease or condition that the drug is designed to treat. At this stage it is important to determine the effectiveness, or efficacy, of the drug. If the drug is no better than placebo then it will not be granted a licence. The side-effect or adverse event profile of the drug is re-examined at this stage, and is particularly pertinent in these patients, who may react more severely to the drug than healthy volunteers. The likelihood and severity of drug interactions is also of great importance in this patient group. Drug interactions – in which the action of one drug interferes with the action of another – can occur if the patient is taking more than one form of medication for the treatment of a comorbid disease or condition. If multiple drugs are administered together, or concomitantly, then the risk of drug interactions is increased.

Phase 3

Phase 3 clinical trials involve between 1000 and 3000 patients diagnosed with the relevant disease or condition. The recruitment of patients and the co-ordination and analysis of the trials is costly, so the pharmaceutical company will not embark on this stage unless they are sufficiently convinced of the therapeutic benefits of their drug. Essentially, phase 3 trials are replications of phase 2 trials but on a larger scale. The duration of the trial depends on the type of drug and the length of time required in order to determine the efficacy of the drug. For example, an antibiotic trial will have a shorter duration than a trial of a drug intended to treat long-term conditions, such as Alzheimer's disease. Acute treatment describes a short-term schedule given over a period of days or weeks, and chronic treatment refers to longer-term treatment schedules, lasting over periods of months or years.

Clinical trials may compare the new drug with an existing drug – a comparative trial – or may simply compare the new drug with no active drug treatment at all – a placebo-controlled trial. The participants who receive a comparator treatment or placebo are termed controls. In placebo-controlled trials, patients are given a placebo – an inert substance with no specific pharmacological activity – in place of the active drug. Patients will be unaware that the substance they are taking is placebo, which will be visually identical to the active treatment. This approach rules out any psychological effects of drug treatment – a patient may perceive that their condition has improved simply through the action of taking a tablet. In order to be considered clinically effective, the experimental drug must produce better results than the placebo.

The clinical trial should be designed in such a way as to limit the degree of bias it carries. The blinding of the trial is one means of eliminating bias. Double-blind trials, in which neither the doctor nor the patient knows which is the real drug and which is the placebo or comparator drug, are the most informative. In single-blind trials, only the patient is unaware of what they are taking, and in open-label trials, all participants are aware of treatment allocation. Conducting the trial across a number of clinics or hospitals, either abroad or in the same country (multicentre trials), further eliminates bias, as does randomisation, the random allocation of patients to treatment groups. At the start of the study, the baseline characteristics of the study population are recorded and are used as a starting point for all subsequent comparisons.

Efficacy is commonly measured by means of primary and secondary endpoints. Endpoints mark a recognised stage in the disease process and are used to compare the outcome in different treatment arms of clinical trials. The endpoint of one trial may be a marker of improvement or recovery whereas another trial may use the deterioration of the patient (morbidity) or death (mortality) to signify the end of the trial. Either way, endpoints represent valid criteria by which to compare treatments. On a similar note, surrogate markers are laboratory measurements of biological activity within the body that provide an indirect measure of the effect of treatment on disease state (e.g. blood pressure and cholesterol levels).

Statistical analysis allows the investigator to draw rational conclusions from clinical trials regarding the effectiveness of their drug. If the patient data generated during the course of a clinical trial are statistically significant, then there is a high probability that the given result, be it an improvement or a decline in the health of the patient, is due to a specific effect of drug treatment, rather than a chance occurrence. The data are put through a number of mathematical procedures that ultimately produce a p-value. This value reflects the probability that the result occurred by chance. For example, if the p-value is less than or equal to 0.05, the result is usually considered to be statistically significant. Such a p-value indicates that there is a 95% probability that the result did not occur by chance. The smaller the p-value, the more significant the result. When quoting clinical findings, the p-value is often given in brackets in order to emphasise the importance of the finding.

Once a drug has progressed through the key stages of development and demonstrated clear efficacy with an acceptable safety profile, the data are collated and the pharmaceutical company will then submit a licence application to the regulatory authorities – a new drug application.

☛ *Someone is always aware of who is taking what in a clinical trial. Whilst neither a doctor nor a patient may be aware of their treatment in a double-blind trial, there is a secure coding system, known only to the investigator, which contains the various treatment allocations.*

Phase 4 (Post-marketing studies)

Phase 4 testing takes place after the drug has been marketed and involves large numbers of patients, sometimes including those groups that may have previously been excluded from clinical trials (e.g. pregnant women and elderly or young patients). These trials are usually open-label, so the patient is aware of what they are taking, without control groups. They provide valuable information regarding the tolerability of the drug, and may reveal any long-term adverse events associated with treatment. Post-marketing surveillance continues throughout the life-span of the drug, and constantly monitors its safety, usage and performance. Doctors are advised to inform the MHRA and the Committee on Safety of Medicines (CSM) of any adverse events they encounter. Patients can also alert the CSM of any adverse events they may experience through their website (*www.yellowcard.gov.uk*).

Editorial

Professor Juliet Compston
Professor of Bone Medicine
University of Cambridge, School of Clinical Medicine

Fractures resulting from osteoporosis are widely recognised as a major cause of morbidity and mortality in the elderly population. It has been estimated that approximately 310,000 osteoporotic fractures occur annually in the UK, with a consequent cost to the health service of £1.7 billion. Over the past two decades major advances have been made in the management of this disease and a number of pharmacological agents have been approved for the reduction of fracture risk in postmenopausal women with osteoporosis. These drugs include the bisphosphonates (alendronate and risedronate), raloxifene, teriparatide and, most recently, strontium ranelate.

In clinical practice, the choice of treatment depends on several factors. Although available interventions appear to be similar in terms of the extent by which they reduce the risk of vertebral fracture, not all of them have been shown to reduce fracture risk at non-vertebral sites, particularly the hip. This is particularly important since a fragility fracture is an independent risk factor for further fractures at any site. Evidence for a reduction in both vertebral and hip fractures in postmenopausal women with osteoporosis is currently available only for alendronate, risedronate and strontium ranelate; hormone replacement therapy (HRT) has been shown to reduce clinical vertebral and hip fractures, albeit in healthy postmenopausal women. In contrast, the reduction in fracture risk with the selective oestrogen receptor modulator (SERM), raloxifene, has only been demonstrated at vertebral sites, and whilst teriparatide was shown to reduce both vertebral and non-vertebral fractures, specific evidence for hip fracture reduction is not available.

Safety and tolerability are major considerations in selecting any treatment, particularly because intervention with these agents is long term, does not produce symptomatic improvement and may be associated with side-effects. The introduction of once-weekly dosing regimens for alendronate and risedronate has proved to be very popular with patients and has improved continuance and compliance, although the dosing instructions may be difficult to follow for some, particularly the frail elderly. Strontium ranelate is taken as granules dissolved in water at bedtime; it has been shown to be well tolerated in clinical trials and, as with the bisphosphonates, serious adverse effects are rare. Raloxifene is taken as a once-daily dose with no specific dosing instructions and is also well tolerated. Although raloxifene may exacerbate vasomotor menopausal symptoms in some patients, the significant protection it offers against breast cancer, which is maintained for up to 8 years of treatment, is an important benefit for some women. The risk–benefit balance of HRT is complex but generally unfavourable

☛ *Remember that the author of this Editorial is addressing her healthcare professional colleagues rather than the 'lay' reader. This provides a fascinating insight into many of the challenges faced by doctors in the day-to-day practice of medicine (see Reader's Guide).*

for the majority, with the exception of women with menopausal symptoms; nevertheless, the increase in absolute risk of stroke, breast cancer and possibly coronary heart disease is small and should not preclude HRT use in women who express an informed preference for this treatment. Finally, treatment with teriparatide was not shown to be associated with serious adverse effects in clinical trials, but the requirement for daily subcutaneous injections may be a disadvantage for some.

Cost-effectiveness of treatment is an increasingly important consideration and is the basis on which the National Institute for Health and Clinical Excellence (NICE) have produced their recent guidance on the secondary prevention of osteoporotic fractures. The costs of alendronate, risedronate, raloxifene and strontium ranelate are broadly similar (around £300 per year), although the recent introduction of generic alendronate should reduce the price of this drug in the future. In contrast, teriparatide is significantly more expensive (approximately £3500 per year), although it is only prescribed for a maximum of 18 months in contrast to the other interventions, for which treatment periods are longer and may even be lifelong.

Since most of the clinical trials of osteoporosis therapy were conducted in women who also received calcium and vitamin D supplements, these supplements should also be used as an adjunct to therapy unless there is evidence of a good dietary calcium intake and an adequate vitamin D status. In addition, appropriate levels of physical activity should be encouraged, with an assessment of the risk of falls and appropriate advice offered where indicated. Physiotherapy has a major role to play in the management of pain given the reduced mobility and lack of confidence in individuals with osteoporotic fractures. A 6–8-week course of calcitonin often proves effective in the acute management of pain following vertebral fracture.

A number of other approaches to osteoporosis treatment are currently in development. These include the use of intravenous bisphosphonates with dosing intervals from once every 3 months to once yearly, subcutaneous injections of an antibody to the osteoclastogenic cytokine RANKL (receptor activator of NFκB ligand) administered at 6-monthly intervals, new selective SERMs and oral formulations of parathyroid hormone. Finally, new approaches to the assessment of fracture risk are also being developed, encompassing both bone mineral density measurements and risk factors that are independent of bone mineral density, for example prior fracture, continuing glucocorticoid therapy and family history of hip fracture.

1. Disease overview – Osteoporosis

Dr Eleanor Bull
CSF Medical Communications Ltd

Summary

Osteoporosis is a disease of skeletal fragility in which bone strength is compromised through the progressive deterioration of bone density and quality. Most common in postmenopausal women as a result of oestrogen deficiency, osteoporosis also affects elderly men as a result of steroid treatment or underlying disease. As the elderly population increases over the next few decades, the incidence of osteoporosis is set to rise. Osteoporosis is known as the 'silent disease' and frequently goes undetected until a fracture occurs. The most common sites for fracture are at the wrist, hip and spine, all of which can have a profound impact on patient mobility, function and quality of life. Hip and spine fractures also increase mortality rates. Fractures may require long-term care, such as orthopaedic management, physiotherapy and pain relief, and can place an enormous burden on healthcare resources.

Introduction

The decade 2000–2010 has been designated the 'Bone and Joint Decade', in recognition of the major burden imposed by musculoskeletal conditions.[1] Osteoporosis is the most common skeletal disorder, and is characterised by the microarchitectural deterioration of skeletal tissue leading to compromised bone strength and increased susceptibility to bone fracture.[2] Osteoporosis is highly prevalent amongst postmenopausal women and is strongly associated with old age in both sexes.

Osteoporosis is sometimes referred to as the 'silent disease' since the deterioration of skeletal tissue proceeds with no obvious clinical sign until fracture occurs. Reduced bone mineral density (BMD) and increased bone fragility as a result of osteoporosis increase susceptibility to fractures that can cause severe pain, disability, restricted mobility and premature death. Osteoporosis is characterised by fractures of the hip, wrist and spine following low-energy trauma, but since the whole skeleton is involved, fractures may occur at any site.[3] Of these, hip fractures are the most serious and are associated with the greatest morbidity, loss of independence and mortality rate.[3] Outward curvature of the thoracic spine region (kyphosis), height loss, unexplained chronic pain and functional difficulties may all be symptomatic of underlying osteoporotic fracture.[3] Thus, the importance of preventing bone loss and diagnosing and treating osteoporosis as early as possible is paramount if this condition is to be controlled adequately and hospitalisation avoided.

Epidemiology

The prevalence of osteoporosis is measured indirectly though the incidence of fractures. Osteoporosis is increasingly common owing to the increasing age of the general population.[1] In the UK, osteoporosis results in over 310,000 fractures each year, including 70,000 hip fractures, 70,000 wrist fraactures, 120,000 vertebral fractures and 50,000 other fractures.[4] Currently, more than 75 million people in Europe, Japan and the USA are affected, with an estimated lifetime risk for wrist, hip and vertebral fracture of around 15% – similar to that of coronary heart disease.[5] The prevalence of fracture varies widely from region to region, with the highest incidence in North America and Europe, particularly Scandinavia, and the lowest incidence in Africa and Asia.[1,6] It is likely, however, that the increased survival of the general population and the urbanisation of these less-developed countries may contribute to a greater global prevalence of the condition in the future.[1]

Osteoporosis predominantly affects females, and in the UK and USA the incidence of hip fracture amongst women is twice that amongst men.[3] The age-standardised prevalence of osteoporosis in England and

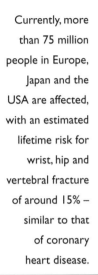

Currently, more than 75 million people in Europe, Japan and the USA are affected, with an estimated lifetime risk for wrist, hip and vertebral fracture of around 15% – similar to that of coronary heart disease.

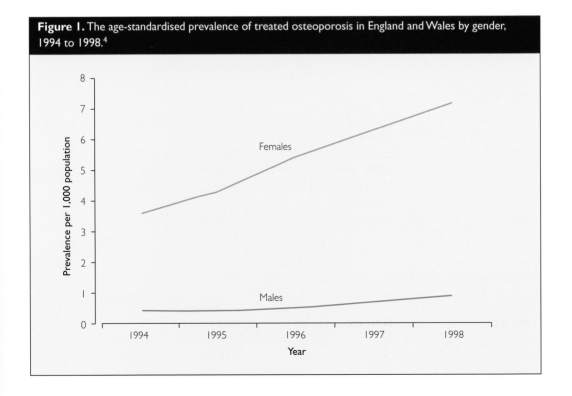

Figure 1. The age-standardised prevalence of treated osteoporosis in England and Wales by gender, 1994 to 1998.[4]

Wales is illustrated in Figure 1.[4] Worldwide, the prevalence of osteoporosis, as defined by the World Health Organization (WHO), is estimated at 5% in women aged 50 years, rising to 50% in women aged 85 years. The incidence is considerably lower in men, with 2.4% of men aged 50 years and 20% of men aged 85 years affected.[1]

Hip fracture

Hip fracture is the most devastating type of osteoporotic fracture, and its incidence is rising by 1–3% per year in most parts of the world. More than three-quarters of all hip fractures occur in women.[3] Worldwide, 1.66 million hip fractures were estimated to have occurred in 1990, with approximately 1.19 million of these in women and 463,000 in men.[1] The number of hip fractures is predicted to increase dramatically over the next few decades, exceeding 6 million cases per year by 2050.[7] There is significant variation in the hip fracture rate between countries, and the rate of fracture is higher in urban than in rural areas.[3]

Vertebral fracture

Vertebral fractures are the most common osteoporotic fractures.[8] It is estimated that one-in-eight men and women in Europe over the age of 50 years have a vertebral deformity, yet only one-third of vertebral fractures are clinically diagnosed.[1] The Chingford Study examined the prevalence of vertebral fracture in 1035 European women aged between 45 and 69 years.[9] Of these, 14.2% had minor vertebral fractures and 1.9% had severe fractures. Bone density, as measured by dual energy X-ray absorptiometry (DXA), was negatively correlated with the incidence of fracture.

Mortality

An Australian study determined that the mortality rate associated with osteoporotic bone fractures is highly dependent on the type of fracture sustained.[10] Between 10 and 20% of women die earlier than expected for their age within the first year of sustaining a hip fracture. At 1 year, hip fracture is associated with 20% mortality whilst 50% of patients are unable to live independently.[1] In a prospective study of 667 men and women with osteoporosis, the mortality rate in patients with one or more vertebral fractures was 4.4-fold greater than that in patients with no vertebral fracture.[11]

> At 1 year, hip fracture is associated with 20% mortality whilst 50% of patients are unable to live independently.

Pathophysiology

Bone remodelling

Bone is comprised of a thick outer shell and a strong inner mesh filled with collagen, calcium and other minerals. The outer shell is referred to as cortical bone and the inner latticework of less dense tissue is known as trabecular bone. Both types of bone contain osteoblasts and osteoclasts.

These are differentiated cells responsible for the process of bone remodelling – the formation and breakdown (or resorption) of bone (Figure 2).[2,12,13] The remodelling of cortical and trabecular bone is an ongoing process and continues after skeletal growth is complete. Of the two types of bone, trabecular bone is the most metabolically active, with a high concentration of osteoblasts and osteoclasts on the surface of trabeculae.

Osteoclasts, derived from haematopoietic progenitor cells, are giant multinucleated cells found alone or in clusters.[2] These cells secrete acid through a proton pump system which dissolves hydroxyapatite crystals in bone and, consequently, exposes the protein matrix, which is subsequently dissolved by digestive enzymes.[2] Osteoblasts are derived from pluripotent precursor cells and, through the production of several bone matrix proteins, lay down a lattice which is ultimately mineralised.[2] Under normal conditions, osteoclasts and osteoblasts provide equivalent levels of bone resorption and new bone formation respectively, maintaining a constant level of bone turnover.

Figure 2. The bone remodelling process.[13]

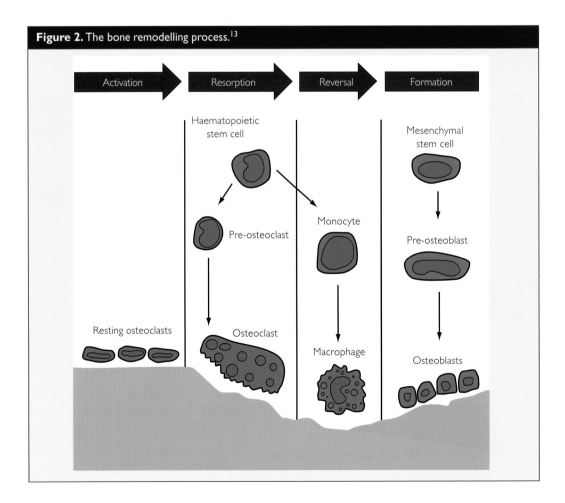

Bone remodelling causing osteoporosis

Osteoporosis is the consequence of an imbalance in the bone remodelling process in which the cellular events of bone resorption are quantitatively larger than those of bone formation.[14] This results in the gradual loss of both cortical and trabecular bone accompanied by a deterioration in their structural integrity.[6] Trabeculae become thinner and perforated, increasingly fragile and less able to tolerate loading.[15] The overall consequence of these pathological changes is reduced skeletal mass and an increased risk of fracture in response to low-energy trauma.[13]

Aetiology

The rate of bone remodelling is governed by genetic and environmental elements. The risk factors for the development of osteoporosis, the most important of which are discussed below, are summarised in Table 1.[1,16,17]

> Osteoporosis is the consequence of an imbalance in the bone remodelling process in which the cellular events of bone resorption are quantitatively larger than those of bone formation.

Table 1. Risk factors for the development of osteoporosis.[1,16,17]

	Risk factor
Genetic	Female gender Maternal family history of hip fracture Caucasian or Asian ethnicity
Demographic	Old age (≥65 years) Low body weight (body mass index <19 kg/m^2) Previous fracture after low-energy trauma
Hormonal	Oestrogen deficiency (early menopause, hysterectomy) Hypogonadism (men)
Disease	Rheumatoid arthritis Hyperthyroidism Serious organ disease (congestive heart failure, renal failure, chronic liver disease, chronic pulmonary disease)
Behavioural	Low calcium intake (<500–850 mg/day) Sedentary lifestyle Vitamin D deficiency Smoking Excessive alcohol consumption
Drug treatment	Glucocorticoids Anticonvulsants High-dose, long-term heparin High-dose methotrexate as cancer therapy

Genetic factors

BMD, skeletal size, geometry and bone turnover may all be under polygenic control.[6,17] It is estimated that up to 60–85% of the variance in BMD is genetically determined.[18] Many of the causative genes have yet to be identified although several chromosomal loci have been proposed.[6] It is possible that, in a small number of cases of osteoporosis, a single inactivating genetic mutation may be responsible for disease development, with the genes for aromatase and the oestrogen receptor being proposed as candidate loci.[18] Polymorphisms of candidate genes including the vitamin D receptor and collagen type 1 α1 genes may also account for some cases of disease.[6]

Oestrogen deficiency

> Oestrogen deficiency is by far the most important contributing factor to osteoporosis and accounts for the high incidence of the disease amongst postmenopausal women.

Oestrogen deficiency is by far the most important contributing factor to osteoporosis and accounts for the high incidence of the disease amongst postmenopausal women or women having undergone a hysterectomy.[14] Oestrogen exerts an inhibitory effect on osteoclast production and so in postmenopausal women in whom oestrogen is deficient, the remodelling balance is disturbed and osteoclastic activity predominates.[19] Thus, the intensity of bone resorption is increased and the rate of bone loss accelerated.[15]

Age

Ageing bone is more susceptible to fractures, due to cumulative cortical bone loss, bone thinning, increased porosity in key regions and bone weakening as a result of repetitive loading.[15,20]

Aside from the quality of ageing bone, the elderly population is more susceptible to fall-induced fractures, as a result of impaired vision, balance and a lower muscle mass relative to younger people.[3,20] Medication for concomitant diseases may also affect balance and cognition.[20]

Smoking and excess alcohol intake

> Long-term exposure to glucocorticoids can suppress bone formation and enhance bone resorption in a dose- and duration-dependent manner.

Smoking may predispose an individual to osteoporosis by inducing an early menopause or by increasing the metabolic breakdown of oestrogen, both of which accelerate bone loss.[14] There is also considerable evidence to suggest that the consumption of excess alcohol may adversely affect bone mass by inhibiting the proliferation of osteoblasts.[21] Alcohol is also associated with protein and/or calcium malnutrition, reduced mobility and hypogonadism, all factors that may increase the risk of osteoporosis.[14]

Glucocorticoids

Long-term exposure to glucocorticoids, used in the treatment of chronic diseases such as asthma, rheumatoid arthritis, chronic obstructive pulmonary disease and ulcerative colitis, can suppress bone formation and enhance bone resorption in a dose- and duration-dependent manner and consequently, may increase the risk of fractures.[22] Bone loss is most pronounced within the first few months of treatment, yet despite this, less than half of glucocorticoid-treated patients are investigated for signs of osteoporosis.[23] In the UK, over 250,000 patients take continuous oral glucocorticoids, yet only 14% receive any therapy to prevent bone loss.[24]

Diagnosis

The measurement of BMD, an indicator of bone strength, is used clinically to diagnose osteoporosis.[16] Currently, the WHO defines the BMD threshold for osteoporosis as at least 2.5 standard deviations below the mean BMD of the young adult (T-score ≤−2.5).[1] These criteria were specifically developed for the spine and/or hip in postmenopausal women but are also likely to apply to men.[13] The BMD threshold values and relative risk of fracture are presented in Table 2. The predictive validity of BMD for bone fracture is considered to be at least as accurate as that of blood pressure for stroke.[25]

At the present time, the assessment of BMD by axial DXA is the diagnostic method of choice for osteoporosis. The differential absorption of two X-ray frequencies by soft tissue and bone provides a measure of bone mass from which the probability of osteoporosis can be judged.[13] The femoral neck and lumbar spine (Figure 3) are the best sites to assess, but peripheral DXA at the distal forearm may also be used.[26] Although the technique is fast and requires only limited exposure to radiation, high cost and limited access to axial DXA equipment may restrict its widespread use.[27] Quantitative ultrasound is an alternative means of quantifying fracture risk and measures the broadband attenuation and speed of sound at various skeletal sites.[13] Ultrasound is easily accessible, portable, inexpensive and does not involve the use of ionising

> The assessment of BMD by axial DXA is the diagnostic method of choice for osteoporosis.

Severity	T-score	Fracture risk	Action
Normal	>−1	Low	Lifestyle advice
Low BMD (osteopenia)	−1 to −2.5	Above average	Lifestyle advice, calcium and vitamin D supplements
Osteoporosis	<−2.5	High	Lifestyle advice, calcium and vitamin D supplements, pharmacological treatment
Severe osteoporosis	<−2.5 and one or more fractures	High	Lifestyle advice, calcium and vitamin D supplements, pain control, exclude secondary causes, pharmacological treatment and consider referral to a specialist

Table 2. Diagnosis of osteoporosis.

BMD, bone mineral density.
T-score relates to absolute fracture risk as defined by the World Health Organization.

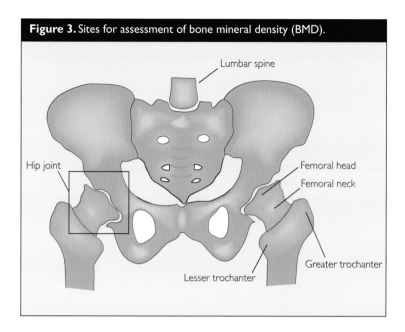

Figure 3. Sites for assessment of bone mineral density (BMD).

radiation.[13] However, it cannot be used to diagnose osteoporosis or to monitor the effects of treatment.[28]

The identification of susceptible patients through risk factor analysis can help identify those at highest risk of fracture or who require DXA scanning. Previous fragility fracture, a maternal history of hip fracture and an increased risk of falling are all factors that may predispose to fracture. Adults who sustain a fracture are 50–100% more likely to have a further fracture, and many will refracture within 1 year.[29]

X-rays are an insensitive method of diagnosing osteoporosis, although they are the method of choice for diagnosing fractures, including vertebral fractures. Routine chest X-rays may identify vertebral deformities but unfortunately these are not currently reported by most radiologists, missing an important opportunity to identify people with asymptomatic vertebral deformities who may be at high risk of future vertebral fractures.[26]

Secondary causes of osteoporosis may account for around 40% of disease cases in men.[13] Common causes include hypogonadism, steroid use, alcohol abuse, malignant diseases, osteomalacia, hyperthyroidism and hyperparathyroidism.[13] These conditions should be excluded by assessment of full blood count, erythrocyte sedimentation rate, serum calcium and serum parathyroid hormone levels and by performing liver function and thyroid tests in appropriate patients.[13]

Socioeconomic impact

The cost of treating osteoporosis, and the fractures sustained as a direct consequence of the condition, represents a major economic burden to the NHS.[3] From the patient's perspective, the chronic pain, restricted mobility, loss of independence and frequent admission to long-term care associated with bone fracture can have devastating effects on quality of life. In the UK, the annual cost of providing social care and support for patients sustaining fractures is estimated at £1.7 billion.[30]

Nearly all patients are hospitalised following a hip fracture and most undergo surgical repair or surgical replacement of the joint.[1] This costs the NHS over £940 million annually.[31] In England, between 1997 and 1998, there were 44,500 and 11,800 NHS hospital admissions for women and men, respectively, for fracture of the femur and hip in people aged 45 years and over.[31] If the cost of treating a fractured hip is considered to be around £4,800 and one-in-five of these patients require long-term residential care, costing £19,000 per year, the economic impact of this condition is considerable.[31]

> The chronic pain, restricted mobility, loss of independence and frequent admission to long-term care associated with bone fracture can have devastating effects on quality of life.

Key points

- Osteoporosis is the most common skeletal disorder, affecting more than 75 million people in Europe, Japan and the USA.

- Postmenopausal women are most commonly affected although prevalence is high in elderly patients of both sexes.

- Osteoporosis is characterised by an imbalance in bone remodelling, in which bone resorption by osteoclasts outweighs new bone formation by osteoblasts.

- Known as the 'silent disease', osteoporosis only becomes apparent once bone fractures are sustained as a result of underlying bone fragility.

- Hip, wrist and vertebral fractures are the most common fractures and impact heavily on mobility, independence and quality of life.

- BMD, as measured by DXA, is used to diagnose osteoporosis, defined as a T-score of −2.5 or less.

- Oestrogen deficiency, old age, glucocorticoids, concomitant disease and lifestyle factors all heavily influence the development of osteoporosis.

References

A list of the published evidence which has been reviewed in compiling the preceding section of *BESTMEDICINE.*

1 Woolf A, Pfleger B. Burden of major musculoskeletal conditions. *Bull World Health Organ* 2003; **81**: 646–56.

2 Inzerillo A, Zaidi M. Osteoporosis: trends and intervention. *Mt Sinai J Med* 2002; **69**: 220–31.

3 Cummings S, Melton L. Epidemiology and outcomes of osteoporotic fractures. *Lancet* 2002; **359**: 1761–7.

4 National Osteoporosis Society. What is osteoporosis? *www.nos.org.uk*

5 Kai M, Anderson M, Lau E. Exercise interventions: defusing the world's osteoporosis time bomb. *Bull World Health Organ* 2003; **81**: 827–30.

6 Mueller G, Russell R. Osteoporosis: pathogenesis and clinical intervention. *Biochem Soc Trans* 2003; **31**: 462–4.

7 Hauselmann HJ, Rizzoli R. A comprehensive review of treatments for postmenopausal osteoporosis. *Osteoporos Int* 2003; **14**: 2–12.

8 Quandt SA, Thompson DE, Schneider DL, Nevitt MC, Black DM. Effect of alendronate on vertebral fracture risk in women with bone mineral density T scores of –1.6 to –2.5 at the femoral neck: the Fracture Intervention Trial. *Mayo Clin Proc* 2005; **80**: 343–9.

9 Spector T, McCloskey E, Doyle D, Kanis J. Prevalence of vertebral fracture in women and the relationship with bone density and symptoms: the Chingford Study. *J Bone Miner Res* 1993; **8**: 817–22.

10 Center J, Nguyen T, Schneider D, Sambrook P, Eisman J. Mortality after all major types of osteoporotic fracture in men and women: an observational study. *Lancet* 1999; **353**: 878–82.

11 Jalava T, Sarna S, Pylkkanen L *et al.* Association between vertebral fracture and increased mortality in osteoporotic patients. *J Bone Miner Res* 2003; **18**: 1254–60.

12 Raisz L. Local and systemic factors in the pathogenesis of osteoporosis. *N Engl J Med* 1988; **318**: 818–28.

13 Compston J, Rosen C. *Fast Facts – Osteoporosis.* 3rd edn. Oxford: Health Press, 2002.

14 Hunter D, Sambrook P. Bone loss. Epidemiology of bone loss. *Arthritis Res* 2000; **2**: 441–5.

15 Seeman E. Pathogenesis of bone fragility in women and men. *Lancet* 2002; **359**: 1841–50.

16 Martens MG. Risk of fracture and treatment to prevent osteoporosis-related fracture in postmenopausal women. A review. *J Reprod Med* 2003; **48**: 425–34.

17 Hansen LB and Vondracek SF. Prevention and treatment of nonpostmenopausal osteoporosis. *Am J Health Syst Pharm* 2004; **61**: 2637–56.

18 Ralston S. Genetic determinants of susceptibility to osteoporosis. *Curr Opin Pharmacol* 2003; **3**: 286–90.

19 Bonn D. New ways with old bones. Osteoporosis researchers look for drugs to replace hormone replacement therapy. *Lancet* 2004; **363**: 786–7.

20 Ettinger MP. Aging bone and osteoporosis: strategies for preventing fractures in the elderly. *Arch Intern Med* 2003; **163**: 2237–46.

21 Klein R. Alcohol-induced bone disease: impact of ethanol on osteoblast proliferation. *Alcohol Clin Exp Res* 1997; **21**: 392–9.

22 McIlwain HH. Glucocorticoid-induced osteoporosis: pathogenesis, diagnosis, and management. *Prev Med* 2003; **36**: 243–9.

23 Walsh L, Wong C, Pringle M, Tattersfield A. Use of oral corticosteroids in the community and the prevention of secondary osteoporosis: a cross sectional study. *BMJ* 1996; **313**: 344–6.

24 Eastell R, Reid D, Compston J *et al.* A UK Consensus Group on management of glucocorticoid-induced osteoporosis: an update. *J Intern Med* 1998; **244**: 271–92.

25 Royal College of Physicians and Bone and Tooth Society for Great Britain. Osteoporosis – Clinical guidelines for prevention and treatment. London: Royal College of Physicians, 1999.

26 *Management of Osteoporosis – Quick Reference Guide 71.* Edinburgh: Scottish Intercollegiate Guidelines Network, 2003. *www.sign.ac.uk*

27 Hodson J, Marsh J. Quantitative ultrasound and risk factor enquiry as predictors of postmenopausal osteoporosis: comparative study in primary care. *Lancet* 2003; **326**: 1250–1.

28 National Osteoporosis Society. *Position Statement on the use of Quantitative Ultrasound in the Management of Osteoporosis.* Bath, 2001. *www.nos.org.uk*

29 Klotzbuecher C, Ross P, Landsman P, Abbott TR, Berger M. Patients with prior fractures have an increased risk of future fractures: a summary of the literature and statistical synthesis. *J Bone Miner Res* 2000; **15**: 721–39.

30 Woolf A, Akesson K. Preventing fractures in elderly people. *BMJ* 2003; **327**: 89–95.

31 Bailey K, Majeed A. Trends in the treatment of osteoporosis and types of drug treatments prescribed in general practice in England and Wales, 1994 to 1998. *Health Statistics Quarterly:* National Statistics Office, 2002.

Acknowledgements

Figure 2 is adapted from Compston and Rosen, 2002.[13]

2. Management options – Osteoporosis

Dr Anna Palmer
CSF Medical Communications Ltd

Summary

The management of osteoporosis encompasses both its prevention
and its treatment. Modifiable lifestyle risk factors for osteoporosis
include poor diet, lack of exercise, excessive alcohol intake and
smoking. Ensuring a plentiful supply of fresh fruits and vegetables
in the diet is thought to contribute to an increase in alkalinity and
to minimise leaching of calcium from the bones. In addition, an
adequate intake of calcium and vitamin D is essential for optimal
bone health throughout life. In elderly individuals, in particular, good
nutrition is essential for the maintenance of a normal bodyweight,
whilst appropriate measures should be taken to reduce the risk of
accidents which may lead to hip fracture. A wide array of
pharmacological interventions is currently available for both the
treatment and prevention of osteoporosis. These include the
bisphosphonates, calcitonin, parathyroid hormone (teriparatide),
selective oestrogen receptor modulators (raloxifene) and
strontium ranelate. Calcium and vitamin D supplements should be
given when any of these drugs are prescribed. Hormone
replacement therapy (HRT) is no longer considered to be a first-
line option for the treatment of osteoporosis due to concerns
regarding its links to heart disease and breast cancer, though it may
still be used where alternative treatments are considered to be
unsatisfactory. The first-line option for the prevention and
treatment of osteoporosis is the bisphosphonates – alendronate,
risedronate and etidronate. These agents are effective in reducing
bone resorption, increasing bone mineral density (BMD) and
reducing the incidence of fractures. Raloxifene is recommended as
an alternative to the bisphosphonates and this drug has also been
shown to be effective in increasing BMD and reducing fracture
rates. Teriparatide and strontium ranelate are more recently

introduced therapies which have anabolic properties on bone formation and proven efficacy in reducing fracture risk, with both drugs currently licensed for the treatment of postmenopausal osteoporosis.

Management of osteoporosis – objectives

The primary objective of osteoporosis treatment is to prevent first and subsequent fracture.

The primary objective of osteoporosis treatment is to prevent first and subsequent fracture. This may be achieved through the implementation of preventative lifestyle strategies or through lifestyle and appropriate pharmacological interventions following a positive diagnosis (Table 1). An algorithm for the management of osteoporosis has been produced by the Royal College of Physicians and includes pharmacological therapy for both prophylaxis and treatment of the disease (Figure 1).[1] In the context of osteoporosis management, the term 'prevention' is defined as prevention of bone loss in postmenopausal women with osteopenia (BMD T-score between –1 and –2.5) whilst 'treatment' refers to reduction in fracture risk in postmenopausal women with diagnosed osteoporosis.[1] The Royal College of Physicians guidelines were published before the introduction of newer antiosteoporotic agents (including teriparatide and strontium ranelate) although the National Institute for Health and Clinical Excellence (NICE) has recently produced some guidance on the use of these agents.[2] Teriparatide is currently

Table 1. Antifracture efficacy of treatment recommendations in postmenopausal women, as defined by the Royal College of Physicians.[1]

Intervention	Vertebral	Non-vertebral	Hip
Alendronate	A	A	A
Calcitonin	A	B	B
Calcitriol	A	A	–
Calcium	A	B	B
Calcium and vitamin D supplementation	–	A	A
Cyclic etidronate	A	B	B
Hip protectors	–	–	A
HRT	A	A	B
Physical exercise	–	B	B
Raloxifene	A	–	–
Risedronate	A	A	A
Vitamin D	B	B	B

A–C denotes level of recommendation, A being highest. Recommendations based on level of evidence: meta-analyses and randomised controlled clinical trials rated highest. HRT, hormone replacement therapy. NB: No advice regarding the efficacy of strontium ranelate and teriparatide were included in the Royal College of Physicians clinical guidelines for prevention and treatment of osteoporosis.

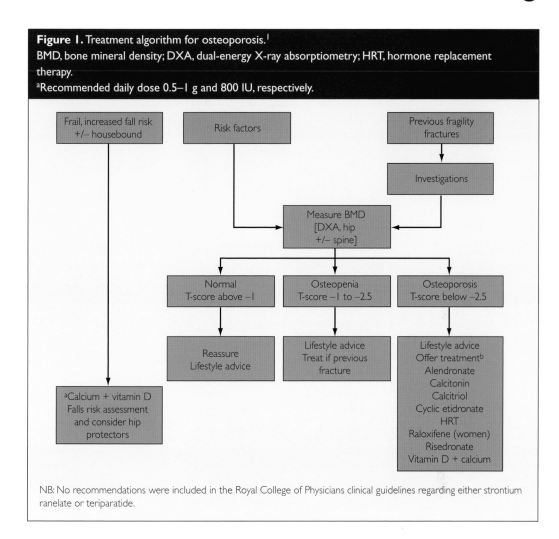

Figure 1. Treatment algorithm for osteoporosis.[1]
BMD, bone mineral density; DXA, dual-energy X-ray absorptiometry; HRT, hormone replacement therapy.
[a]Recommended daily dose 0.5–1 g and 800 IU, respectively.

NB: No recommendations were included in the Royal College of Physicians clinical guidelines regarding either strontium ranelate or teriparatide.

recommended as a second-line option for the treatment of osteoporotic women aged over 65 years, who are at high risk of fracture and who have shown a poor response or inability to tolerate bisphosphonate therapy. The data regarding the clinical and cost-effectiveness of strontium ranelate are currently undergoing review.

Preventive measures and lifestyle changes

Adopting a healthy lifestyle, particularly stopping smoking, engaging in exercise, eating a good diet and reducing excessive alcohol intake, can slow the rate of bone loss. These changes are discussed in detail in the following sections.

Calcium and vitamin D supplementation

Calcium and vitamin D are essential for optimum bone health throughout life, and supplementation with both nutrients has been shown to improve BMD and to reduce fracture risk.[3,4]

> Adopting a healthy lifestyle, particularly stopping smoking, engaging in exercise, eating a good diet and reducing excessive alcohol intake, can slow the rate of bone loss.

Increasing calcium
intake either
through the
diet or by
supplementation
may slow the rate
of bone loss.

Increasing calcium intake either through the diet or by supplementation may slow the rate of bone loss, particularly in the elderly and in those patients with a low calcium intake, but should not be viewed as a substitute for other bone-sparing therapies in patients with established osteoporosis.[5] Current evidence indicates that the risk for fragility fracture is greatest in those who consume under 400 mg of calcium daily.[6] Therefore, efforts to ensure that the population receives adequate calcium intake are likely to prove beneficial in reducing the incidence of new osteoporotic fractures. Calcium and vitamin D supplementation is always advised for those diagnosed with osteoporosis (unless they are receiving adequate levels from dietary sources), and increasing dietary intake is an important strategy for the prevention of the disease.

Vitamin D, given either alone or in combination with oral calcium supplements, should be administered routinely to frail elderly patients in residential care or nursing homes, in whom calcium and/or vitamin D deficiency is common due to poor dietary intake, reduced absorption or a lack of exposure to sunshine (resulting in impaired vitamin D synthesis in the skin).[5] The term vitamin D refers to a group of compounds including ergocalciferol (calciferol, vitamin D_2), colecalciferol (vitamin D_3), dihydrotachysterol, alfacalcidol and calcitriol. A twice-daily supplement with calcitriol (0.25 µg) is recommended for the management of postmenopausal osteoporosis.[1] Daily supplementation with 1.2 g of calcium and 800 IU of colecalciferol over 3 years has been shown to reduce the risk of hip fracture substantially in frail elderly nursing home patients.[7] However, studies evaluating vitamin D supplementation in elderly patients living in the community have failed to replicate these findings, perhaps as a result of higher baseline vitamin D levels in this population.[8] A twice-yearly intramuscular injection of 150,000–300,000 IU may be the most convenient and cost-effective way to maintain sufficient vitamin D levels in this patient population. Inadequate levels of vitamin D can result in secondary hyperparathyroidism and an increased risk of osteomalacia and fracture.[9] There is also some evidence that low vitamin D status results in increased postural sway and muscle weakness, which increases the risk of falling and therefore the likelihood of fracture.

Calcium and vitamin D supplements should be given to those patients treated with bone-sparing therapies, including the bisphosphonates, selective oestrogen receptor modulators (SERMs) and teriparatide, where dietary intake of these nutrients is insufficient.

Diet and nutrition

The majority of epidemiological studies linking calcium with bone health are based on the consumption of milk and other dairy products, yet calcium is available from a wide array of dietary sources.[6] A varied diet rich in dairy products, bony fish, dark green vegetables, tofu, beans and pulses should be sufficient to maintain a daily calcium intake of greater than 400 mg/day. Table 2 illustrates the calcium content of those

Table 2. Calcium content of a selection of food products.[10]

Calcium content (mg/100 g of foodstuff)	Food type[a]
<100	Tinned tuna (in oil)
	Soya milk
	Oranges (fresh)
	Baked beans
	Green/French beans
	Olives in brine
	Cottage cheese
	Dried apricots
	Tinned salmon
100–400	Muesli
	Semi-skimmed milk (100 mL)
	Steamed tofu
	Yoghurt (low fat)
	Spinach or watercress
	Pizza (cheese and tomato)
	Milk chocolate
	Tinned pilchards (in tomato sauce)
	Camembert
>400	Tinned sardines (oil or tomato sauce)
	Cheddar cheese
	Fried whitebait
	Sesame seeds

[a]Foods are arranged in order of calcium content, from lowest to highest, thus sesame seeds are the richest source of dietary calcium amongst this selection of foodstuffs.

foods highest in calcium, though many calcium-fortified beverages, such as soya milk or orange juice, may also be useful in boosting daily calcium intake.[10]

The naturally occurring plant products, phyto-oestrogens are of potential interest for nutritional prevention of osteoporosis.[6] These compounds include soya-derived isoflavones (genistein and daidzein) and lignans derived from cereals, fruits and vegetables. Animal studies have shown that these compounds have weak oestrogenic effects and can prevent bone loss. However, their potential has yet to be explored fully in large-scale human studies. Similarly, ipriflavone is a synthetic derivative of the natural isoflavones and is found in soya, red clover and other food sources but again, its efficacy remains controversial.[11] There is also evidence for a role of the essential fatty acids, gamma-linolenic acid and eicosapentaenoic acid, in maintaining or increasing bone mass.[12] Supplementation with these fatty acids has been shown to enhance calcium absorption and increase calcium deposition in bone. Evening primrose oil is a good source of gamma-linolenic acid whilst oily fish or fish oil supplements are the most common sources of eicosapentaenoic acid. A beneficial role of fluoride in increasing BMD has been reported but, on the whole, the evidence is inconclusive and, most tellingly, a reduction in fracture risk secondary to increased fluoride intake has not been demonstrated.[5] Studies have also demonstrated that vitamin K supplementation may improve bone density and reduce the risk for fracture.[11]

Excessive consumption of animal-derived protein has been linked to an increased incidence of bone fracture.[6] Animal-derived protein is rich in sulphur-containing amino acids which contribute to an acidic environment in the body that, in turn, leads to an increased loss of calcium from the skeleton. These concerns have led to the hypothesis that a lower consumption of animal protein and increased consumption of fruits and vegetables (which are believed to reduce the systemic 'acid load') may be beneficial for bone health.[13] However, trials to date have failed to demonstrate a clear benefit to bone health of a lactovegetarian diet. This lack of an effect could be a simple function of the acidic nature of many cheeses and grains (widely consumed in most lactovegetarian diets) counteracting the beneficial effects of increased fruits and vegetables. Further investigation in this area would be of great interest. There is also significant interest in the way in which the electrolytes, sodium and potassium, impact upon the progression of osteoporosis.[6] Sodium intake is a stronger determinant of urinary calcium excretion (i.e. involving calcium loss from bones) than calcium intake, whilst a high intake of sodium has been shown to be deleterious to bone health.[6] In contrast, studies have shown that supplementation with potassium bicarbonate neutralises an acidic environment and reduces urinary calcium excretion. Therefore, an increased consumption of dietary potassium (via an increased intake of fruits and vegetables) is likely to be beneficial to bone health.[6]

Other dietary concerns that have arisen in the field of osteoporosis prevention regard alcohol, caffeine and excessive consumption of vitamin A.[6] Alcoholism is an established risk factor for osteoporosis but there is no consistent evidence that moderate alcohol consumption increases osteoporosis risk. Caffeine is not associated with any increased risk for bone loss or fracture.[5] Evidence from some studies has indicated that excessive intake of vitamin A (> 1500 μg retinol equivalents) may contribute to low BMD and increased fracture risk, but not all studies have confirmed this link.[14] This level of dietary vitamin A would most commonly be derived from highly enriched supplements such as cod liver oil (which contains 1200 μg vitamin A in a 10 mL dose) and whilst controversy persists regarding the precise role of vitamin A in bone health it may be prudent that older people avoid excessively high doses of pure cod liver oil.[10]

In general, the current evidence would suggest that adopting a diet which has reduced levels of sodium, increased levels of potassium

An increased consumption of dietary potassium (via an increased intake of fruits and vegetables) is likely to be beneficial to bone health.

combined with plentiful fresh fruit and vegetables is not detrimental to bone health and may well be beneficial. Furthermore, maintaining a healthy bodyweight is also important, since a low body mass index (BMI) is positively associated with an enhanced risk of osteoporosis.[6]

Avoid risk and reduce impact of falls

The risk of sustaining a fragility fracture increases with advancing age. Consequently, efforts to minimise the potential for, and impact of, falls in the elderly represents a relatively straightforward initiative to reduce fracture risk. The risk of a potentially damaging fall may be reduced by correcting eye problems such as cataracts, avoiding slippery floor surfaces and installing adequate lighting. Energy-absorbing hip protectors can be worn by the patient to minimise the impact of a fall and reduce the likelihood of fracture. A recent meta-analysis of elderly people has indicated that the use of hip protectors was effective in reducing fracture rates in institutionalised individuals (hip fracture rate 4.8 *vs* 11.0% for hip protectors and control, respectively; $p<0.05$) but were ineffective in those living in the community.[15] However, compliance may be poor since these devices can be cumbersome and uncomfortable, and they are also expensive since several pairs are needed for each patient.[16]

Minimise use of glucocorticoids

In light of the strong association between glucocorticoid treatment and the increased incidence of osteoporosis, the lowest possible dose of glucocorticoid should be used for the shortest period of time, and adjunctive therapy with bone-sparing drugs should be considered as recommended in joint guidelines from the Royal College of Physicians, the Bone and Tooth Society and the National Osteoporosis Society (Figure 2).[17] Since the rate of bone loss is greatest during the first 3–12 months of glucocorticoid use, bone-sparing therapy should be initiated at the same time as glucocorticoid therapy where appropriate.[17]

Exercise

Regular, weight-bearing and resistance exercise is important throughout life for maximising peak bone mass and preventing bone loss. Physical stress can reduce bone loss by stimulating bone growth and preserving bone mass, in addition to strengthening muscle. Resistance exercise, where heavier loads are lifted slowly, is most effective for preserving bone mass but is obviously not suitable in some patients who already have osteoporosis. Individually tailored exercise programmes, which include Tai Chi and yoga, have been shown to be particularly useful in preventing falls in the elderly. Good bone-building exercises include running, skipping, aerobics, tennis and brisk walking, and a minimum of 20 minutes of exercise at least three-times a week is a common recommendation.[10]

Adopting a diet which has reduced levels of sodium, increased levels of potassium combined with plentiful fresh fruit and vegetables is not detrimental to bone health and may well be beneficial.

Regular, weight-bearing and resistance exercise is important throughout life for maximising peak bone mass and preventing bone loss.

Figure 2. Management of glucocorticoid-induced osteoporosis in men and women.[17]
BMD, bone mineral density; DXA, dual-energy X-ray absorptiometry.
[a]In patients with previous fragility fracture: full blood count, erythrocyte sedimentation rate, bone and liver function tests, serum creatinine, serum thyroid-stimulating hormone.
[b]General measures include minimising the dose of glucocorticoids, considering alternative routes of administration or alternate formulations (i.e. budesonide which is reported to have bone-sparing properties) and prescription of alternative immunosuppressive agents. In addition, adequate calcium intake, good nutrition, maintenance of normal body weight, smoking cessation, avoidance of excessive alcohol consumption and engaging in physical activity should all be encouraged, and fall risk assessments performed for at-risk patients.

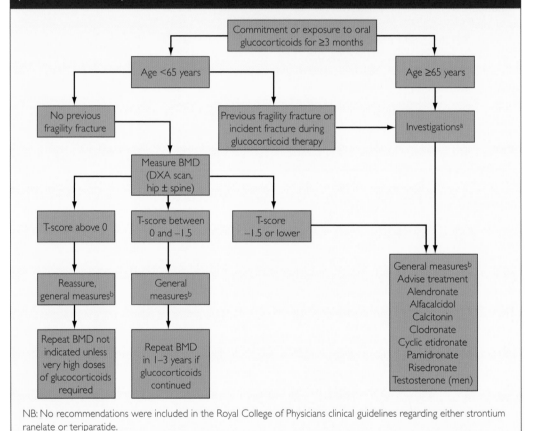

NB: No recommendations were included in the Royal College of Physicians clinical guidelines regarding either strontium ranelate or teriparatide.

Complementary and alternative medicine

The use of complementary and alternative medicine in the treatment or prevention of osteoporosis is not widespread and there is no clear evidence to suggest that either herbal, homeopathic or traditional Chinese remedies are superior to currently recommended pharmacological and lifestyle intervention strategies. However, it is worthwhile to briefly describe those complementary therapies which are believed to augment the management of osteoporosis, and which the patient may encounter.

Traditional Chinese medicine is aimed towards early disease prevention and its methods are composed of a combination of acupuncture and herbal remedies.[18] According to Chinese medicine there is a strong relationship between the kidney and the skeletal system and thus, kidney tonifying herbs are used to prevent bone loss whilst acupuncture techniques are centred upon points which stimulate kidney energy.[11] Other Chinese herbal remedies are thought to act by increasing oestrogen levels via their natural phyto-oestrogen components.[18] Those most commonly encountered include black cohosh, angelica, cypress, hops, pomegranate husk, sage, ginseng, licorice, horsetail, stinging nettle, knotweed, hemp nettle and maërl. Many of these remedies are also utilised in the practice of herbal medicine and those most commonly used in the treatment of osteoporosis are described in more detail below.

Several herbal remedies are widely recommended by professional herbalists for the treatment and/or prevention of osteoporosis based on the ability of these herbs to balance hormones and benefit bone health.[11] Black cohosh (*Cimicifuga racemosa*) and red clover (*Trifolium pratense*) both contain phyto-oestrogens which help to combat bone loss. Black cohosh has long been used by Native Americans for treating musculoskeletal disorders and has also been widely used in Europe for the treatment of menstrual and menopausal symptoms. Other herbal components proposed to be of value in the management of osteoporosis include horsetail (*Equisetum arvense*), oat straw (*Avena sativa*), wild yam (*Dioscorea villosa*), kelp (*Fucus vesiculosus*) and chaste tree (*Vitex agnus castus*).[11] The stems of the horsetail plant are rich in silica which helps repair broken bones and form collagen. The tubers of wild yams contain diosgenin which is a steroid-like substance involved in progesterone production, though there is little evidence for any hormonal activity of wild yam itself in the treatment of osteoporosis.

The evidence for the majority of alternative and complementary therapies is largely anecdotal and is derived from historical and traditional beliefs. This situation is slowly changing as alternative remedies are increasingly examined in placebo-controlled randomised clinical trials in order to define their effects more clearly. However, to date, insufficient rigorous scientific evidence is available to enable informed opinion of the suitability of these remedies in the treatment of osteoporosis. Thus, their use should be approached with caution and with the guidance of professional practitioners in both Western medicine and the therapy in question. Consultation with a GP is particularly important to ensure that these therapies do not harmfully interact with any existing medications that the patient may already be receiving.

> The evidence for the majority of alternative and complementary therapies is largely anecdotal and is derived from historical and traditional beliefs.

Pharmacological treatment

The currently available treatments for osteoporosis are very effective in preventing bone loss and reducing fracture risk. Anabolic agents such as parathyroid hormone (teriparatide) stimulate new bone formation by continually activating osteoblasts.[19] In contrast, inhibitors of bone resorption reduce osteoclastic activity, resulting in stabilisation or small increases in bone mass.[20] These compounds include the bisphosphonates, SERMs and calcitonin. A recently introduced compound, strontium ranelate, has a unique mechanism of action that targets both bone resorption and bone formation, resulting in increased bone mass.[21]

HRT was previously considered to be the main treatment for postmenopausal women with osteoporosis. However, the increased risk of heart disease and breast cancer associated with its use has led to it no longer being recommended for the long-term prevention or treatment of osteoporosis.[20] Nevertheless, its use may still be considered in situations where other therapies are contraindicated, cannot be tolerated or evoke no response.[22] Testosterone supplementation may be considered in hypogonadal men who are receiving oral glucocorticoid therapy.[17]

Bisphosphonates

The bisphosphonates (e.g. alendronate, risedronate [detailed reviews of these drugs are presented in this edition of *BESTMEDICINE*], and etidronate) are stable chemical analogues of inorganic pyrophosphate, characterised by a phosphorus-carbo-phosphorus bond.[5,23] Etidronate (administered cyclically and intermittently with calcium), alendronate and risedronate are now licensed in the UK for both the treatment and prevention of postmenopausal and glucocorticoid-induced osteoporosis.[22] Other bisphosphonates (i.e. pamidronate and clodronate) are also utilised in the treatment of cancer to preserve bone strength and in other diseases of the bone such as Paget's disease. The bisphosphonates show a strong affinity for bone apatite and prevent bone resorption by inhibiting recruitment of osteoclasts and promoting apoptosis.[5] The incidence of vertebral fractures in postmenopausal women with osteoporosis has been shown to be reduced by 40–49% over 3 years following treatment with bisphosphonates.[5] Vertebral fracture risk is rapidly reduced following as little as 6–12 months of treatment. Hip and other non-vertebral fractures are also reduced. In general, the side-effect profile of these drugs is favourable, although there is controversy regarding the extent of the association between alendronate treatment and upper gastrointestinal adverse experiences.[24] The bioavailability of these compounds following oral administration is poor, and therefore they should be taken on an empty stomach, and the recommendations of the manufacturer of each drug should be adhered to.[5,22] Once-weekly preparations of some of these drugs are now available and these offer improved convenience for the patient, potentially improving their compliance to treatment, and therefore their treatment outcomes.

SERMs

Raloxifene is a benzothiopene compound which competitively inhibits the action of oestrogen in the breast and endometrium yet acts as an oestrogen agonist in bone and lipid metabolism.[5] This highly specific mechanism of action makes raloxifene an ideal candidate for the treatment of osteoporosis. The Multiple Outcomes of Raloxifene Evaluation (MORE) study reported a 30–50% reduction in the incidence of vertebral, but not non-vertebral, fractures following raloxifene treatment, which was also accompanied by a significant 70% reduction in the risk of breast cancer.[25,26] However, raloxifene has been associated with an increased risk of venous thromboembolism and may also worsen vasomotor symptoms.[5,20] The results of the Raloxifene Use for The Heart (RUTH) study are widely anticipated in order to clarify whether raloxifene reduces or increases the risk of heart disease, following reports of the positive correlation of HRT treatment with heart disease.

Calcitonin

Calcitonin is an endogenous peptide, produced by thyroid C cells, which directly inhibits osteoclast activity thereby reducing bone resorption.[5] Clinical studies have shown that BMD is increased following calcitonin treatment. Reductions in new vertebral fractures have also been reported with calcitonin, though these effects are less pronounced than those associated with the bisphosphonates.[1] Salmon-derived calcitonin is ten-times more potent than the human form and is therefore the most common formulation used in clinical practice.[22] Currently, only parenteral calcitonin is licensed for use in postmenopausal osteoporosis. The salcatonin formulation is recommended at a daily dose of 100 U daily with coadministration of calcium (600 mg) and vitamin D (400 IU). Tolerance of calcitonin can be poor, with side-effects including nausea, diarrhoea and flushing which can be avoided, in part, by the use of an intranasal spray.[5] The expense and inconvenience of administration mean that calcitonin is used less commonly than the bisphosphonates.

Parathyroid hormone

Teriparatide, a recombinant form of human parathyroid hormone, is indicated for the treatment of established postmenopausal osteoporosis.[22] By increasing the proliferation of osteoblast progenitor cells and reducing the death rate of mature osteoblasts, teriparatide directly promotes bone formation.[20] Teriparatide must be administered daily by subcutaneous injection, which necessitates the training of the patient with regard to injection technique, whilst treatment should not exceed a maximum of 18 months.[22] Side-effects may include gastrointestinal upset, depression, urinary disorders and muscle cramps, and teriparatide is contraindicated in patients with severe renal impairment.

Strontium ranelate

Strontium ranelate was recently introduced in the UK to reduce the risk of vertebral and hip fractures in postmenopausal women with osteoporosis.[21] The compound comprises organic ranelic acid and two atoms of stable non-radioactive strontium. In contrast to agents such as the SERMs and bisphophonates, which act by inhibiting bone resorption and anabolic agents such as parathyroid hormone which increase bone formation, pharmacological studies have demonstrated that strontium ranelate has a novel dual mechanism of action resulting in a decrease in bone resorption and an increase in bone formation, thereby resulting in increased bone mass. Clinical studies have demonstrated a relative risk reduction of 49% in the incidence of new vertebral fractures after the first year of treatment and a 41% risk reduction after 3 years of treatment (both p<0.001 vs placebo).[27] The relative risk of non-vertebral fractures (including hip fractures) was also shown to be reduced after treatment with strontium ranelate, whilst BMD increased at the lumbar spine and at the femoral neck.[28] Strontium ranelate has a favourable safety profile; the only significant side-effects reported at a greater frequency than placebo in controlled clinical trials were diarrhoea and nausea, which were generally transient and disappeared within 3 months of treatment initiation.

Key points

- The management of osteoporosis may be tackled both directly and prophylactically. Appropriate lifestyle and pharmacological intervention may prevent the onset of osteoporosis in those women at highest risk whilst similar strategies are also effective in stabilising bone mass in those already diagnosed with osteoporosis.

- An adequate intake of dietary calcium and vitamin D is essential for optimal bone function and should be monitored and optimised in patients with osteoporosis. This may be either via dietary advice or by supplementation where necessary.

- Lifestyle modification for the prevention of osteoporosis should include plentiful consumption of fruits and vegetables and foods rich in potassium, essential fatty acids and phyto-oestrogens, in addition to regular weight-bearing exercise.

- Excessive consumption of sodium, vitamin A and alcohol should be avoided and smoking should be discouraged. All of these factors are believed to be detrimental to bone health.

- There are a variety of complementary therapies which are purported to improve bone health. However, there is a lack of scientific evidence to support these claims and it is advisable to follow professional medical advice prior to their use.

- Pharmacological intervention with bisphosphonates (alendronate, risedronate and etidronate) is the recommended first-line therapy for both the treatment and prevention of osteoporosis.

- Other pharmacological therapies for the treatment of osteoporosis include raloxifene, calcitonin, and the more recently introduced teriparatide and strontium ranelate. The latter two therapies are distinguished by their bone promoting activities in contrast to the antiresorptive mechanism of action of the older agents.

References

A list of the published evidence which has been reviewed in compiling the preceding section of *BESTMEDICINE*.

1 Royal College of Physicians and Bone and Tooth Society for Great Britain. *Osteoporosis – Clinical guidelines for prevention and treatment.* London: Royal College of Physicians, 2005.

2 Bisphosphonates (alendronate, etidronate, risedronate), selective oestrogen receptor modulators (raloxifene) and parathyroid hormone (teriparatide) for the secondary prevention of osteoporotic fragility fractures in postmenopausal women. Technology Appraisal 87. National Institute for Health and Clinical Excellence. January 2005. *www.nice.org.uk*

3 Shea B, Wells G, Cranney A *et al.* Calcium supplementation on bone loss in postmenopausal women. *Cochrane Database Syst Rev* 2004: CD004526.

4 Boonen S, Rizzoli R, Meunier PJ *et al.* The need for clinical guidance in the use of calcium and vitamin D in the management of osteoporosis: a consensus report. *Osteoporos Int* 2004; **15**: 511–19.

5 Delmas P. Treatment of postmenopausal osteoporosis. *Lancet* 2002; **359**: 2018–26.

6 Prentice A. Diet, nutrition and the prevention of osteoporosis. *Public Health Nutr* 2004; **7**: 227–43.

7 Chapuy M, Arlot M, Delmas P, Meunier P. Effect of calcium and cholecalciferol treatment for three years on hip fractures in elderly women. *BMJ* 1994; **308**: 1081–2.

8 Lips P, Graafmans W, Ooms M, Bezemer P, Bouter L. Vitamin D supplementation and fracture incidence in elderly persons. A randomized, placebo-controlled clinical trial. *Ann Intern Med* 1996; **124**: 400–6.

9 Lips P. Vitamin D deficiency and secondary hyperparathyroidism in the elderly: consequences for bone loss and fractures and therapeutic implications. *Endocr Rev* 2001; **22**: 477–501.

10 National Osteoporosis Society. 2005. What is osteoporosis ? *www.nos.org.uk*

11 University of Maryland Medical System. *www.umm.edu*

12 Kettler DB. Can manipulation of the ratios of essential fatty acids slow the rapid rate of postmenopausal bone loss? *Altern Med Rev* 2001; **6**: 61–77.

13 New SA. Intake of fruit and vegetables: implications for bone health. *Proc Nutr Soc* 2003; **62**: 889–99.

14 Barker ME, Blumsohn A. Is vitamin A consumption a risk factor for osteoporotic fracture? *Proc Nutr Soc* 2003; **62**: 845–50.

15 Sawka AM, Boulos P, Beattie K *et al.* Do hip protectors decrease the risk of hip fracture in institutional- and community-dwelling elderly? A systematic review and meta-analysis of randomized controlled trials. *Osteoporos Int* 2005. Epub ahead of print.

16 Patel S, Ogunremi L, Chinappen U. Acceptability and compliance with hip protectors in community-dwelling women at high risk of hip fracture. *Rheumatology* 2003; **42**: 769–72.

17 Bone and Tooth Society, National Osteoporosis Society, Royal College of Physicians. *Glucocorticoid-induced Osteoporosis: Guidelines for Prevention and Treatment.* London: Royal College of Physicians, 2002.

18 Xu H, Lawson D. Theories and practice in prevention and treatment principles in relation to Chinese herbal medicine and bone loss. *J Tradit Chin Med* 2004; **24**: 88–92.

19 Compston J, Rosen C. *Fast Facts – Osteoporosis.* 3rd edn. Oxford: Health Press, 2002.

20 Bonn D. New ways with old bones. Osteoporosis researchers look for drugs to replace hormone replacement therapy. *Lancet* 2004; **363**: 786–7.

21 Servier Laboratories Ltd. Protelos® (strontium ranelate). *Summary of product characteristics.* Slough, November, 2004.

22 *British National Formulary (BNF) 49.* London: British Medical Association and Royal Pharmaceutical Society of Great Britain. March 2005.

23 Mueller G, Russell R. Osteoporosis: pathogenesis and clinical intervention. *Biochem Soc Trans* 2003; **31**: 462–4.

24 Biswas PN, Wilton LV, Shakir SA. Pharmacovigilance study of alendronate in England. *Osteoporos Int* 2003; **14**: 507–14.

25 Cauley J, Norton L, Lippman M *et al.* Continued breast cancer risk reduction in postmenopausal women treated with raloxifene: 4-year results from the MORE trial. Multiple outcomes of raloxifene evaluation. *Breast Cancer Res Treat* 2001; **65**: 125–34.

26 Cummings S, Eckert S, Krueger K *et al.* The effect of raloxifene on risk of breast cancer in postmenopausal women: results from the MORE randomized trial. Multiple Outcomes of Raloxifene Evaluation. *JAMA* 1999; **281**: 2189–97.

27 Delmas PD. Clinical effects of strontium ranelate in women with postmenopausal osteoporosis. *Osteoporos Int* 2004 (E-pub ahead of print).

28 Reginster JY, Deroisy R, Jupsin I. Strontium ranelate: a new paradigm in the treatment of osteoporosis. *Drugs Today (Barc)* 2003; **39**: 89–101.

Acknowledgements

Figure 1 is adapted from The Royal College of Physicians, 2005.[1]

Figure 2 is adapted from The Royal College of Physicians, 2002.[17]

PATIENT NOTES
Dr Pam Brown

We now know that osteoporosis is preventable and treatable, and that treatment can improve even advanced disease.

Introduction

Osteoporosis is a bone disease that affects the whole of the skeleton, making the bones thin and more fragile, and therefore more likely to break (fracture). Unless the disease is treated, the bones continue to get thinner with time; one fracture makes other fractures more likely. It was previously believed that osteoporosis was a natural consequence of growing old, and that nothing could be done to stop it damaging bones. We now know that osteoporosis is preventable and treatable, and that treatment can improve even advanced disease. However, since it is impossible to rebuild badly damaged bones and make them as strong as they were originally, the earlier the disease is tackled, the better. Although lifestyle changes can help prevent osteoporosis, most people who have had fractures will need drug treatment to reduce the risk of further fractures.

How common is osteoporosis?

Osteoporosis is common, with one-in-two women over the age of 50 years, and one-in-five men, affected. Osteoporosis is important because of the fractures that it causes – more than 310,000 fractures are reported each year in the UK, including 70,000 hip fractures, 70,000 Colles (wrist) fractures, 120,000 vertebral (spine) fractures and 50,000 other fractures. The numbers of fractures continue to increase year on year, out of proportion to the increase in the elderly population in the UK. Osteoporosis costs around £1.7 billion annually; however this does not take into consideration the terrible burden of pain, disability and loss of life and independence that is associated with untreated disease.

Colles (wrist) fractures usually occur in younger women aged 50–60 years, with spinal fractures more common in those in their 60s and 70s, whilst hip fractures affect mainly people in their 70s and 80s. Osteoporotic fractures are often called 'fragility' fractures, meaning they resulted from a fairly minor injury – usually falling from a standing height or less, such as slipping on an icy pavement. Spinal fractures usually result from a normal activity such as lifting shopping bags or turning over in bed, rather than a fall.

Fractures cause pain and disability; they interfere with people's ability to walk, dress and shop, and hence often result in loss of independence, causing people to rely on family or friends for help. Hip fractures are the most severe consequence of osteoporosis, resulting in admission to hospital and an operation.

*Repeated
fractures result
in loss of height
and the back
becomes stooped.*

One-in-five elderly people who suffer a hip fracture die within the first 6 months, representing 14,000 deaths each year in the UK. Although around 80% of women can walk independently before their hip fracture, 1 year afterwards only 15–20% can do so, whilst less than 10% can climb stairs unaided even though 60% were able to do this before their fracture.

Vertebral fractures can cause severe back pain radiating around the chest or abdomen. Repeated fractures result in loss of height and the back becomes stooped, producing a 'kyphosis'. When this occurs, it is difficult for the person to stand upright or expand their lungs fully, and it can interfere with digestion. Since back pain is so common, it can be very difficult for doctors and people with osteoporosis to know that they have had a spinal fracture. Surprisingly, around one-third of vertebral fractures cause no symptoms at all, another third cause back pain but the fracture is not diagnosed, with only the remaining third being diagnosed. Those who have had a previous osteoporotic fracture are much more likely to have another. Twenty per cent of people with a vertebral fracture break another spinal bone within 1 year of the initial fracture.

Breaking a bone in later life is an important event, and should encourage the person to find out whether they need treatment for osteoporosis. For people aged under 75 years, a dual-energy X-ray absorptiometry (DXA) scan will be needed to confirm the diagnosis of osteoporosis. If there is a long waiting list for a scan, drug treatment can be started whilst waiting for the diagnosis, and stopped later if it is not needed. Unfortunately, DXA scans are still not available in all parts of the UK, which is far from ideal. Plain X-rays are good for diagnosing fractures, but are not good at predicting who has osteoporosis, as more than one-third of the bone mass needs to be lost before thinning of the bones can be diagnosed by X-ray.

How does osteoporosis occur?

Although we think of bones as solid and unchanging, they are continuously broken down and replaced, like most other parts of our bodies. Throughout the skeleton, bone-eating cells (osteoclasts) break down small areas of bone, and bone-building cells (osteoblasts) fill the areas with new bone. Early in life, the bone building cells work harder than the bone-eating cells and the skeleton gets bigger and denser. In midlife, bone breakdown and building occur at about the same rate, and the amount of bone stays fairly constant. However, later in life, and in those who are losing bone, the bone-eating cells remove more bone than the bone-building cells can replace, bone is slowly lost, and osteoporosis develops. As osteoporosis deteriorates, the cross struts of the bones that help give them strength get eaten away, making the bones even more fragile.

The amount of bone in the skeleton reaches a peak (the 'peak bone mass') in an individual's early 20s. By the mid-30s slow loss of bone begins in both men and women and continues for the remainder of life. In women, a rapid phase of bone loss is superimposed on this, lasting for about 5–10 years from the time of the menopause. Peak bone mass for an individual is thought to be genetically determined, but lifestyle factors such as poor diet, lack of exercise, smoking or late onset of periods in girls can all interfere with achieving peak bone mass. Exercising or dieting too much so that periods stop can also decrease the peak bone mass achieved. An individual's risk of osteoporosis later in life depends on the peak bone mass achieved, the time when bone loss begins and the rate at which it is lost later in life.

Who is most at risk of osteoporosis?

The highest risk of osteoporosis is in those who have had one or more fractures, those taking steroid tablets, the frail elderly (particularly those living in residential or nursing homes) and those who had an early menopause (before the age of 45 years). Elderly people who fall are also at a high risk of fractures.

Women whose mothers experienced a hip fracture before the age of 75 years, anyone who smokes, drinks alcohol heavily, is immobile, underweight (body mass index [BMI] <19 kg/m^2 [calculated by dividing your weight in kilograms by the square of your height in metres]), or has a condition such as coeliac disease that reduces the normal absorption of calcium from the diet, are at increased risk of osteoporosis.

What can you do to help reduce your risk of osteoporosis?

Although most people who have had fractures will need drug treatment, some simple changes to your lifestyle can also help reduce your risk. The good news is that these lifestyle changes also help reduce the risk of heart disease, stroke, diabetes and some cancers.

Studies have shown that eating a diet rich in fruit and vegetables, which are high in potassium, magnesium and vitamin K, may improve bone density and reduce hip fracture rates. High caffeine intake, particularly if combined with low calcium intake, may result in increased hip fracture rates. Smoking has a direct damaging effect on bone, and women who smoke tend to have their menopause at an earlier age than non-smokers, resulting in bone loss occurring earlier. One or two alcoholic drinks per day may be beneficial for bones, but more than 14 units per week increases the risk of osteoporosis (one unit is half a pint of beer, one glass of wine or one measure of spirits).

Some simple changes to your lifestyle can also help reduce your risk.

The advice on the type of exercise that is needed to protect bones has changed recently. It is now recognised that only vigorous weight-bearing exercise such as jumping, skipping, jogging, and resistance exercise can help to improve bone density. Brisk walking protects against heart disease, and staying active may reduce the risk of falls, but these are not enough on their own to protect against bone loss. Resistance exercise, with slow lifting of relatively heavy weights can increase bone density by 1–5% but only improves the bones that are being stressed. All types of exercise need to be carried out regularly and over the long-term to be effective. If you already have osteoporosis or have had a fracture, do not start any exercise programme without talking to your doctor as these types of exercise may increase your risk of further fractures.

Only vigorous weight-bearing exercise such as jumping, skipping, jogging, and resistance exercise can help to improve bone density.

3. Drug review – Alendronate (Fosamax®)

Dr Anna Palmer
CSF Medical Communications Ltd

Summary

Alendronic acid (alendronate) is one of the most widely prescribed drugs for the prevention and treatment of osteoporosis. Alendronate belongs to a family of drugs called the bisphosphonates and it acts primarily by inhibiting the resorption (breakdown) of bone. Secondary to this, alendronate also inhibits new bone formation. Daily or weekly dosing with alendronate has consistently been shown to increase bone mineral density (BMD) at the spine, various sites at the hip and throughout the whole body, although it has less consistent effects at the forearm. In addition, alendronate reduces biochemical markers of bone turnover including those which are indicative of bone formation and those which are a surrogate for bone resorption. These effects have been observed most often in postmenopausal women with osteoporosis but also occur in women with normal bone mass, in men with osteoporosis and in men or women suffering from glucocorticoid-induced osteoporosis. The effects of alendronate on bone turnover are apparent after just a few months of therapy, whilst significant increases in BMD are observed from between 6 months and 1 year after initiating alendronate therapy. These beneficial effects have been reported to persist over 10 years of therapy. Alendronate has an excellent safety and tolerability profile, which is generally not different to placebo treatment. In particular, accumulating evidence indicates that alendronate, when administered according to manufacturer's instructions (which aim to ensure minimal oesophageal exposure), the incidence of upper gastrointestinal adverse events is not different to that observed with placebo treatment.

Introduction

Alendronate is an oral antiresorptive agent licensed in the UK for the treatment and prevention of osteoporosis (and glucocorticoid-induced osteoporosis) in either a daily (5 or 10 mg) or weekly (70 mg) dose.

Alendronate is an oral antiresorptive agent licensed in the UK for the treatment and prevention of osteoporosis, including that induced by glucocorticoids, and the rarer occurrence of osteoporosis in men. A simpler weekly dosing regimen of alendronate (70 mg) has been introduced to improve patient compliance in the long-term treatment of postmenopausal women with osteoporosis. Along with etidronate and risedronate, alendronate is a member of the bisphosphonate drug class. These drugs inhibit bone resorption, and increase BMD by altering both the activation and function of osteoclasts – the cells responsible for the breakdown of bone. Alendronate is approved for use in over 80 countries worldwide and, in 2003/04, 61% of prescriptions for bisphosphonates in England were for alendronate.[1,2]

The primary goal of treatment for osteoporosis is to reduce the risk of fractures by decreasing bone loss and increasing bone mass of normal quality.[3] Preclinical studies have shown that alendronate is able to increase bone mass and bone strength with no evidence of a decrease in bone quality.[3,4] The following review will summarise the pharmacology of alendronate and the major findings from a wealth of clinical trials examining its potential for the treatment and prevention of osteoporosis.

Pharmacology

Chemistry

The chemistry of alendronate is of essentially academic interest and most healthcare professionals will, like you, skip this section.

As a bisphosphonate, alendronate is an analogue of pyrophosphate in which the central oxygen atom has been substituted by carbon (Figure 1). Currently, no known enzymes are able to cleave the phosphorus–carbon–phosphorus bond, which forms the framework for all the bisphosphonate compounds. This is likely to explain the stability and lack of metabolism that characterises this class of drugs.[5]

Mechanism of action

As explained in detail in the subsequent Pharmacokinetics section, alendronate is cleared rapidly from plasma and sequestered within bone at sites of high metabolic activity.[2] These sites tend to be composed of

Figure 1. Structure of alendronate (alendronic acid; monosodium 4-amino-1-hydroxybutylidene bisphosphonate).

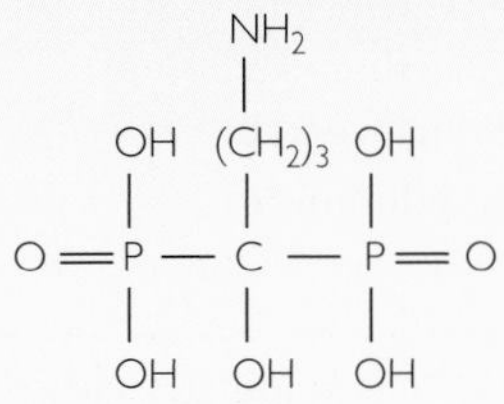

trabecular bone, which is characterised by high rates of turnover. Alendronate binds to hydroxyapatite (a calcium phosphate compound), which is exposed at sites of bone resorption and is mobilised and taken up by osteoclasts, thereby reducing the resorptive activity of these cells. Any remaining alendronate that is not taken up by osteoclasts is encased within newly formed bone and is then incorporated within the bone matrix where it becomes pharmacologically inactive. The pharmacological activity of this deposited alendronate is renewed when the process of bone resorption removes the outer layers of bone, bringing the molecule back to the surface where it interacts with osteoclasts again.

The processes of bone resorption and bone formation are tightly coupled and consequently any effect on one process will invariably affect the other. Thus, there is evidence to show that, although the primary effect of alendronate is to inhibit osteoclast bone resorption, in time the drug will also begin to inhibit bone formation.[2]

In order to increase resistance to fracture there must be an increase in bone strength which may occur via improved mineralisation, enhanced microarchitectural organisation or increased volume of bone.[4] Alendronate reduces bone turnover thereby increasing the time available for bone mineralisation. In addition, a recent examination of bone biopsies taken from both placebo- and alendronate-treated postmenopausal women with osteoporosis has shown that alendronate therapy increases trabecular bone volume and trabecular thickness.[6] Therefore, alendronate appears to increase BMD, improve bone strength and reduce fracture risk by means of increasing bone mineralisation, and possibly by increasing bone volume (although this requires corroboration in further trials), rather than affecting any alterations in bone architecture.[4]

Molecular mechanisms

The molecular targets by which the bisphosphonates mediate their effects have been progressively defined in greater detail.[5] Alendronate and other nitrogen-containing bisphosphonates inhibit farnesyl diphosphate synthase, an enzyme involved in cholesterol biosynthesis and protein isoprenylation. The alendronate-mediated inhibition of protein isoprenylation predominantly results in effects on small signalling molecules (GTPases). These small GTPases are vital for regulating a variety of osteoclast cellular functions including cytoskeletal function, formation of the ruffled border and apoptosis. The presence of a ruffled border, which itself is highly dependent on cytoskeletal function, is a hallmark of an active osteoclast. Disruption of both of these processes by alendronate inhibits osteoclast bone resorption. Furthermore, a secondary action of alendronate appears to be the induction of apoptosis, which decreases the number of osteoclasts and thus suppresses bone resorption over the longer term.

Overall, these mechanisms combine to cause an increase in bone mass and mineralisation, which are both attributable to a reduction in bone turnover. A steady state is gradually achieved and the rate of change

> Alendronate binds to hydroxyapatite, which is exposed at sites of bone resorption and is mobilised and taken up by osteoclasts, thereby reducing the resorptive activity of the osteoclast.

> A secondary action of alendronate appears to be the induction of apoptosis, which decreases the number of osteoclasts and thus suppresses bone resorption over the longer term.

of BMD mediated by alendronate appears to decline after the third year of therapy.[5]

Dosage and administration

The current recommended doses of alendronate for the treatment and prevention of osteoporosis in men and women in the UK are outlined in Table 1.[7] Studies performed in rats have indicated that similar reductions of bone loss can be achieved whether alendronate was administered daily, alternate daily, twice weekly or once weekly.[8] This study provided the rationale for weekly dosing with alendronate (Table 1). Alendronate should be taken in strict accordance with manufacturer's instructions, which aim to facilitate adequate drug delivery and absorption from the stomach whilst minimising exposure to the oesophagus, thereby reducing any associated irritation and consequent adverse reactions. Alendronate (5, 10 or 70 mg) should be taken in the morning with plenty of water (at least 200 mL) and prior to consumption of food, drinks (other than water) or other oral medications. Alendronate should not be chewed. The patient should be in an upright position to take the drug, and should remain so for at least 30 minutes thereafter. Patients should not eat or drink during this period.[7]

☛ *The pharmacokinetics of a drug are of interest to healthcare professionals because it is important for them to understand the action of a drug on the body over a period of time.*

Pharmacokinetics

Absorption and distribution

Alendronate has very poor oral bioavailability and absorption is further compromised by coingestion with food, due to the formation of insoluble complexes.[2] When administered after an overnight fast and 2 hours before a standardised breakfast, the oral bioavailability of alendronate (dose range 5–80 mg) was 0.7% in women and 0.6% in men. The bioavailability of alendronate is reduced by 85–90% if taken up to 2 hours after breakfast, but bioavailability is less affected (reduced by ~40%) when alendronate is taken between 30 minutes and 1 hour

Table 1. Recommended doses of alendronate.[7]

Alendronate dose	Indication
5 mg daily	• Prevention of osteoporosis in postmenopausal women • Treatment and prevention of glucocorticoid-induced osteoporosis in men, premenopausal women and postmenopausal women receiving hormone replacement therapy
10 mg daily	• Treatment of osteoporosis in postmenopausal women • Treatment of osteoporosis in men • Treatment and prevention of glucocorticoid-induced osteoporosis in postmenopausal women not receiving hormone replacement therapy
70 mg weekly	• Treatment of osteoporosis in postmenopausal women

prior to breakfast. Bioavailability of alendronate, 10 mg, was also reduced by approximately 60% after coadministration with coffee and orange juice (in comparison with water) in healthy postmenopausal women. The low bioavailability of alendronate and consequent low penetration into cells contributes to its favourable safety profile.[8]

Our understanding of the distribution of alendronate in humans is largely extrapolated from studies in rats and supported by clinical urinary excretion data.[2] Plasma concentrations following therapeutic doses are exceedingly low and predominantly below the limit of detection. An intravenous dose (1 mg/kg) of alendronate administered to rats was distributed widely throughout the soft tissue of the body, followed by either elimination in the urine or rapid redistribution to the skeleton. The concentration present in non-calcified tissues fell from 63% at 5 minutes post-administration to 5% after 1 hour. The mean steady state volume of distribution, exclusive of bone, is at least 28 L and human plasma protein binding (predominantly to albumin) is around 78%. As the concentration of alendronate in soft tissue slowly decreases, so its concentration in bone gradually rises. Five minutes after intravenous administration of alendronate to rats, 30% of the dose resides in bone, whilst by 1 hour levels had risen to between 60 and 70%. Furthermore, the distribution of alendronate within bone is determined by the rate of bone turnover. Thus, greater deposition occurs at sites with greater blood flow and bone resorptive activity, such as trabecular bone.[2,4,7]

Metabolism and elimination

In common with other bisphosphonates, alendronate does not appear to be metabolised in animals or humans.[2] The major routes for clearance of alendronate from the plasma are via deposition in bone and urinary excretion. Renal clearance was found to average 4.26 L/hour. A negligible amount of the drug (<0.2%) was detected in faeces after intravenous administration. Following distribution of alendronate from plasma to soft tissue to bone, the drug is slowly released from the skeleton with a multiphasic pattern of elimination. A detailed elimination profile of alendronate has been obtained from intravenous dosing of radiolabelled alendronate, 10 mg, administered to 12 patients with metastatic breast cancer.[2] Approximately 45% of the dose was excreted in urine in the first 8 hours post-dose whilst only around 5% was excreted in the following 64 hours. This drop in urinary excretion is thought to correlate with sequestration of alendronate in the skeleton. Approximately one-third of the alendronate initially retained within bone is renally excreted over the first 6 months whilst subsequent excretion is much slower. The terminal elimination half-life of alendronate (10.5±2.65 years) was estimated using renal clearance data collected over 18 months following intravenous administration of alendronate to 11 patients.[2,4,7]

The distribution of alendronate within bone is determined by the rate of bone turnover. Greater deposition occurs at sites with greater blood flow and bone resorptive activity, such as trabecular bone.

In common with other bisphosphonates, alendronate does not appear to be metabolised in animals or humans.

Clinical efficacy

Study design and outcome measures

The majority of studies investigating the clinical efficacy of alendronate in osteoporosis utilise the World Health Organisation (WHO) diagnostic criteria for osteoporosis for recruitment purposes.[9] This is described in greater detail in the Disease Overview section of this edition of *BESTMEDICINE*. Briefly, these criteria define reduced bone density (indicative of osteoporosis) in terms of a T-score of less than or equal to –2.5, measured at the lumbar spine or femoral neck of the hip. Common exclusion criteria that are applied in clinical trials include the presence of disorders of bone or mineral metabolism, recent history of major upper gastrointestinal disease, presence of other serious disease, low bodyweight and previous or current treatment with other osteoporosis drugs, corticosteroids, anticonvulsants or regular aspirin.[10]

Current European directives require that patients taking part in clinical trials for new osteoporosis therapies must have adequate intakes of calcium and vitamin D.[11] This is due to the vital role that these nutrients play in general bone health and the necessity for adequate levels of these nutrients for the optimal effect of antiresorptive therapies. Thus, most clinical trials will provide supplements to subjects (commonly calcium carbonate, 500 mg, and vitamin D, 250 IU) in order to maintain dietary intakes of calcium above 1 g/day.

The measurement of BMD, at present, is central to the diagnosis, research and management of osteoporosis.[12] There are several different methods currently available for the measurement of this parameter including single photon absorptiometry and single-energy X-ray absorptiometry. These both measure BMD in the appendicular bones (those relating to limbs), whilst dual photon absorptiometry, dual-energy X-ray absorptiometry (DXA) and quantitative computed tomography measure BMD mainly in the axial skeleton (bones of the trunk). Unless otherwise specified in the text, BMD refers to areal BMD expressed in grams per square centimetre, measured by DXA.

Biochemical markers of bone metabolism are often measured in clinical trials in order to assess the response to antiresorptive therapy, although there is still a lack of consensus on their value in predicting an individual patient's risk of fracture.[13] A persuasive rationale for their use in monitoring bone turnover, as an alternative to regular monitoring of BMD, is that the small changes in BMD which manifest after a year or more of bisphosphonate therapy are only slightly larger than the precision error of DXA (1–3%), the most commonly used instrument for the measurement of BMD.[14] Thus, a 3% increase in BMD may represent a real increase in bone density but may also simply be indicative of instrument variability. Markers of bone formation include bone-specific serum alkaline phosphatase (BSAP; in contrast, total serum alkaline phosphatase is a less sensitive marker of bone formation), serum intact N-terminal propeptide of type 1 procollagen (P1NP) and osteocalcin.[15] Markers of bone resorption are generally related to collagen degradation and include urinary levels of hydroxyproline,

> The measurement of BMD is central to the diagnosis, research and management of osteoporosis.

deoxypyridinoline, cross-linked N-telopeptides of type 1 collagen (NTX) and cross-linked C-terminal telopeptides of type 1 collagen (CTX).[13,14]

Frequency and magnitude of dose

Several studies have investigated the optimum dosing schedule for alendronate based on early observations from animal studies which have indicated that weekly dosing is as effective and well tolerated as daily dosing.[8] The efficacy and safety of once-weekly alendronate, 70 mg (n=519), twice-weekly alendronate, 35 mg (n=369), and daily alendronate, 10 mg (n=370), was compared in a year-long, double-blind, multicentre study of postmenopausal women (aged 42–95 years) with osteoporosis (T-score ≤2.5 in either the lumbar spine or femoral neck).[16] All three regimens elicited similar increases in BMD at all sites tested and similar alterations in biochemical markers of bone formation and resorption. All treatment regimens were well tolerated with a similar incidence of upper gastrointestinal adverse events. The study was extended for a further year and, despite significant increases in BMD with all treatment regimens, there remained no difference between the groups (Table 2).[9] Similarly, there remained no difference in markers of bone resorption or formation (NTX and BSAP, respectively) between the three groups in the second year. Upper gastrointestinal adverse events occurred in 29.3, 29.0 and 30.0% of patients in the once-weekly, twice-weekly and once-daily treatment groups. Furthermore, the incidence rates of clinical fracture were similar amongst the different treatment groups. Therefore, these data corroborate those reported after 1 year of alendronate therapy.[9,16]

A further study examined patient preference for once-weekly (70 mg) or once-daily alendronate (10 mg) in 266 postmenopausal women in a randomised, open-label, crossover design.[17] The treatment periods were each of 4 weeks in duration, separated by a 1-week washout phase. The majority of the study group preferred the once-weekly regimen (86.4%;

Table 2. Mean percentage changes from baseline in bone mineral density (BMD) after 2 years of alendronate therapy with different dosage regimens.[9]

Site	Changes from baseline in BMD (%)		
	Alendronate, 10 mg, once daily	Alendronate, 35 mg, twice weekly	Alendronate, 70 mg, once weekly
Spine	7.4	7.0	6.8
Total hip	4.3	4.3	4.1
Femoral neck	3.5	3.5	3.3
Trochanter	6.1	6.2	5.9
Total body	1.6	1.6	1.8

NB: All changes represent significant increases from baseline (p≤0.001).

p<0.001) and found it to be more convenient (89%; p<0.001) and more likely to support long-term compliance (87.5%; p<0.001) than the once-daily dosing schedule. Overall, these studies suggest that weekly dosing with alendronate offers equivalent efficacy, greater convenience, improved compliance and a lower risk of upper gastrointestinal symptoms compared with daily administration.[18]

The optimum dose of alendronate for prevention of osteoporosis by stabilisation of BMD was examined in a 3-year study in 447 postmenopausal women with a baseline bone density within two standard deviations (–2 SD) of the normal range.[19] Women were randomly assigned to receive either placebo or alendronate (1, 5, 10 or 20 mg/day). Patients in the 20 mg/day group received this dose for 2 years, followed by placebo for the third year. The effects of these different treatment regimens are illustrated in Figure 2. Although alendronate, 1 mg, was shown to attenuate the loss of bone mass observed with placebo, only the higher doses of alendronate actively increased BMD. A similar pattern was observed in terms of the effects of treatment on biochemical markers of bone turnover (i.e. NTX, deoxypyridinoline, BSAP and osteocalcin), where alendronate, 5, 10 and 20 mg, exhibited similar effects whilst alendronate, 1 mg, had minimal effects. These data support the use of alendronate, 10 mg, as the optimal daily therapeutic dose for treating pre-existing osteoporosis whilst the 5 mg dose appears to be optimal for stabilisation of bone mass in patients at risk of developing osteoporosis.

Bone density and fracture risk at hip, spine and forearm

In the 1990s, two randomised, double-blind, placebo-controlled studies of identical design were conducted to determine the clinical efficacy of oral alendronate therapy in postmenopausal osteoporosis.[3] The results of these studies were combined for publication. A total of 881 postmenopausal women (T-score ≤–2.5; mean age 64 years; 16.5 years post menopausal; body mass index [BMI] 24 kg/m^2) were randomised to receive alendronate, 5, 10 or 20 mg/day, or placebo, for 3 years. Patients receiving alendronate, 20 mg/day, received this dose for 2 years, followed by 5 mg/day in the third year. The BMD at the lumbar spine, hip (femoral neck and trochanter), forearm and in the total body were determined using DXA, whilst fractures were detected using yearly digitised radiographs. Mean baseline BMD (data combined for alendronate groups) did not differ between the different treatment groups or according to the type of DXA instrument used.

Significant increases in BMD were observed at the spine, hip and in the total body with all three doses of alendronate, compared with significant reductions recorded in the placebo group. Relative to placebo, alendronate, 10 mg, mediated an 8.8% increase in BMD of the spine, a 5.9 and 7.8% increase at the femoral neck and trochanter, respectively and a 2.5% increase for total body. At 2 years, the 10 mg dose of alendronate had increased BMD by the same extent as the 20 mg dose

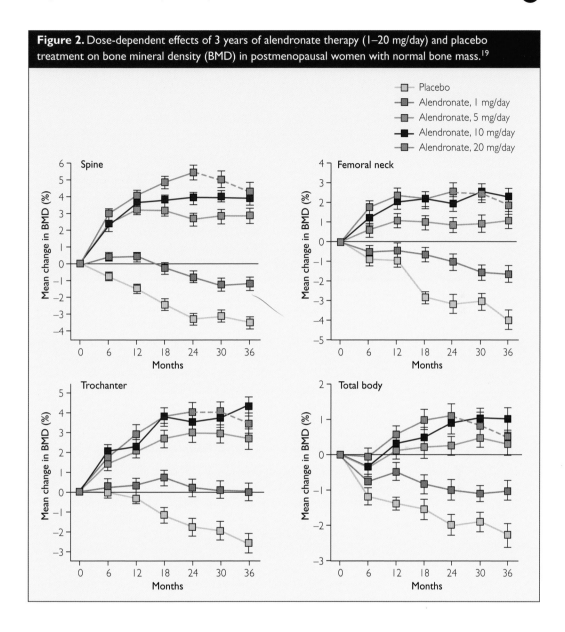

Figure 2. Dose-dependent effects of 3 years of alendronate therapy (1–20 mg/day) and placebo treatment on bone mineral density (BMD) in postmenopausal women with normal bone mass.[19]

but increased BMD by a significantly greater extent than the 5 mg dose at all skeletal sites measured. In the third year of treatment, only the 10 mg dose of alendronate mediated significant increases in BMD at the same sites. Also, in the forearm (a site consisting almost entirely of cortical bone), a 2.2% greater BMD was observed with alendronate, 10 mg, than with placebo ($p<0.001$). The risk of new vertebral fractures was reduced by alendronate, in comparison with placebo, and this reduction in risk remained after stratification for age (less than or more than 65 years) or in the presence or absence of previous vertebral fractures. The percentage of women with new vertebral fractures was 2.9% after 5 mg alendronate, 2.8% after 10 mg alendronate and 4.1% after 20/5 mg

Daily treatment
with alendronate
progressively
increases the
BMD of the spine,
hip, forearm and
total body, and
reduces the risk
of vertebral
fractures, the
progression of
spinal deformity
and height loss in
postmenopausal
women with
osteoporosis.

alendronate ($p<0.05$ *vs* placebo [6.2%]). Amongst the women with new vertebral fractures, the proportion with two or more fractures was lower in the combined alendronate group (18%) than in the placebo group (68%). Increases in the spine deformity index were less common in the alendronate group (reported in 33% of women) than in the placebo group (41% of women; $p<0.05$). Amongst the women with new vertebral fractures, a pronounced loss of stature was observed in those receiving placebo treatment (23.3 mm), compared with a much less profound loss in height following alendronate treatment (5.9 mm). In contrast, women without new vertebral fractures demonstrated much smaller height losses, which were similar between the active treatment and placebo groups (2.8 and 3.3 mm, respectively). Alendronate treatment also conferred a reduced incidence of non-vertebral fractures compared with placebo (8.5 *vs* 10.7%, respectively), though the study was not sufficiently powered to detect differences between the treatment groups in this regard. Alendronate was well tolerated and the most common side-effects considered by the investigators to be treatment-related were abdominal pain, musculoskeletal pain, nausea, dyspepsia, constipation and diarrhoea.[3]

In summary, data from this study indicate that daily treatment with alendronate progressively increases the BMD of the spine, hip, forearm and total body, and reduces the risk of vertebral fractures, the progression of spinal deformity and height loss in postmenopausal women with osteoporosis.

The Fracture Intervention Trial

The Fracture Intervention was a landmark investigation conducted into the effects of alendronate on fracture frequency in postmenopausal women with low bone mass.[10] This double-blind, placebo-controlled trial was conducted over 3 or 4 years with alendronate administered at 5 mg/day for the first 2 years increasing to 10 mg/day at the end of the second year. A total of 6459 women were randomised to treatment and divided into two groups: those with existing vertebral fractures at baseline (n=2027, treatment duration 3 years) and those without vertebral fractures (n=4432, treatment duration 4 years). The majority of participants (82%) had baseline dietary calcium intakes of less than 1 g/day and were given a daily supplement containing 500 mg calcium carbonate and 250 IU vitamin D. The criteria for enrolment into the study included: age between 55 and 80 years; postmenopausal status of at least 2 years; femoral neck BMD of at least 0.68 g/cm^2. In the population with pre-existing vertebral fractures at baseline, the presence of fracture was indicative of osteoporosis. In contrast, in women without pre-existing vertebral fractures the mean T-score was –1.6, which though representative of a reduced BMD, is not necessarily indicative of osteoporosis (in fact, only approximately one-third of women in the trial had a T-score $\leq$–2.5). Thus, this study did not employ standard recruitment criteria (T-score $\leq$ –2.5), although the effects of baseline BMD on alendronate efficacy were specifically examined.[20] The primary endpoints determined in this trial were BMD (assessed by DXA), and both clinically evident fractures (i.e. those that came to medical attention and were reported to study centres by participants) and those confirmed radiographically (morphometric) fractures. Compliance rates in this study were good; at the final study visit, 87% of patients were still receiving placebo and 89% remained on alendronate, whilst follow-up radiographs were obtained for 98% of patients. The data arising from the various aspects of the Fracture Intervention Trial are discussed in detail below.

Efficacy in women with pre-existing vertebral fractures

The earliest published results from the Fracture Intervention Trial concerned the effects of alendronate in the 2027 women with pre-existing vertebral fractures (defined as any ratios of vertebral height being more than three standard deviations [–3 SD] below the population norm).[21] A new morphometric vertebral fracture was defined as a decrease of 20%, and at least 4 mm, in vertebral height from the baseline radiograph.

Treatment with alendronate was associated with a significant increase in mean bone mass compared with placebo ($p<0.001$ at all sites). Specifically, bone mass increased at the femoral neck (4.1% difference from placebo), total hip (4.7%), posterior–anterior lumbar spine (6.2%), trochanter (6.1%), whole body (1.8%), lateral spine (6.8%) and proximal forearm (1.6%). Of the 1946 participants for whom follow-up radiographs were obtained, 8% of alendronate-treated women experienced new vertebral fractures, compared with 15% in the placebo arm (Table 3). Alendronate treatment also reduced the incidence of multiple new vertebral fractures compared with placebo (≥2 fractures: 0.5 *vs* 4.9%, respectively; ≥4 fractures: 0 *vs* 1.3%, respectively). Overall, the risk of new radiographic vertebral fractures was 47% lower with alendronate than with placebo ($p<0.001$). In terms of clinical fractures, fewer women treated with alendronate suffered clinical vertebral fractures (2.3%) compared with placebo (5.0%; $p<0.001$). Fewer alendronate-treated women reported fractures at the hip and wrist compared with those receiving placebo, though the incidence of clinical fractures at other sites was similar in the two treatment groups (Table 3). Furthermore, alendronate treatment resulted in less pronounced height loss (6.1 mm) over the 3 years of follow-up than placebo treatment (9.3 mm; $p<0.001$). Finally, the incidence of adverse events, including upper gastrointestinal problems, was similar in the placebo and treatment groups, as was the proportion of women discontinuing due to adverse events (7.6 *vs* 9.6% for alendronate *vs* placebo; $p=0.123$). However, whilst the incidence of gastrointestinal events was low it is important to note that peptic-ulcer disease and dyspepsia were part of the exclusion criteria employed in this study.

A *post hoc* analysis of this study was performed in order to investigate the effects of alendronate therapy on the daily consequences of back pain, resulting from pre-existing vertebral fractures, in the same group of postmenopausal women.[22] Vertebral fractures are the most common

> Alendronate treatment resulted in less height loss over the 3 years of follow-up than placebo treatment.

Table 3. Percentage of women with at least one new fracture of the types indicated.[20,21]

Fracture type	Women with new fracture(s) (%)			
	Vertebral fracture at baseline[21]		No vertebral fracture at baseline[20]	
	Placebo	Alendronate	Placebo	Alendronate
Clinical fractures				
Any clinical	18.2	13.6	14.1	12.3
Any non-vertebral	14.7	11.9	13.3	11.8
Hip	2.2	1.1	1.1	0.9
Wrist	4.1	2.2	3.2	3.7[c]
Other clinical[a]	9.9	9.8	10.2	8.2*
Vertebral fractures[b]				
≥1	15.0	8.0	3.8	2.1*
≥2	4.9	0.5	0.5	0.2

[a]Includes fractures of the hand, finger, shoulder, ankle, toes etc.
[b]Morphometric fractures defined by radiographic findings alone.
[c]The relative risk for this data pair is >1 (i.e. risk of fracture is higher with alendronate than with placebo) whereas the relative risk for all other data sets is <1 (i.e. risk of fracture is lower with treatment).
*$p<0.05$ vs placebo.

Alendronate reduces the risk of several types of fracture, increases BMD and reduces the functional limitations resulting from back pain secondary to vertebral fracture.

osteoporotic fracture and a history of previous vertebral fracture is an important risk factor for future fractures.[23] The presence of vertebral fractures is associated with a substantial increase in back pain, functional limitation, loss of height and disability. The most pronounced effect of alendronate in this analysis was a 63% reduction in the number of bed-rest days experienced over 3 years due to back pain in comparison with placebo (1.9 vs 5.1 days; $p<0.001$).[22] Alendronate also reduced the number of days of limited activity due to back pain (61.8 days) in comparison with placebo (73.2 days; $p<0.05$). However, the number of days of moderate or severe back pain, though slightly reduced by alendronate, was not significantly different between the two groups (moderate pain: 185.6 vs 191.3 days, $p=0.53$; severe pain: 32.4 vs 37.2 days, $p=0.07$; for alendronate and placebo, respectively).

Thus, in postmenopausal women with low bone mass and pre-existing vertebral fractures, alendronate reduces the risk of several types of fracture, increases BMD and reduces the functional limitations (bed-rest days and limited activity) resulting from back pain secondary to vertebral fracture.

Efficacy in women without pre-existing vertebral fractures

Although vertebral fractures are an extremely common feature of postmenopausal osteoporosis, the majority of postmenopausal women with low BMD will not have pre-existing fractures. The effect of alendronate treatment (4 years, dose described previously [see page 38]) was examined in 4432 women, without pre-existing vertebral fractures, from the Fracture Intervention Trial cohort described previously.[20] At baseline, 37% of women had femoral neck T-scores of ≤–2.5, 32% had T-scores between –2.0 and –2.5, and 31% had T-scores between –1.5 and –2.0.

In comparison with placebo, alendronate treatment increased the average BMD at all measured sites (Figure 3; $p<0.001$). The alendronate-mediated increases in BMD did not differ between subgroups of women with different baseline bone densities (i.e. T-score: ≤2.5, –2.0 to –2.5, or –1.5 to –2.0). The primary endpoint of this study was the incidence of clinical fractures which, after 48 months of treatment, occurred in a smaller proportion of alendronate-treated than placebo-treated women (Table 3). A small reduction in the proportion of women with hip fractures was observed with alendronate (0.9%) compared with placebo (1.1%; relative hazard 0.79).[a] Fractures at sites other than the spine, hip or wrist also occurred in fewer alendronate-treated women than placebo-treated patients (relative hazard 0.79). However, a greater number of women suffered fractures of the wrist in the alendronate group than in the placebo group (Table 3).

In contrast to the changes in BMD, which increased by a similar extent regardless of baseline BMD, alendronate mediated much greater reductions in clinical fracture risk in those women with lower BMD at

> The primary endpoint of this study was the incidence of clinical fractures which, after 48 months of treatment, occurred in a smaller proportion of alendronate-treated than placebo-treated women.

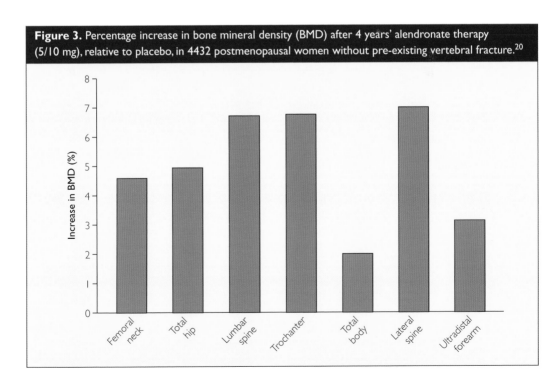

Figure 3. Percentage increase in bone mineral density (BMD) after 4 years' alendronate therapy (5/10 mg), relative to placebo, in 4432 postmenopausal women without pre-existing vertebral fracture.[20]

---

[a]The interpretation of a relative hazard, for example, of 0.79 is a reduction in risk of 21%.

Alendronate
reduced the risk
of hip fractures by
a much greater
extent in those
women with low
baseline BMD.

baseline (T-score $\leq$ –2.5). In women with the lowest baseline BMD, clinical fractures occurred in 13.1% of alendronate-treated women and in 19.6% of placebo-treated women (difference of 6.5%; relative hazard 0.64). By contrast, there was no apparent benefit of alendronate on clinical fracture risk in women with higher baseline BMD (T-score –1.5 to –2.5). In addition, alendronate reduced the risk of hip fractures by a much greater extent in those women with low baseline BMD (1.0 *vs* 2.2% for alendronate *vs* placebo; relative hazard 0.44). Finally, alendronate reduced the incidence of new radiographically defined vertebral fractures (Table 3), and mediated a smaller reduction in stature (7.0 mm height loss) than placebo over the 4 years of treatment (8.5 mm height loss; *p*<0.001). Tolerability was similar in the two groups.

In summary, 4 years of alendronate therapy decreases the risk of all clinical fractures, hip fractures, vertebral fractures and deformities in postmenopausal women with low BMD of the hip but with no existing vertebral fractures at baseline.

Efficacy in women both with and without vertebral fractures

A further subgroup analysis of the Fracture Intervention Trial data set out to determine the relative effect of alendronate therapy on fracture risk in women with pre-existing vertebral fractures (vertebral fracture group) compared with those without existing fracture and with T-score less than –2.5 (low BMD group).[24] The study cohort consisted of a total of 3658 postmenopausal women. Additional objectives of this analysis were to examine the effects of alendronate in both groups of women combined and to determine the time course of effect of alendronate.

Due to the *post hoc* nature of this analysis, there were several statistically significant differences in baseline characteristics of the two populations (including age, years since menopause and baseline BMD), though these were small and were considered unlikely to impact on the interpretations of this analysis. Alendronate consistently reduced the risk of all types of fracture (relative risk: 0.1–0.88 according to site) in both the vertebral fracture and the low BMD arms of the study. Figure 4 illustrates the risk reduction mediated by alendronate in the combined group of women from both the vertebral fracture and low BMD arms of the study. This demonstrates that some reduction in risk is apparent for all types of fracture from as early as 1 year of therapy. The only difference apparent between the two arms of the study was in the incidence of new vertebral fractures. Women in the vertebral fracture group experienced a higher incidence of new vertebral fractures and a greater reduction in fracture risk in response to alendronate treatment. For example, in the vertebral fracture arm, the annual fracture rate of clinical vertebral fractures was 1.77 in the placebo group and 0.82 in the alendronate group, corresponding to a relative risk reduction of 54%. In the low BMD group, the corresponding relative risk reduction was 16% (annual fracture rates: 0.41 and 0.35, respectively). This trend was also apparent with regard to the projected numbers needed to treat (NNT) with alendronate for 5 years to prevent a selected type of fracture. The

Women in
the vertebral
fracture group
experienced a
higher incidence
of new vertebral
fractures and a
greater reduction
in fracture risk
in response
to alendronate.

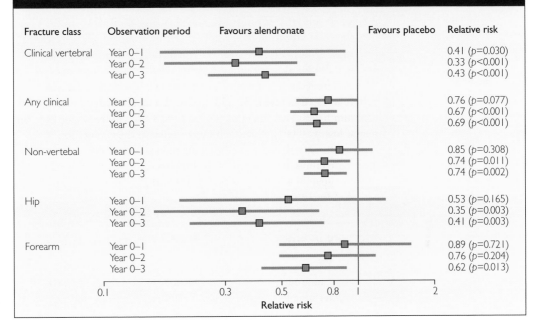

Figure 4. Cumulative reductions in fracture risk in years 1, 2 and 3 of the Fracture Intervention Trial amongst women with vertebral fractures or femoral neck bone mineral density (BMD) T-scores of less than −2.5 at baseline.[24]

NNT was 8 in the vertebral fracture arm and 29 in the low BMD arm, reflecting the greater relative efficacy of alendronate in women with existing vertebral fractures and the greater prevalence of new vertebral fractures in this group.

In summary, alendronate treatment for 3 or 4 years provides benefits to postmenopausal women whose osteoporosis is defined either by the pre-existence of vertebral fractures or by the measured presence of low BMD. Alendronate reduces the risk of new fractures of the spine, hip or wrist in both groups, though the effects on new vertebral fracture risk are magnified in women with existing vertebral fractures.

An additional recently published *post hoc* analysis of the Fracture Intervention Trial data has demonstrated that alendronate was also effective in reducing the risk of both radiographic and clinical vertebral fracture in a subgroup of women with a T-score of between −1.6 and −2.5 at the femoral neck.[25] This subgroup of women was a combined group including women with and without baseline vertebral fracture who can be defined as suffering from osteopenia rather than osteoporosis.

Prediction of future fracture risk

Data from the Fracture Intervention Trial have also been used to determine whether the risk of future fracture may be directly related to changes in BMD or bone turnover.[13,26] The relationship between the magnitude of change in BMD (following alendronate therapy) and the reduction in risk of new vertebral fractures was determined in a *post hoc*

Alendronate treatment for 3 or 4 years provides benefits to postmenopausal women whose osteoporosis is defined either by the pre-existence of vertebral fractures or by the measured presence of low BMD.

analysis of 2984 women.[26] Despite the established role of low BMD as a predictor of increased fracture risk and a diagnostic marker for osteoporosis, few studies have determined whether the degree of change in BMD directly relates to the extent of future fracture risk. Data were categorised into three groups according to whether increases in BMD at 12 and 24 months were zero, less than 3% or at least 3%. Women with the largest increase in BMD (≥3%) had the lowest incidence of new vertebral fractures. At 24 months, there was a clear relationship between BMD measured at the spine, femoral neck or total hip and the risk of a new vertebral fracture (Figure 5). At the 12-month time point, this correlation was weaker and was not apparent with BMD measured at the femoral neck. The fact that the risk of fracture cannot solely be explained in terms of change in BMD is supported by the results of a long-term follow-up study of 9704 women (aged >65 years) in which

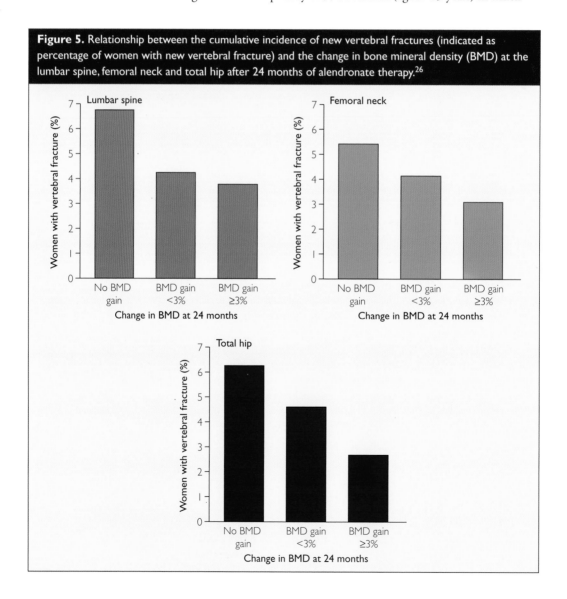

Figure 5. Relationship between the cumulative incidence of new vertebral fractures (indicated as percentage of women with new vertebral fracture) and the change in bone mineral density (BMD) at the lumbar spine, femoral neck and total hip after 24 months of alendronate therapy.[26]

only 10–44% of fractures were attributable to the presence of osteoporosis (as defined by a T-score ≤–2.5).[27] Indeed, it is currently debated whether BMD measurement represents the best method with which to guide diagnosis and treatment of osteoporosis and to predict fracture risk.[28]

Biochemical markers of bone formation (BSAP and P1NP) and bone resorption (CTX) were measured in serum samples taken at baseline and after 1 year of alendronate (n=3105) or placebo treatment (n=3081) in the Fracture Intervention Trial with the objective of determining whether these markers could be used to directly predict future fracture risk.[13] Mean baseline levels of all three markers were not different between alendronate and placebo-treated women, and all markers fell by between 31 and 59% after 1 year of alendronate therapy (Table 4). The smaller reductions observed in placebo-treated women were presumed to be an effect of calcium and vitamin D supplementation. In the placebo group compared with the alendronate group, a greater number of women (no statistical analyses performed) suffered spinal fracture (217 *vs* 119 women, respectively), non-spinal fracture (426 *vs* 360 women) and hip fracture (46 *vs* 26 women). Regression analysis showed that, in the alendronate group, the greatest reductions in BSAP were associated with the greatest reductions in subsequent spine, hip and non-spine fracture whilst women with the smallest change in BSAP suffered the greatest number of subsequent fractures. No such association was observed in the placebo group. Furthermore, each standard deviation reduction in the percentage change in BSAP was associated with 26% reductions in the risk of fracture of the spine, 11% reductions in risk of non-spine fractures and 39% reductions in risk of fracture of the hip. There were also significant associations between changes in P1NP and CTX and reductions in spinal fracture, though the association with non-spinal and hip fracture was not significant.

Thus, greater reductions in markers of bone turnover associated with alendronate therapy are associated with fewer hip, spine and non-spine fractures. Of the biochemical markers measured in this study, BSAP correlates most closely with future fracture risk. There is also a

> Greater reductions in markers of bone turnover associated with alendronate therapy are associated with fewer hip, spine and non-spine fractures.

Table 4. Changes in biochemical markers of bone turnover after 1 year of alendronate or placebo treatment in postmenopausal women.[13]

Biochemical marker	Alendronate (n=3105)		Placebo (n=3081)	
	Baseline value	Change from baseline (%)	Baseline value	Change from baseline (%)
BSAP (ng/mL)	13.7	–31.1	13.8	–8.4
P1NP (ng/mL)	51.4	–50.9	51.7	–9.6
CTX (pmol/L)	3327	–59.2	3313	–30.6

BSAP, bone-specific alkaline phosphatase; P1NP, N-terminal propeptide of type 1 procollagen; CTX, cross-linked C-terminal telopeptides of type 1 collagen.

relationship between the degree of change in BMD and subsequent fracture risk such that women who demonstrate the greatest alendronate-mediated increases in BMD have the lowest odds of suffering future vertebral fracture.

Long-term alendronate therapy

For the prevention of osteoporosis

Postmenopausal women are at high risk of developing osteoporosis and thus, well-tolerated preventative therapy is an attractive avenue of investigation. A cohort of 160 postmenopausal women with normal baseline bone mass (spinal BMD no more than two standard deviations above or below the healthy normal mean [mean baseline BMD at the spine 0.93 g/cm^2]; aged 40–59 years; 6–36 months' postmenopausal) were recruited to three alendronate dosing regimens: alendronate, 5 mg/day, for 5 years (5 mg group); placebo for 3 years then alendronate, 5 mg/day, for 2 years (placebo/5 mg group); and alendronate, 20 mg, for 2 years followed by 1 year of placebo and 2 years of no treatment (20 mg/placebo group).[29] The first 3 years of placebo treatment in women in the placebo/5 mg group resulted in progressive reductions in BMD at the spine, femoral neck, trochanter, total body and forearm whilst the subsequent 2 years of alendronate, 5 mg, mediated increases in BMD at all of the sites, with the exception of the forearm (Figure 6). Overall, there was no increase from baseline in BMD at the 5 year endpoint in the women in this group. No improvement in BMD of the forearm (at either one-third distal or ultra distal sites) was observed with any of the alendronate regimens employed. Women in either the alendronate, 5 mg group, or the 20 mg/placebo group all displayed increased BMD at the spine, femoral neck and trochanter in the first 3 years of therapy. At this point, BMD appeared to plateau in both groups but remained above baseline levels at the spine (increases at year 5: 2.5% in 5 mg group and 2.8% in 20 mg/placebo group; both $p<0.001$ from baseline) and trochanter (3.2 and 2.5%, respectively; both $p<0.01$ from baseline) but declined to baseline values at the femoral neck. The total body BMD remained at baseline levels (i.e. was considered not stabilised) throughout the study in both the 5 mg and 20 mg/placebo groups. This study also evaluated the biochemical markers of bone turnover, NTX and CTX, which fell by between 70 and 80% in the 5 mg and 20 mg/placebo groups in the first year of treatment and thereafter remained stable unless treatment was withdrawn at which point levels began to rise again.

A further randomised, placebo-controlled study – the Early Postmenopausal Intervention Cohort – examined lower doses of alendronate (2.5 or 5 mg/day) in postmenopausal women with normal bone density (baseline spine BMD ≥0.8 g/cm^2; aged 45–59 years).[30] At baseline, 585 women were randomised to treatment, of whom 52.1% completed the 6-year study. Of the 280 patients who discontinued therapy at some point during the course of the study, 22% withdrew due to adverse events. A progressive loss was observed in bone density with placebo treatment at all measured sites. As observed in previous studies

NTX and CTX fell by between 70 and 80% in the first year of treatment and then remained stable unless treatment was withdrawn.

of shorter duration and in women with osteoporosis, the most pronounced improvements in BMD with alendronate were observed at the lumbar spine and total hip. Relative to placebo, alendronate, 2.5 mg, increased BMD at the spine by 4.7% and at the total hip by 3.7%, whilst alendronate, 5 mg, provided respective increases of 6.6 and 4.9% (all $p<0.001$ compared with baseline). The effects of alendronate, 5 mg, were significantly greater than those mediated by the 2.5 mg dose ($p<0.001$ for the spine and $p<0.01$ for the hip). Up until the fourth year of the study, small increases in total body BMD were observed with alendronate, 5 mg, but at years five and six, total body BMD declined in both alendronate groups such that the final change in BMD represented a reduction in bone mass from baseline of –1.3% with the 2.5 mg dose and –0.4% with the 5 mg dose. In comparison with a final reduction in total body BMD of 3.7% in the placebo group, this represents a degree of stabilisation in bone density loss. Alendronate at both doses attenuated the loss in BMD at the forearm but did not completely prevent it. Mean levels of NTX decreased in all treatment groups, including placebo, over the course of this study. The most profound decrease in NTX occurred during the initial 6 months of therapy (~25% with placebo but ~50% and ~60% with alendronate, 2.5 mg and 5 mg, respectively). Thereafter, a more gradual decline in NTX was observed, and the final reductions from baseline were 37.9% with placebo, 63.9% with alendronate, 2.5 mg, and 68.0% with the 5 mg dose of alendronate ($p<0.001$ both alendronate groups *vs* placebo).

The incidence of adverse events was not significantly different between the three treatment groups, and the lowest incidence of fracture occurred in the alendronate, 5 mg, group (8.9, 10.3 and 11.5% for

> The most pronounced improvements in BMD with alendronate were observed at the lumbar spine and total hip.

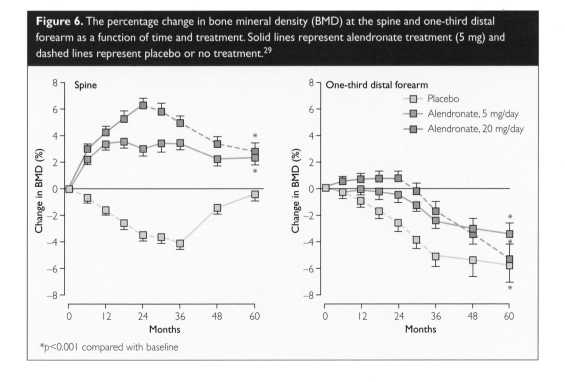

Figure 6. The percentage change in bone mineral density (BMD) at the spine and one-third distal forearm as a function of time and treatment. Solid lines represent alendronate treatment (5 mg) and dashed lines represent placebo or no treatment.[29]

*$p<0.001$ compared with baseline

alendronate, 5 and 2.5 mg, and placebo, respectively; no significant differences reported).

In summary, alendronate appears to be an effective strategy for the preservation of bone mass in postmenopausal women with normal baseline bone density.

For the treatment of osteoporosis

Long-term treatment with alendronate has also been examined in women with postmenopausal osteoporosis to determine safety, tolerability and continuing effects on bone activity and bone mineral density. In addition, discontinuation of alendronate therapy has been examined to determine the optimum period of treatment and to determine for how long changes in BMD are maintained following treatment withdrawal. This is particularly interesting given that alendronate, once sequestered within the skeleton, is eliminated very slowly (with a half-life of over 10 years [see Pharmacokinetics]). Following an initial 3-year double-blind, placebo-controlled, randomised trial of alendronate in 994 postmenopausal women with osteoporosis, a further 4-year open-label extension phase was conducted in which all patients received alendronate, 5 or 10 mg/day.[31] The continued use of placebo was no longer considered ethical after the first 3 years of the study in light of the convincing evidence for alendronate's ability to reduce the risk of fracture. Three hundred and fifty women were included in this 7-year study with a mean spinal BMD of 0.71 g/cm^2 at baseline. The total lumbar spine BMD increased by 11.4% after 7 years of alendronate, 10 mg, and by 8.2% with the lower dose (5 mg). Increases in hip BMD appeared to plateau after 3 years of treatment. By year seven, alendronate, 5 mg, had increased BMD at the femoral neck by 2.6% and at the trochanter by 5.6% whilst alendronate, 10 mg, elicited respective increases of 4.9 and 9.5%. In common with the long-term studies described above, the greatest reductions in biochemical markers of bone turnover (NTX and BSAP) occurred during the first 6 months of treatment and were then maintained for the remainder of the study. Discontinuation of alendronate resulted in small, non-significant declines in BMD at the hip, and small but significant reductions in BMD in the total body and forearm. Alendronate withdrawal also resulted in small increases in urinary NTX and serum BSAP.[31]

A further study examined the effects of alendronate treatment administered over 10 years in 247 postmenopausal women with osteoporosis (mean baseline characteristics: spine BMD 0.7 g/cm^2; age 63 years; 16 years' postmenopausal; BMI 24 kg/m^2; 18–31% with pre-existing vertebral fractures).[32] The mean increases in BMD after 10 years of alendronate, 10 mg/day, were 13.7% at the lumbar spine, 10.3% at the trochanter, 5.4% at the femoral neck, 6.7% at the proximal femur, 2.9% for total body and 1.0% at the distal one-third forearm compared with baseline (Figure 7). With the exception of the forearm (0.8% decrease in BMD), increases in BMD also occurred, but were of lesser magnitude, with the 5 mg/day dose of alendronate. A third group of

Alendronate appears to be an effective strategy for the preservation of bone mass in postmenopausal women with normal baseline bone density.

The total lumbar spine BMD increased by 11.4% after 7 years of alendronate, 10 mg, and by 8.2% with the lower dose (5 mg).

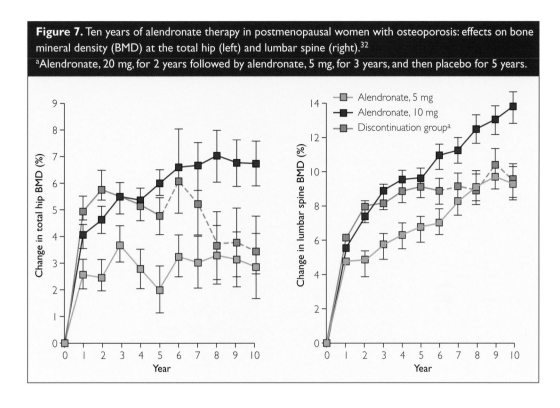

Figure 7. Ten years of alendronate therapy in postmenopausal women with osteoporosis: effects on bone mineral density (BMD) at the total hip (left) and lumbar spine (right).[32]
[a]Alendronate, 20 mg, for 2 years followed by alendronate, 5 mg, for 3 years, and then placebo for 5 years.

women received alendronate, 20 mg/day, for the first 2 years and then 5 mg/day for 3 years, followed by placebo treatment for 5 years (defined as the discontinuation group). Women in this group experienced increases in BMD at year ten from baseline and these were of similar magnitude to those mediated by the 5 mg dose at the lumbar spine (9.3% in both groups), trochanter (5.3 and 4.8% for discontinuation groups *vs* alendronate, 5 mg) and total hip (3.4 and 2.9%, respectively). Mean levels of NTX and BSAP declined dramatically during the first year of treatment and remained stable over the 10 years of continuing treatment. The smallest height loss from the sixth to the tenth year occurred in alendronate, 10 mg group (5.6 mm), though this was not significantly different from that observed in the alendronate, 5 mg group (7.2 mm), or the discontinuation group(7.0 mm). The incidence of all adverse events was similar in all three groups, though the lowest incidences of upper gastrointestinal events and oesophageal events were observed in the alendronate, 5 mg group (14.1 and 1.3%, respectively; alendronate, 10 mg group: 27.9 and 2.3%, respectively; discontinuation group: 24.1% and 7.2%).

The therapeutic effects of alendronate upon BMD, therefore, appear to persist over a 10-year period with no loss of safety or tolerability whilst discontinuation of treatment does not result in any acceleration of bone loss or any increase in the rate of bone turnover. Rather, discontinuation of alendronate results in a gradual loss of the effects of the drug which manifests as a slow decrease in BMD and a gradual return to baseline levels of bone activity. These conclusions are

The therapeutic effects of alendronate upon BMD, therefore, appear to persist over a 10-year period with no loss of safety or tolerability.

corroborated in an interim report from a long-term extension of the Fracture Intervention Trial.[33] In the UK, there are no recommendations regarding the optimal treatment period for alendronate therapy and, as treatment remains well tolerated, there appears to be no rationale for premature treatment discontinuation.

Comparative studies

Alendronate *vs* oestrogen therapy

Hormone replacement therapy (HRT) is no longer a first-line treatment option for either prevention or treatment of osteoporosis due to an association with increased risk of breast cancer and recent controversy regarding its effects upon cardiovascular risk.[34] Several studies have compared the effect of alendronate with that of oestrogen (sometimes in combination with progestin) in preventing the onset of osteopororis in healthy postmenopausal women.[35–39] One of the largest of these studies was derived from the Early Postmenopausal Intervention Cohort (described previously) in which 1609 women (aged 45–59 years; baseline spine BMD ≥0.8 g/cm^2) were randomised to receive oral alendronate (2.5 or 5 mg/day), open-label oestrogen–progestin, or placebo, for 4 years.[35,36] The regimen of oestrogen–progestin given to participants differed between the US and European cohorts, such that the US women received 0.625 mg/day of continuous conjugated equine oestrogens plus 5 mg/day of medroxy-progesterone acetate whilst in Europe, women received micronised 17β-estradiol, 1–2 mg/day, and norethisterone acetate, 1 mg/day, administered sequentially according to a monthly cycle. The effects of these therapies on BMD are illustrated in Figure 8, which shows that the European oestrogen–progestin regimen mediated the greatest increases in BMD at all time points and at all measured sites. Alendronate, 5 mg, was more effective than the 2.5 mg dose, with both the US and European oestrogen–progestin regimens being significantly more effective than alendronate, 5 mg/day, in promoting BMD at the spine (US: $p<0.001$ *vs* alendronate, 5 mg; Europe: $p<0.05$) and forearm ($p<0.001$ both regimens *vs* alendronate, 5 mg). The European oestrogen–progestin regimen also mediated greater increases in total body BMD compared with alendronate, whilst both regimens mediated similar changes to alendronate, 5 mg, at the hip. Similar decreases in NTX, osteocalcin and BSAP were observed in all treatment groups and all were significantly reduced in comparison with placebo ($p<0.001$). The percentage of drug-related adverse events was greater in the combined oestrogen–progestin group (88%) in comparison with all the other treatment groups.[36]

Whilst the above study indicates that oestrogen–progestin therapy is more effective than the low 'preventative' dose of alendronate (5 mg), other studies have shown that the efficacy of oestrogen–progestin is not markedly different from alendronate when administered at 10 mg/day.[37,38] For example, 2 years of treatment in hysterectomised postmenopausal women (n=425) with either alendronate, 10 mg/day, or conjugated equine oestrogen, 0.625 mg/day, resulted in similar increases in BMD at

Figure 8. Mean percentage change in bone mineral density (BMD) at the spine, hip, total body and forearm in postmenopausal women treated with low-dose alendronate (2.5 or 5 mg/day), oestrogen–progestin or placebo.[36]

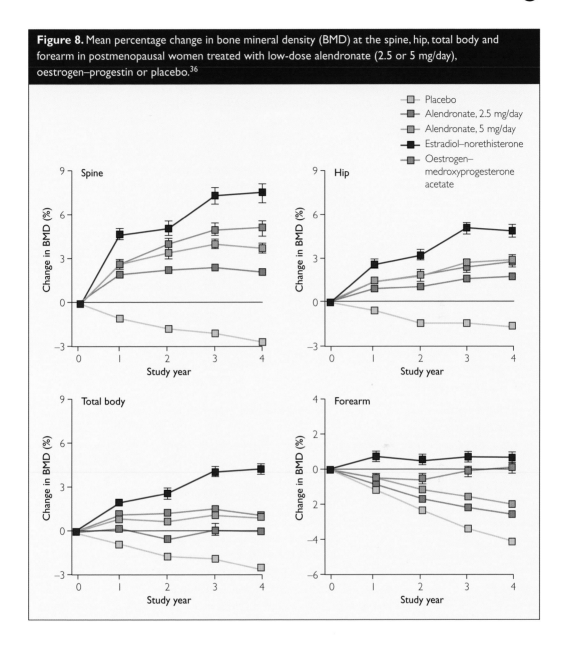

the lumbar spine (6.0 and 6.0%, respectively), total hip (4.0 and 3.4%), femoral neck (2.9 and 2.6%), trochanter (5.9 and 4.3%) and total body (1.3 and 1.7%).[37] Furthermore, alendronate, 10 mg, stimulated a greater reduction in urinary NTX than did the conjugated oestrogens (61 and 52% reductions, respectively) though reductions in BSAP did not differ between the two groups. The tolerability profile of both active treatment groups and the placebo group was favourable, though conjugated oestrogen treatment was associated with more reports of breast pain and weight gain.

Withdrawal of oestrogen, alendronate or both?

Alendronate has been examined in combination with oestrogen in a number of studies, as has the effect of the withdrawal of HRT.[37–39] In comparison with the results given above for treatment with either alendronate or conjugated oestrogen, 2 years of combined therapy (alendronate, 10 mg, and conjugated equine oestrogen, 0.625 mg) mediated greater increases in BMD than either of the single therapies at the spine (8.3%), total hip (4.7%), femoral neck (4.2%), trochanter (6.5%) and total body (2.0%).[37] Combination therapy was also effective in a further double-blind placebo-controlled trial conducted over 2 years but, in this case, the between-group differences were not significant.[38] The primary aim of this trial was to determine the effects of discontinuation of alendronate, oestrogen, or a combination of both treatments on bone turnover and density.[38] The principal finding from this study was that the accelerated bone loss associated with withdrawal of oestrogen therapy (which has been widely reported) is attenuated by co-therapy with alendronate. The losses in BMD observed at 3 years after discontinuation of oestrogen at year two were 4.5% at the spine, 1.8% at the hip, 2.4% at the femoral neck and 2.4% at the trochanter. In contrast, women who discontinued treatment with either alendronate or combined alendronate and oestrogen showed no significant change in BMD at any of the skeletal sites measured. Similarly, discontinuation of oestrogen therapy was associated with the greatest rebound increase in NTX and BSAP in comparison with discontinuation of either oestrogen–alendronate or alendronate alone. Thus, smaller overall decreases in NTX from baseline occurred in the oestrogen discontinuation group (15%; $p<0.01$), compared with overall decreases of 39 and 38%, in the alendronate and combination discontinuation treatments, respectively ($p<0.001$ from baseline). For comparison, continuous 3-year treatment with combination therapy mediated an overall decrease in NTX of 75%. Similar trends were reported for BSAP.

Overall, these data demonstrate the beneficial effects on bone density and bone turnover of adding alendronate to existing oestrogen therapy. Importantly, these benefits of alendronate addition even extend into the period following discontinuation of treatment.

> The accelerated bone loss associated with withdrawal of oestrogen therapy (which has been widely reported) is attenuated by cotherapy with alendronate.

Alendronate *vs* raloxifene

Raloxifene is a selective oestrogen receptor modulator (SERM), which inhibits bone resorption via specific agonistic effects on oestrogen receptors. A randomised, double-blind, multicentre study directly compared the effects of alendronate (70 mg once weekly) with raloxifene (60 mg daily) in 487 postmenopausal women with low BMD at the hip or spine (mean baseline values: T-score –2.9; age 62 years; BMI 25.5 kg/m^2; 15 years' postmenopausal).[40] Both treatments resulted in increases from baseline in BMD over the 12-month treatment period but alendronate elicited significantly greater increases than raloxifene. Thus, the mean percentage increase in BMD at the lumbar spine was 4.8% for alendronate and 2.2% for raloxifene ($p<0.001$), whilst at the hip,

> Both treatments resulted in increases in BMD over the 12-month treatment period but alendronate elicited significantly greater increases than raloxifene.

alendronate mediated increases of 2.2–2.9% compared with increases of 0.8–1.0% with raloxifene ($p<0.001$). Alendronate also provoked significantly greater changes to biochemical markers of bone formation and resorption. Thus, treatment with alendronate was associated with 68 and 51% reductions in NTX (measured and expressed relative to creatinine) and BSAP, in contrast to respective reductions of 27 and 11.9% with raloxifene. The incidence of all adverse events was similar between the groups, but raloxifene was associated with a greater incidence of drug-related upper gastrointestinal events (22%) and vasomotor adverse experiences (7.9%) in comparison with alendronate (15.4 and 2.4%, respectively; $p<0.05$).

This study demonstrated a greater effect of alendronate, when compared with raloxifene, in reducing bone density and biochemical markers of bone turnover in women with postmenopausal osteoporosis. A further comparative study of alendronate and raloxifene is currently underway which aims to determine the relative efficacy of both compounds on fracture outcome in a large group (~3000) of postmenopausal women with osteoporosis (Evista and Alendronate Comparison [EVA] trial).[41] Results of the EVA study are keenly anticipated.

Alendronate *vs* calcitonin

Calcitonin is an additional antiresorptive agent licensed in the UK for the treatment of postmenopausal osteoporosis. Two years of treatment with alendronate (10 and 20 mg) was compared with intranasal salmon calcitonin (100 IU/day) in 286 postmenopausal osteoporotic women. Alendronate was shown to be superior to calcitonin both in terms of increasing BMD and reducing bone turnover.[42] No differences were observed between the two doses of alendronate. The minor effects of calcitonin on spine, femoral neck and trochanter BMD were not significantly different from either baseline or placebo whereas alendronate mediated significant increases in BMD of similar magnitude to those reported elsewhere in this review. In addition, both doses of alendronate decreased total serum alkaline phosphatase and serum osteocalin by similar extents whilst calcitonin had no effect.

> Alendronate was shown to be superior to calcitonin both in terms of increasing BMD and reducing bone turnover.

Alendronate *vs* teriparatide

Teriparatide is a recombinant version of the amino-terminal fragment of human parathyroid hormone and is thought to increase new bone formation by promoting osteoblast cell numbers. It is available in the UK as a subcutaneous injection (recommended daily dose 20 µg) for the treatment of postmenopausal osteoporosis. Several studies have directly compared the efficacy of teriparatide with that of alendronate.[43,44]

A randomised, double-blind trial of 146 postmenopausal women (T-score $\leq$–2.5; aged 30–85 years) compared alendronate (10 mg/day) with teriparatide (40 µg, once daily) for up to 17 months.[43] Teriparatide treatment results in marked increases in BMD at the lumbar spine, femoral neck, total hip and total body, which were significantly greater than those observed with alendronate (all $p<0.001$). Teriparatide increased both the bone mineral content (by 15.1%) and the projected bone area (by 1.29 cm^2) components of BMD at the lumbar spine by a greater extent than alendronate (6.6% and 0.49 cm^2 increases, respectively; both $p<0.001$ in favour of teriparatide). Increases in BMD at the trochanter, however, were of the same magnitude in the alendronate and teriparatide groups. Neither alendronate nor teriparatide altered BMD at the ultradistal forearm, whilst at the one-third distal radius, teriparatide mediated a significant decrease in BMD ($p<0.001$) but alendronate had no effect. Consistent with the divergent mechanisms of action of the two drugs, alendronate mediated decreases in levels of NTX and BSAP whilst teriparatide increased the concentration of both (by 160 and 100% at month 12, respectively). Moreover, teriparatide was associated with a lower frequency of non-vertebral fracture than alendronate of 4.1% compared with 13.7% ($p<0.05$). Both therapies were generally well tolerated. Teriparatide treatment was associated with transient elevations in serum calcium, though these were asymptomatic.

In summary, teriparatide appears to be superior to alendronate in increasing BMD at the femoral neck and lumbar spine and in reducing the incidence of non-vertebral fracture, though this superiority did not extend to the forearm or the trochanter. Despite the improved efficacy of teriparatide over the short-term in comparison with alendronate, it is important to be aware that the current UK license for teriparatide restricts its use to short-term therapy only (i.e. a maximum of 18 months) and that current National Institute for Health and Clinical Excellence (NICE) guidelines report that it is a less cost-effective option than bisphosphonate therapy.[1]

Alendronate in combination with parathyroid hormone

The combination of two effective treatments with non-overlapping mechanisms of action may intuitively be predicted to provide greater benefits than either agent alone. However, several studies have shown that the combination of alendronate with parathyroid hormone may actually be less effective than either monotherapy.[44,45]

One study has examined the effect of the full-length (1–84 amino acid) parathyroid hormone (100 μg/day), either alone or in combination with alendronate (10 mg/day) in 238 postmenopausal women with osteoporosis.[44] BMD was assessed by DXA and additional measurements of volumetric BMD (measured in g/cm^3) and bone geometry were assessed using quantitative computed tomography. Parathyroid hormone, alendronate and the combination of the two all increased BMD at the lumbar spine whilst only alendronate or the combination increased BMD at the total hip and femoral neck. Volumetric BMD at the trabecular spine was increased by the greatest extent with parathyroid hormone (25.5%), whilst the other two treatments increased this

---

Teriparatide appears to be superior to alendronate in increasing BMD at the femoral neck and lumbar spine and in reducing the incidence of non-vertebral fracture, though this superiority did not extend to the forearm or the trochanter.

Several studies have shown that the combination of alendronate with teriparatide may actually be less effective than either monotherapy.

parameter by similar extents (12.9% with combination therapy and 10.5% with alendronate). Volumetric density of cortical bone at the hip was reduced by parathyroid hormone (−1.7%; $p<0.001$ *vs* combination), increased by alendronate (1.2%) and unchanged by combination therapy (+0.1%). Cortical volume was also unchanged by combination therapy but was increased by both alendronate and parathyroid hormone. In terms of biochemical markers of bone turnover, P1NP (a marker of bone formation) and CTX (a marker of bone resorption) were increased by parathyroid hormone, decreased by alendronate and decreased by a lesser extent with the combination treatment.

Thus, this study provides no evidence of synergy between parathyroid hormone and alendronate. The lack of advantage of this combination is supported by results from a further small clinical trial conducted in men with low BMD.[45] It is unclear whether these data extrapolate to the combination of teriparatide with alendronate but, at present, there is no evidence to suggest that this combination would provide additional beneficial. Indeed, the biochemical data on bone turnover suggest that concurrent use of alendronate attenuates the beneficial effects of parathyroid hormone in promoting bone formation.

Alendronate in comparison with other bisphosphonates

Risedronate and etidronate are additional members of the bisphosphonate class that are licensed in the UK. Whilst alendronate and risedronate are considered first-line options for the treatment of osteoporosis, etidronate may be considered if these are unsuitable or intolerable.[46]

Alendronate has been compared with risedronate in two large, randomised, double-blind studies in postmenopausal women with low bone mass.[47,48] A weekly regimen of alendronate (70 mg/week), a daily regimen of risedronate (5 mg/day) and a double-dummy placebo treatment were compared in 549 postmenopausal women (mean age 69 years; mean 21 years postmenopausal; T-score ≤ −2.5) given over 12 months.[48] The percentage reductions in BMD mediated by the two treatment groups are summarised in Table 5. In summary, these data indicate that alendronate treatment was superior to risedronate in terms of the changes in BMD at the spine, femoral neck, trochanter and total hip. Biochemical markers of bone turnover, NTX and BSAP, were reduced by both alendronate (−52 and −40%; $p<0.001$ *vs* baseline) and risedronate (−32 and −24%; $p<0.001$ *vs* baseline) but these reductions were significantly greater in the alendronate group ($p<0.001$). Both therapies were well tolerated and caused a similar incidence of adverse events.

An additional study has compared the effects on alendronate and risedronate when both drugs were administered in a weekly regimen (alendronate, 70 mg/week; risedronate, 35 mg/week) to women with postmenopausal osteoporosis.[47] This 12-month trial included 1053 patients with a mean age of 65 years, who were on average

> Alendronate treatment was superior to risedronate in terms of the changes in BMD at the spine, femoral neck, trochanter and total hip.

Table 5. Comparative effects of alendronate and risedronate on the percentage change in bone mineral density (BMD) at the spine and hip in comparison with placebo.[48]

Treatment	Change in BMD (%)			
	Lumbar spine	Femoral neck	Trochanter	Total hip
Placebo	0.09	−0.08	−0.65	−0.17
Risedronate (5 mg/day)	2.80*	1.44*	0.90**	0.93*
Alendronate (70 mg/week)	4.75*†	2.23*‡	3.27*†	2.70*†

*$p<0.001$, **$p<0.05$ vs baseline
†$p<0.001$, ‡$p<0.05$ vs risedronate

18.5 years postmenopausal. In common with the previous study, alendronate mediated greater increases in BMD at the trochanter, femoral neck, lumbar spine and total hip than did risedronate therapy. The treatment differences between the two therapies were 1.4% at the hip trochanter, 1.1% at the total hip, 0.7% at the femoral neck and 1.2% at the lumbar spine. Significant differences in BMD between the treatment groups were observed as early as the 6-month time point at the total hip, femoral neck and lumbar spine. Significant reductions in NTX, CTX, BSAP and P1NP were observed with both treatments by 3 months of therapy ($p<0.001$ from baseline). However, alendronate mediated a significantly greater reduction than risedronate in all of these markers after 3 months of treatment ($p<0.001$) and these differences were sustained at the 12-month endpoint of the trial (reductions at 12 months: NTX: −53 *vs* −40%; CTX: −78 *vs* 54%; BSAP: −41 *vs* −28%; P1NP: −64 *vs* −48%; all $p<0.001$ for alendronate *vs* risedronate and for both in comparison with baseline).

The efficacy of alendronate and etidronate has been compared in a randomised, controlled, open-label clinical trial in 140 postmenopausal women with vertebral osteoporosis (aged 60–82 years; mean hip BMD 0.7 g/cm^2).[49] This 12-month trial comprised four treatment groups of continuous alendronate (10 mg/day), cyclical alendronate (10 mg daily for 3-month on/off cycles), cyclical etidronate (400 mg for 14 days, then calcium carbonate, 500 mg, for 76 days; repeated in 3-monthly cycles), or calcitriol (250 ng twice daily). Increases in BMD at the spine and total hip were observed in all three bisphosphonate groups ($p<0.01$) but not in the calcitriol group. The greatest increases were observed with continuous alendronate (5.7% increase in BMD at the spine and 2.6% increase at the hip) whilst the respective increases with cyclical alendronate and cyclical etidronate were similar (4.1 and 4.9%, respectively, at the spine; 1.6 and 2.0%, respectively, at the total hip). Significant reductions in bone turnover were noted in all treatment groups with the greatest reductions observed with continuous alendronate treatment.

In summary, these data indicate that alendronate promotes greater increases in BMD and greater reductions in markers of bone turnover than either risedronate or etidronate. However, and as previously discussed in this review, it is thus far unproven whether these outcome measures relate directly to tangible clinical benefits and there remains a lack of evidence regarding the relative efficacies of the three bisphosphonates in reducing fracture risk.

Efficacy in special populations

Glucocorticoid-induced osteoporosis

Glucocorticoids are used widely in the treatment of inflammatory diseases of all kinds. However, osteoporosis is a common complication of long-term glucocorticoid therapy.[50] Following high-dose glucocorticoids, loss of bone density from sites such as the vertebrae can be rapid and may lead to fractures within months.

The combined results of two double-blind, placebo-controlled, multicentre trials into the effects of alendronate (5 and 10 mg) for the prevention and treatment of glucocorticoid-induced osteoporosis were combined for publication.[51] The total study group comprised 560 men and women, aged 17–83 years, who required long-term therapy (≥1 year) with oral glucocorticoids (≥7.5 mg/day prednisone or equivalent) and were recruited regardless of their baseline BMD. Treatment with alendronate, 5 or 10 mg, for 48 weeks, significantly increased BMD at the lumbar spine (2.9%), trochanter (2.7%) and femoral neck (1.0%), whilst total body BMD was increased only in the 10 mg alendronate group (0.7%; all comparisons, $p<0.001$ vs baseline). The alendronate-mediated increases in BMD did not differ according to either the glucocorticoid dose or the duration of glucocorticoid treatment. Levels of NTX and BSAP were decreased by 60 and 27%, respectively, with alendronate therapy. There was a slight but non-significant difference in the incidence of morphometrically defined vertebral fractures between the placebo and treatment groups (3.7 vs 2.3% for placebo and alendronate, respectively).

These and other data lend support to a role for alendronate in the prevention and treatment of glucocorticoid-induced osteoporosis in men and women.[50,51]

Efficacy in men

Alendronate is licensed for the treatment and prevention of osteoporosis in men. Osteoporosis is less common in males yet still represents a serious and debilitating condition. Two hundred and forty-one men (aged 31–87 years; femoral neck T-score ≤–2.0; 50% with vertebral fractures at baseline) were randomised to receive alendronate, 10 mg, or placebo for 2 years in a double-blind fashion.[52] Alendronate treatment resulted in increases in BMD at all measured sites from as early as 6 months and these effects were not dependent upon serum free testosterone levels at baseline. The increases in BMD mediated by

> Alendronate promotes greater increases in BMD and greater reductions in markers of bone turnover than either risedronate or etidronate.

> The alendronate-mediated increases in BMD did not differ according to either the glucocorticoid dose or the duration of glucocorticoid treatment.

alendronate after 2 years were 7.1% at the lumbar spine, 2.5% at the femoral neck, 4.3% at the trochanter, 3.1% at the total hip and 2.0% at the total body (all $p<0.001$ vs baseline). Alendronate also reduced NTX (by 59%; $p<0.001$) and BSAP (by 38%; $p<0.001$) over the study period from baseline and these were significantly different from the smaller decreases (9 and 5%, respectively) observed with placebo. A non-significant increase in height of 0.6 mm was observed in alendronate-treated men whereas men in the placebo group suffered a loss in height of 2.4 mm ($p<0.001$ vs baseline). There was little difference in fracture rates between the two groups, but the incidence of vertebral fractures (assessed by quantitative morphometric methods) was significantly reduced in the alendronate group (0.8%) compared with the placebo group (7.1%; $p<0.05$). The tolerability profile of alendronate was reported to be favourable in this patient population with a similar incidence of adverse events and no difference in study withdrawals between treatment groups. Alendronate therefore appears to be a valuable treatment option for the amelioration of bone loss and prevention of fracture in men diagnosed with osteoporosis.

> Alendronate appears to be a valuable treatment option for the amelioration of bone loss and prevention of fracture in men diagnosed with osteoporosis.

Efficacy in the elderly

The effect of alendronate has been specifically evaluated in older women with osteoporosis since this population carries the greatest risk for fracture.

The first study set out to determine the dose effect of alendronate (1, 2.5 and 5 mg/day) in osteoporotic women aged between 60 and 69 years (n=135) or 70 and 85 years (n=224).[53] Alendronate at all three doses mediated increases in BMD from baseline at the spine, hip, total body and one-third forearm. However, only the 2.5 mg and 5 mg doses mediated significant increases in comparison with placebo. Dose-dependent decreases in urinary deoxypyridinoline, NTX/creatinine, serum osteocalcin and total serum alkaline phosphatase were also observed. The magnitude of all of these changes is consistent with results described previously in this review. However, there were no differences in any outcome between the older and younger women in this study.

A second study has determined the efficacy of alendronate (10 mg/day) and HRT (0.625 mg/day conjugated equine oestrogen with or without medroxyprogesterone, 2.5 mg/day), or a combination of both, in a group of 373 community-dwelling older women (65–90 years [mean age 72 years]; mean baseline total hip T-score –1.3) of whom 34% were diagnosed with osteoporosis and the remainder were osteopenic.[54] In common with the study by Greenspan et al. described previously,[38] this study also demonstrated that combination treatment with oestrogen and alendronate provides slightly greater increases in BMD (at the hip and spine) than either therapy alone in this older patient population. Changes in BMD were found not to be consistently related to baseline age. However, the proportion of patients responding (i.e. a change in BMD at the spine or hip greater [more positive] than –1.0%) was greatest in women younger than 70 years (93%) compared with those between 70 and 75 years (88%) or those older than 75 years

> Changes in BMD were found not to be consistently related to baseline age.

(80%; $p<0.01$). No treatment differences or age-related changes in safety or tolerability were reported.

In conclusion, alendronate is well tolerated and effectively improves BMD and decreases bone turnover in an older population of postmenopausal women, although the effects of alendronate on fracture frequency in this population remain to be determined.

Efficacy in diabetic patients

There is little information regarding the effects of alendronate on bone mass in diabetic patients. A subset of patients derived from the Fracture Intervention Trial were classified as having type 2 diabetes by self-report at baseline or follow-up.[55] The 297 women recruited to the diabetic arm of this study included those who had received a diagnosis of diabetes since the age of 30 years, used insulin or hypoglycaemic medications, or demonstrated a random non-fasting glucose value of more than 11 mmol/L. These criteria may have resulted in the inclusion of some women with late onset type 1 diabetes and some who were not actually diabetic. Alendronate (5 mg for 2 years and then 10 mg for 1 year) was given to 148 women in the diabetic arm and the remainder were given placebo. Further comparisons were performed against non-diabetic alendronate- and placebo-treated women from the original Fracture Intervention Trial.

Alendronate mediated significant increases in BMD at the lumbar spine (6.6%), total hip (2.4%), femoral neck (2.6%), trochanter (4.1%) and intertrochanter (1.8%) of diabetic women ($p<0.001$ vs placebo or baseline). These increases were non-significantly lower than those reported in the 2825 non-diabetic alendronate-treated women from the original study group (lumbar spine 7.5%, total hip 3.1%, femoral neck 3.4%, trochanter 4.9% and intertrochanter 2.4%). However, it was noted that diabetic women treated with placebo lost more bone than non-diabetic women at the total hip (-1.9 vs -1.2%; $p<0.05$) and intertrochanter (-2.3 vs -1.5%; $p<0.05$). No difference was found between diabetic and non-diabetic women in biochemical markers of bone loss.

Thus, this study indicates that alendronate elicits similar increases in BMD and changes in bone turnover in diabetic women with low bone density as in a non-diabetic osteoporotic population.

> Alendronate elicits similar increases in BMD and changes in bone turnover in diabetic women with low bone density as in a non-diabetic osteoporotic population.

Meta-analyses

The effect of alendronate on bone density and fracture rates has been examined in a meta-analysis of 11 randomised controlled trials which included a total of 12,855 postmenopausal women.[56] Two of the included trials dealt with osteoporosis prevention, and the remainder (including the Fracture Intervention Trial) involved women with low baseline BMD. The results demonstrate a reduction in relative risk of both vertebral and non-vertebral fractures with alendronate treatment at daily doses of 5–40 mg, although smaller effect sizes were observed with the 5 mg dose of alendronate than with doses ranging from 10 to 40 mg.

In addition, similar reductions in fracture risk were observed for 'non-osteoporotic' fractures (i.e. those in which the relative risk of fracture was less than 1.5 in a previous study) and for 'osteoporotic' fractures such as those at the hip, wrist and forearm. The pooled estimate of relative risk for vertebral fractures with alendronate was 0.52 whilst that for hip fracture was 0.63. The analysis also reported significant improvements in bone density with alendronate treatment at all sites measured ($p<0.01$), again with greater responses observed at doses of 10 mg and more.

The same authors have also performed a meta-analysis of the data regarding seven different osteoporosis treatments: calcium, vitamin D, HRT, alendronate, risedronate, raloxifene and calcitonin.[57] Significant reductions ($p<0.05$) in pooled relative risk for vertebral fracture were reported for alendronate (relative risk 0.52), raloxifene (0.60), vitamin D (0.63), etidronate (0.63), risedronate (0.64) and calcitonin (0.79) whilst only alendronate and risedronate demonstrated significant reductions in relative risk for non-vertebral fracture (0.51 and 0.73, respectively; both $p<0.01$). In terms of percentage change in BMD at the lumbar spine, all therapies except vitamin D mediated significant changes ($p<0.01$) but the largest effects were observed with alendronate and HRT (weighted mean differences 7.48 and 6.76, respectively; both $p<0.01$). Alendronate and HRT also mediated the greatest weighted mean differences in BMD at the combined hip (4.24 and 4.12, respectively; both $p<0.01$).

These analyses indicate that alendronate is effective in improving BMD and reducing fracture risk at a range of measured skeletal sites in postmenopausal women. Furthermore, of a range of alternative treatment options for osteoporosis, only alendronate and risedronate significantly reduced the risk for non-vertebral fracture. Direct head-to-head comparator studies are necessary in order to confirm or refute these findings.

Safety and tolerability

Adverse events

It is apparent from the studies described previously, and from other reviews regarding the safety profile of alendronate, that this antiresorptive agent is an effective and well-tolerated therapy for the prevention and treatment of osteoporosis.[58,59] Indeed, one could predict the favourable tolerability profile of alendronate based on its low bioavailability, low extraskeletal uptake, lack of metabolism and its rapid elimination by excretion in the urine.[58]

One of the major concerns regarding the bisphosphonates as a class, however, is their potential to cause irritation in the upper gastrointestinal tract. This property has been specifically examined for alendronate in several studies.[21,60–62] A large, open-label investigation into the tolerability of alendronate was carried out in 11,916 patients (89.1% female; mean age 69 years) using prescription-event monitoring with data collected from GPs in the UK via questionnaire.[60] A total of 457 events deemed to be adverse reactions to alendronate were reported

Of a range of alternative treatment options for osteoporosis, only alendronate and risedronate significantly reduced the risk for non-vertebral fracture.

You are strongly urged to consult your doctor before taking, stopping or changing any of the products reviewed or referred to in BESTMEDICINE or any other medication that has been prescribed or recommended by your doctor.

in 2.8% of the cohort with the most common adverse events reported being nausea/vomiting (0.4%), unspecified gastrointestinal events (0.4%), abdominal pain (0.3%) and dyspepsia (0.3%). The most common reason for discontinuing alendronate (24.5% of the cohort discontinued treatment) was dyspeptic conditions (6.3% of cohort), which comprised dyspepsia, oesophagitis, oesophageal reflux, duodenitis, gastritis and heartburn. However, tolerability data from other large-scale, randomised placebo-controlled trials indicated that a high incidence of gastrointestinal events occurred with both placebo and alendronate treatment in a further population of postmenopausal women.[21] Results from the entire cohort of 6459 women enrolled into the Fracture Intervention Trial revealed that the incidence of upper gastrointestinal adverse events was not different between alendronate and placebo treatment (Table 6). Dyspepsia was the most commonly reported adverse event in this category occurring in 18.2% of alendronate- and 19.1% of placebo-treated patients. This safety analysis also illustrated that the incidence of upper gastrointestinal adverse events was not elevated in patients at higher risk of this type of event, such as older women, women with a history of gastrointestinal disorders or those with a history of non-steroidal anti-inflammatory drug use. This and other studies have highlighted the fact that the incidence of gastrointestinal adverse events appears to be fairly high in a population of older postmenopausal women and this may account for the widely held perception that alendronate therapy is associated with gastrointestinal irritation.[21,62,63] This point is well illustrated in a multicentre, double-blind study of

Table 6. The incidence of upper gastrointestinal adverse events in postmenopausal women enrolled in the Fracture Intervention Trial and treated for 3 years with alendronate or placebo.[21]

Adverse events	Incidence (%)	
	Placebo (n=3223)	Alendronate (n=3236)
Any upper gastrointestinal event	46.2	47.5
Type of event		
Dyspepsia	19.1	18.2
Abdominal pain	13.1	13.7
Nausea	11.8	10.9
Vomiting	3.1	3.4
Acid reflux	6.1	6.6
Gastritis	2.3	2.5
Gastric ulcer	0.8	0.8
Oesophagitis	0.4	0.7
Oesophageal ulcer	0.2	0.2
Duodenal ulcer	0.3	0.1
Peptic ulcer	0.4	0.3

This analysis
revealed that
there was no
difference
between
alendronate and
placebo in the
incidence
of upper
gastrointestinal
adverse
experiences.

alendronate therapy in 172 postmenopausal women (mean age 67 years) who had previously discontinued treatment with alendronate due to upper gastrointestinal symptoms.[63] After a washout period of 1 month, these patients were re-randomised to treatment with either alendronate, 10 mg, or placebo for 8 weeks. Following this re-challenge, the incidence of upper gastrointestinal adverse events was 27.3% with alendronate and 28.6% with placebo, and discontinuation due to this type of adverse event was 14.8% with alendronate and 16.7% with placebo.

The general safety profile of alendronate was closely monitored in a group of 2027 postmenopausal women with pre-existing vertebral fractures participating in the Fracture Intervention Trial.[21] Study withdrawal due to adverse events was not different between alendronate- and placebo-treated groups (7.6 *vs* 9.6%, respectively; *p*=0.123) whilst hospitalisations due to adverse events were more common in the placebo group (29.9%) than in the alendronate group (24.5%; *p*<0.01). The difference in hospitalisations was largely a function of more placebo-treated women being admitted to hospital for treatment of fractures. Death occurred in 2.3% of the alendronate-treated and 2.1% of the placebo-treated patients (*p*=0.687). Again, there was no difference between alendronate and placebo in the incidence of upper gastrointestinal events (41.3 *vs* 40.0%, respectively; *p*=0.67).

Finally, the effect of long-term treatment with alendronate on bone safety has been reviewed, and it was concluded that, according to current knowledge, alendronate mediates only beneficial effects upon bone health.[64]

Cautions

Alendronate is not licensed for use in children and the drug has not been studied in this population. No dosage adjustments are required in the elderly. Alendronate is not recommended for use in patients with renal impairment whose creatinine clearance is below 35 mL/minute due to lack of clinical experience in this patient population. In patients with creatinine clearance greater than 35 mL/minute no dosage adjustments are necessary.[7]

The bisphosphonates as a class have the potential to initiate irritation of the upper gastrointestinal mucosa and as such caution should be exercised when prescribing alendronate to patients with disorders of the upper gastrointestinal tract including dysphagia, oesophageal disease, gastritis, duodenitis, ulcers, active gastrointestinal bleeding or prior surgery of the upper gastrointestinal tract. The physician and patient should also be alert to signs of oesophageal irritation including dysphagia, pain on swallowing, retrosternal pain or new or worsening heartburn. These symptoms may be indicative of an oesophageal reaction and alendronate should be discontinued and other aetiologies considered.

Disorders of mineral metabolism (particularly hypocalcaemia, vitamin D deficiency or hypoparathyroidism) should be corrected before alendronate therapy is initiated. Also, alternative causes of osteoporosis other than oestrogen deficiency, ageing and glucocorticoid use (such as hyperthyroidism, hyperparathyroidism, osteomalacia or hypogonadism) should be excluded prior to initiating treatment with alendronate. Finally, it is imperative that an adequate intake of calcium and vitamin D is maintained concomitantly with alendronate therapy and, thus, any deficiency should be corrected by increasing dietary intake or with appropriate supplements.

Contraindications

The use of alendronate is contraindicated in patients suffering from abnormalities of the oesophagus or other factors which delay oesophageal emptying (e.g. stricture or achalasia). Other contraindications include the inability to stand or sit upright for at least 30 minutes (required for correct drug administration), hypocalcaemia, pregnancy, breast feeding and hypersensitivity to any component of the product.[7]

Pharmacoeconomics

The effect of alendronate therapy on healthcare utilisation and healthcare costs associated with fracture incidence has been examined in a further study based on data derived from the Fracture Intervention Trial.[65] The proven benefits of alendronate in reducing the incidence of clinical fractures were hypothesised to be associated with substantial reductions in fracture-related healthcare costs. From the 2027 women enrolled into the vertebral fracture arm of the Fracture Intervention Trial, 9.5% used healthcare services for fracture-related purposes. The majority of women experiencing fracture of the hip used healthcare facilities (97%) compared with 30% of women who experienced new vertebral fractures. The mean costs per patient were calculated, in US dollars, for visits to the emergency room, hospital stays and rehabilitation subsequent to fractures of the hip, vertebrae, wrist or other sites. Significant differences between placebo and alendronate treatment were found in terms of emergency room visits, hospital stays and total costs associated with fractures of the hip. The reductions in hip fracture-related hospital costs indicate potential savings of over 50% with alendronate treatment in comparison with placebo (costs per patient per event: US $132 vs 312 for alendronate vs placebo, respectively; $p<0.05$). Thus, these cost savings would represent a substantial reduction in the extensive burden upon healthcare services as the prevalence of osteoporosis in an increasingly elderly population continues to grow.

Current guidelines from NICE recommend treatment with bisphosphonates to women aged over 65 years with fragility fracture and women aged between 50 and 64 years with T-score below –3.2 or with a T-score below –2.5 and with additional risk factors (i.e. a history of systemic corticosteroid use or a history of maternal hip fracture).[1] These recommendations are based on data which show that the cost per quality-adjusted life-year (QALY) gained with alendronate reduces with age, from £54,313 at age 50 to £24,777 at 65 years, with a cost saving predicted by the age of 80 years.

> The reductions in hip fracture-related hospital costs indicate potential savings of over 50% with alendronate treatment in comparison with placebo.

Key points

- Alendronate is a member of the bisphosphonate class of compounds which increases bone density by inhibition of bone resorption.

- Daily alendronate oral therapy is licensed for either the stabilisation or increase of BMD in postmenopausal women, osteoporotic men, or in men and women with glucocorticoid-induced osteoporosis. Weekly alendronate therapy is indicated for the treatment of postmenopausal osteoporosis.

- Studies have shown that alendronate increases BMD at the spine, hip and total body, and also reduces biochemical markers of bone resorption and formation.

- Alendronate has been shown to reduce the incidence of clinical fractures in a large cohort of postmenopausal women in the Fracture Intervention Trial.

- The beneficial effects of alendronate on bone mass persist over 10 years of therapy.

- In comparison with other therapies for osteoporosis, alendronate is more effective than either raloxifene or calcitonin, and is similar in efficacy to HRT.

- In comparison with alendronate, teriparatide induces greater increases in BMD over the short-term ($\leq$18 months) but is currently ten-times as costly as alendronate and, unlike alendronate, is not licensed for long-term therapy.

- In comparison with other bisphosphonates, alendronate appears to exert greater increases in BMD than either risedronate or etidronate.

- Alendronate has an excellent safety profile and, despite a widespread perception that the drug causes irritation of the upper gastrointestinal tract, clinical studies have reported an equal incidence of these events with alendronate and placebo when the drug is administered according to manufacturer's instructions.

References

A list of the published evidence which has been reviewed in compiling the preceding section of *BESTMEDICINE*.

1   National Institute for Clinical Excellence. Bisphosphonates (alendronate, risedronate), selective oestrogen receptor modulators (raloxifene) and parathyroid hormone (teriparatide) for the secondary prevention of osteoporotic fragility fractures in postmenopausal women. Technology Appraisal 87. National Institute for Health and Clinical Excellence. January 2005. *www.nice.org.uk*

2   Porras AG, Holland SD, Gertz BJ. Pharmacokinetics of alendronate. *Clin Pharmacokinet* 1999; **36**: 315–28.

3   Liberman UA, Weiss SR, Broll J *et al*. Effect of oral alendronate on bone mineral density and the incidence of fractures in postmenopausal osteoporosis. The Alendronate Phase III Osteoporosis Treatment Study Group. *N Engl J Med* 1995; **333**: 1437–43.

4   Sharpe M, Noble S, Spencer CM. Alendronate: an update of its use in osteoporosis. *Drugs* 2001; **61**: 999–1039.

5   Reszka AA, Rodan GA. Nitrogen-containing bisphosphonate mechanism of action. *Mini Rev Med Chem* 2004; **4**: 711–19.

6   Recker R, Masarachia P, Santora A *et al*. Trabecular bone microarchitecture after alendronate treatment of osteoporotic women. *Curr Med Res Opin* 2005; **21**: 185–94.

7   Merck Sharp & Dohme Ltd. Fosamax® (alendronate sodium). *Summary of product characteristics*. Hertfordshire, 2004: 1–9.

8   Rodan GA, Seedor JG, Balena R. Preclinical pharmacology of alendronate. *Osteoporos Int* 1993; **3(Suppl 3)**: S7–12.

9   Rizzoli R, Greenspan SL, Bone G, 3rd *et al*. Two-year results of once-weekly administration of alendronate 70 mg for the treatment of postmenopausal osteoporosis. *J Bone Miner Res* 2002; **17**: 1988–96.

10 Black DM, Reiss TF, Nevitt MC *et al*. Design of the Fracture Intervention Trial. *Osteoporos Int* 1993; **3**: S29–39.

11 Boonen S, Rizzoli R, Meunier PJ *et al*. The need for clinical guidance in the use of calcium and vitamin D in the management of osteoporosis: a consensus report. *Osteoporos Int* 2004; **15**: 511–19.

12 Ravn P, Overgaard K, Huang C *et al*. Comparison of bone densitometry of the phalanges, distal forearm and axial skeleton in early postmenopausal women participating in the EPIC Study. *Osteoporos Int* 1996; **6**: 308–13.

13 Bauer DC, Black DM, Garnero P *et al*. Change in bone turnover and hip, non-spine, and vertebral fracture in alendronate-treated women: the fracture intervention trial. *J Bone Miner Res* 2004; **19**: 1250–8.

14 Ravn P, Hosking D, Thompson D *et al*. Monitoring of alendronate treatment and prediction of effect on bone mass by biochemical markers in the early postmenopausal intervention cohort study. *J Clin Endocrinol Metab* 1999; **84**: 2363–8.

15 Garnero P, Shih WJ, Gineyts E, Karpf DB, Delmas PD. Comparison of new biochemical markers of bone turnover in late postmenopausal osteoporotic women in response to alendronate treatment. *J Clin Endocrinol Metab* 1994; **79**: 1693–700.

16 Schnitzer T, Bone HG, Crepaldi G *et al*. Therapeutic equivalence of alendronate 70 mg once-weekly and alendronate 10 mg daily in the treatment of osteoporosis. Alendronate Once-Weekly Study Group. *Aging (Milano)* 2000; **12**: 1–12.

17 Simon JA, Lewiecki EM, Smith ME *et al*. Patient preference for once-weekly alendronate 70 mg versus once-daily alendronate 10 mg: a multicenter, randomized, open-label, crossover study. *Clin Ther* 2002; **24**: 1871–86.

18 Sambrook P. Once weekly alendronate. *Drugs Today (Barc)* 2003; **39**: 339–46.

19 McClung M, Clemmesen B, Daifotis A *et al*. Alendronate prevents postmenopausal bone loss in women without osteoporosis. A double-blind, randomized, controlled trial. Alendronate Osteoporosis Prevention Study Group. *Ann Intern Med* 1998; **128**: 253–61.

20 Cummings SR, Black DM, Thompson DE *et al*. Effect of alendronate on risk of fracture in women with low bone density but without vertebral fractures: results from the Fracture Intervention Trial. *JAMA* 1998; **280**: 2077–82.

21 Black D, Cummings SR, Karpf DB *et al*. Randomised trial of effect of alendronate on risk of fracture in women with existing vertebral fracture. *Lancet* 1996; **348**: 1535–41.

22 Nevitt MC, Thompson DE, Black DM *et al*. Effect of alendronate on limited-activity days and bed-disability days caused by back pain in postmenopausal women with existing vertebral fractures. Fracture Intervention Trial Research Group. *Arch Intern Med* 2000; **160**: 77–85.

23 Lippuner K. Medical treatment of vertebral osteoporosis. *Eur Spine J* 2003; **12(Suppl 2)**: S132–41.

24 Black DM, Thompson DE, Bauer DC *et al*. Fracture risk reduction with alendronate in women with osteoporosis: the Fracture Intervention Trial. FIT Research Group. *J Clin Endocrinol Metab* 2000; **85**: 4118–24.

25 Quandt SA, Thompson DE, Schneider DL, Nevitt MC, Black DM. Effect of alendronate on vertebral fracture risk in women with bone mineral density T scores of –1.6 to –2.5 at the femoral neck: the Fracture Intervention Trial. *Mayo Clin Proc* 2005; **80**: 343–9.

26 Hochberg MC, Ross PD, Black D *et al*. Larger increases in bone mineral density during alendronate therapy are associated with a lower risk of new vertebral fractures in women with postmenopausal osteoporosis. Fracture Intervention Trial Research Group. *Arthritis Rheum* 1999; **42**: 1246–54.

27 Stone KL, Seeley DG, Lui LY *et al.* BMD at multiple sites and risk of fracture of multiple types: long-term results from the Study of Osteoporotic Fractures. *J Bone Miner Res* 2003; **18**: 1947–54.

28 Heaney RP. Is the paradigm shifting? *Bone* 2003; **33**: 457–65.

29 Ravn P, Weiss SR, Rodriguez-Portales JA *et al.* Alendronate in early postmenopausal women: effects on bone mass during long-term treatment and after withdrawal. Alendronate Osteoporosis Prevention Study Group. *J Clin Endocrinol Metab* 2000; **85**: 1492–7.

30 McClung MR, Wasnich RD, Hosking DJ *et al.* Prevention of postmenopausal bone loss: six-year results from the Early Postmenopausal Intervention Cohort Study. *J Clin Endocrinol Metab* 2004; **89**: 4879–85.

31 Tonino RP, Meunier PJ, Emkey R *et al.* Skeletal benefits of alendronate: 7-year treatment of postmenopausal osteoporotic women. Phase III Osteoporosis Treatment Study Group. *J Clin Endocrinol Metab* 2000; **85**: 3109–15.

32 Bone HG, Hosking D, Devogelaer JP *et al.* Ten years' experience with alendronate for osteoporosis in postmenopausal women. *N Engl J Med* 2004; **350**: 1189–99.

33 Ensrud KE, Barrett-Connor EL, Schwartz A *et al.* Randomized trial of effect of alendronate continuation versus discontinuation in women with low BMD: results from the Fracture Intervention Trial long-term extension. *J Bone Miner Res* 2004; **19**: 1259–69.

34 Bonn D. New ways with old bones. Osteoporosis researchers look for drugs to replace hormone replacement therapy. *Lancet* 2004; **363**: 786–7.

35 Hosking D, Chilvers CE, Christiansen C *et al.* Prevention of bone loss with alendronate in postmenopausal women under 60 years of age. Early Postmenopausal Intervention Cohort Study Group. *N Engl J Med* 1998; **338**: 485–92.

36 Ravn P, Bidstrup M, Wasnich RD *et al.* Alendronate and estrogen-progestin in the long-term prevention of bone loss: four-year results from the early postmenopausal intervention cohort study. A randomized, controlled trial. *Ann Intern Med* 1999; **131**: 935–42.

37 Bone HG, Greenspan SL, McKeever C *et al.* Alendronate and estrogen effects in postmenopausal women with low bone mineral density. Alendronate/Estrogen Study Group. *J Clin Endocrinol Metab* 2000; **85**: 720–6.

38 Greenspan SL, Emkey RD, Bone HG *et al.* Significant differential effects of alendronate, estrogen, or combination therapy on the rate of bone loss after discontinuation of treatment of postmenopausal osteoporosis. A randomized, double-blind, placebo-controlled trial. *Ann Intern Med* 2002; **137**: 875–83.

39 Lindsay R, Cosman F, Lobo RA *et al.* Addition of alendronate to ongoing hormone replacement therapy in the treatment of osteoporosis: a randomized, controlled clinical trial. *J Clin Endocrinol Metab* 1999; **84**: 3076–81.

40 Sambrook PN, Geusens P, Ribot C *et al.* Alendronate produces greater effects than raloxifene on bone density and bone turnover in postmenopausal women with low bone density: results of EFFECT (Efficacy of FOSAMAX versus EVISTA Comparison Trial) International. *J Intern Med* 2004; **255**: 503–11.

41 Lufkin EG, Sarkar S, Kulkarni PM *et al.* Antiresorptive treatment of postmenopausal osteoporosis: review of randomized clinical studies and rationale for the Evista alendronate comparison (EVA) trial. *Curr Med Res Opin* 2004; **20**: 351–7.

42 Adami S, Baroni MC, Broggini M *et al.* Treatment of postmenopausal osteoporosis with continuous daily oral alendronate in comparison with either placebo or intranasal salmon calcitonin. *Osteoporos Int* 1993; **3(Suppl 3)**: S21–7.

43 Body JJ, Gaich GA, Scheele WH *et al.* A randomized double-blind trial to compare the efficacy of teriparatide [recombinant human parathyroid hormone (1–34)] with alendronate in postmenopausal women with osteoporosis. *J Clin Endocrinol Metab* 2002; **87**: 4528–35.

44 Black DM, Greenspan SL, Ensrud KE *et al.* The effects of parathyroid hormone and alendronate alone or in combination in postmenopausal osteoporosis. *N Engl J Med* 2003; **349**: 1207–15.

45 Finkelstein JS, Hayes A, Hunzelman JL *et al.* The effects of parathyroid hormone, alendronate, or both in men with osteoporosis. *N Engl J Med* 2003; **349**: 1216–26.

46 *British National Formulary (BNF) 49.* Bisphosphonates and other drugs affecting bone metabolism. London: British Medical Association and Royal Pharmaceutical Society of Great Britain, 2005.

47 Rosen CJ, Hochberg MC, Bonnick SL *et al.* Treatment with once-weekly alendronate 70 mg compared with once-weekly risedronate 35 mg in women with postmenopausal osteoporosis: a randomized double-blind study. *J Bone Miner Res* 2005; **20**: 141–51.

48 Hosking D, Adami S, Felsenberg D *et al.* Comparison of change in bone resorption and bone mineral density with once-weekly alendronate and daily risedronate: a randomised, placebo-controlled study. *Curr Med Res Opin* 2003; **19**: 383–94.

49 Sahota O, Fowler I, Blackwell PJ *et al.* A comparison of continuous alendronate, cyclical alendronate and cyclical etidronate with calcitriol in the treatment of postmenopausal vertebral osteoporosis: a randomized controlled trial. *Osteoporos Int* 2000; **11**: 959–66.

50 Sambrook PN, Kotowicz M, Nash P *et al.* Prevention and treatment of glucocorticoid-induced osteoporosis: a comparison of calcitriol, vitamin D plus calcium, and alendronate plus calcium. *J Bone Miner Res* 2003; **18**: 919–24.

51 Saag KG, Emkey R, Schnitzer TJ *et al.* Alendronate for the prevention and treatment of glucocorticoid-induced osteoporosis. Glucocorticoid-Induced Osteoporosis Intervention Study Group. *N Engl J Med* 1998; **339**: 292–9.

52 Orwoll E, Ettinger M, Weiss S et al. Alendronate for the treatment of osteoporosis in men. N Engl J Med 2000; **343**: 604–10.

53 Bone HG, Downs RW, Jr., Tucci JR et al. Dose-response relationships for alendronate treatment in osteoporotic elderly women. Alendronate Elderly Osteoporosis Study Centers. J Clin Endocrinol Metab 1997; **82**: 265–74.

54 Greenspan SL, Resnick NM, Parker RA. Combination therapy with hormone replacement and alendronate for prevention of bone loss in elderly women: a randomized controlled trial. JAMA 2003; **289**: 2525–33.

55 Keegan TH, Schwartz AV, Bauer DC, Sellmeyer DE, Kelsey JL. Effect of alendronate on bone mineral density and biochemical markers of bone turnover in type 2 diabetic women: the fracture intervention trial. Diabetes Care 2004; **27**: 1547–53.

56 Cranney A, Wells G, Willan A et al. Meta-analyses of therapies for postmenopausal osteoporosis. II. Meta-analysis of alendronate for the treatment of postmenopausal women. Endocr Rev 2002; **23**: 508–16.

57 Cranney A, Guyatt G, Griffith L et al. Meta-analyses of therapies for postmenopausal osteoporosis. IX: Summary of meta-analyses of therapies for postmenopausal osteoporosis. Endocr Rev 2002; **23**: 570–8.

58 Watts N, Freedholm D, Daifotis A. The clinical tolerability profile of alendronate. Int J Clin Pract Suppl 1999; **101**: 51–61.

59 Kherani RB, Papaioannou A, Adachi JD. Long-term tolerability of the bisphosphonates in postmenopausal osteoporosis: a comparative review. Drug Saf 2002; **25**: 781–90.

60 Biswas PN, Wilton LV, Shakir SA. Pharmacovigilance study of alendronate in England. Osteoporos Int 2003; **14**: 507–14.

61 Eisman JA, Rizzoli R, Roman-Ivorra J et al. Upper gastrointestinal and overall tolerability of alendronate once weekly in patients with osteoporosis: results of a randomized, double-blind, placebo-controlled study. Curr Med Res Opin 2004; **20**: 699–705.

62 Bauer DC, Black D, Ensrud K et al. Upper gastrointestinal tract safety profile of alendronate: the fracture intervention trial. Arch Intern Med 2000; **160**: 517–25.

63 Baker DE. Alendronate and risedronate: what you need to know about their upper gastrointestinal tract toxicity. Rev Gastroenterol Disord 2002; **2**: 20–33.

64 Rodan G, Reszka A, Golub E, Rizzoli R. Bone safety of long-term bisphosphonate treatment. Curr Med Res Opin 2004; **20**: 1291–300.

65 Chrischilles EA, Dasbach EJ, Rubenstein LM et al. The effect of alendronate on fracture-related healthcare utilization and costs: the fracture intervention trial. Osteoporos Int 2001; **12**: 654–60.

Acknowledgements

Figure 2 is adapted from McClung et al., 1998.[19]
Figure 3 is adapted from Cummings et al., 1998.[20]
Figure 4 is adapted from Black et al., 2000.[24]
Figure 5 is adapted from Hochberg et al., 1999.[26]
Figure 6 is adapted from Ravn et al., 2000.[29]
Figure 7 is adapted from Bone et al., 2004.[32]
Figure 8 is adapted from Ravn et al., 1999.[36]

4. Drug review – Raloxifene (Evista®)

Dr Eleanor Bull
CSF Medical Communications Ltd

Summary

Raloxifene is a selective oestrogen receptor modulator (SERM) that is currently licensed for the prophylaxis and treatment of osteoporosis in postmenopausal women. Structurally distinct from the other drugs of its class, raloxifene acts as an oestrogen agonist in bone and on serum lipid metabolism, and as an oestrogen antagonist in the breast and the uterus. The Multiple Outcomes of Raloxifene Evaluation (MORE) study, which investigated the clinical consequences of up to 4 years of continuous treatment, showed that raloxifene significantly reduced the incidence of vertebral fractures, preserved bone mass and increased bone mineral density (BMD) in postmenopausal women. In addition to its beneficial effects in bone, raloxifene improved the serum lipid profile and reduced the risk of cardiovascular complications in susceptible patients. The propensity for raloxifene to reduce the incidence of invasive breast cancer amongst postmenopausal women may represent an additional therapeutic application, although currently the drug is not licensed for this purpose. Unlike another SERM, tamoxifen, raloxifene acts as an oestrogen receptor antagonist in uterine tissue, so the risk of endometrial cancer is negligible. Although raloxifene is generally well tolerated, women receiving long-term therapy have an increased risk of developing thromboembolic disease. Hot flushes and leg cramps may also adversely affect patient compliance.

Introduction

The publication of the Women's Health Initiative (WHI) study in 2002, which identified a small but significant risk of coronary heart disease, stroke, pulmonary embolism and breast cancer associated with continuous combined hormone replacement therapy (HRT), restricted the use of such treatments for the management of postmenopausal osteoporosis and instead focused attention on alternative agents. Current antiresorptive treatments of choice include the bisphosphonates (e.g. alendronate, etidronate, risedronate) and raloxifene, a SERM.

A structurally diverse group of compounds, the SERMs (e.g. clomifene, raloxifene, tamoxifen and toremifene) exert selective agonist or antagonist actions on tissues responsive to oestrogen.[1] Unlike HRT, the SERMs interact with specific oestrogen receptors within the body, providing the potential benefits of oestrogen in the skeleton, but avoiding the negative effects of oestrogen in other tissues.[2] Clinically, SERMs decrease the risk of fracture via an oestrogen-agonist effect on bone, and also reduce breast cancer risk via an oestrogen-antagonist effect on the breast tissue. Tamoxifen was the first SERM to be used on a long-term basis for the treatment of breast cancer.[1] Large-scale trials are ongoing to determine the effectiveness of the SERMs against a number of other oestrogen-related diseases including postmenopausal osteoporosis, hormone-dependent cancers and cardiovascular disease.

Raloxifene, launched in the UK in 1998, was the first SERM to be approved for the treatment and prevention of osteoporosis in postmenopausal women.[3] This edition of *BESTMEDICINE* reviews the pharmacological properties of raloxifene and its efficacy in controlled clinical trials, with particular emphasis on the MORE study.

Pharmacology

Chemistry

The chemical structure of raloxifene, a benzothiopene, is illustrated in Figure 1. Structurally distinct from the planar triphenylethylenes (e.g. clomifene, tamoxifen and toremifene), raloxifene contains a flexible 'hinge' region which results in a nearly orthogonal orientation of the basic side chain.[4] These differences in structure may account for the differential tissue selectivity of the SERMs.

> Raloxifene was the first SERM to be approved for the treatment and prevention of osteoporosis in postmenopausal women.

> ☞ The chemistry of raloxifene is of essentially academic interest and most healthcare professionals will, like you, skip this section.

Figure 1. The chemical structure of raloxifene.

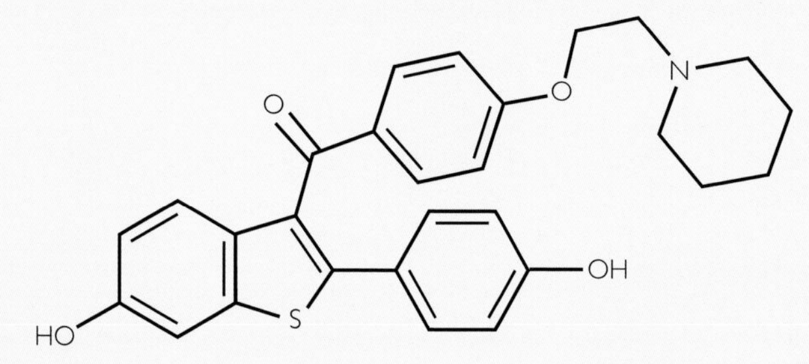

Mechanism of action

Although its exact mechanism of action is not fully understood,
raloxifene is known to act as an oestrogen agonist in the skeleton and on
serum lipid metabolism, whilst acting as an oestrogen antagonist in the
breast and uterus.[3] This profile differs to that of the other SERMs,
including tamoxifen, the skeletal effects of which are less pronounced
(Table 1).[5] Raloxifene displays a high affinity for the oestrogen receptor
($K_d{}^a$ 50 pmol/L), and the oestrogen receptor/raloxifene complex
interacts with an oestrogen-response element to regulate gene
transcription.[4,6] The existence of a tissue-specific oestrogen-response
element that is activated by the raloxifene parent compound and
metabolites of 17β-estradiol has been proposed, and may account for the
tissue-selective oestrogen agonist or antagonist activity of raloxifene.[7]
The tissue selectivity of raloxifene may also originate from the
differential modulation of oestrogen-responsive genes by specific
conformations of the receptor–ligand complex.[4]

> Raloxifene acts as an oestrogen agonist in the skeleton and on serum lipid metabolism, whilst acting as an oestrogen antagonist in the breast and uterus.

Bone-selective activity

The bone preserving and antiresorptive action of oestrogen is mediated
by oestrogen receptors in osteoblasts.[8] It is envisaged that raloxifene,
through binding to these receptors, modulates the expression of a
number of key components of the bone remodelling pathway. Raloxifene
has been shown to:

- upregulate the expression of transforming growth factor (TGF)-β3,
  an important regulator of bone remodelling[9]

Table 1. Significant biological effects of the selective oestrogen receptor modulators (SERMs) and hormone replacement therapy (HRT) in postmenopausal women.[5]

	Lipids	Breast	Bone	Oestrogenic effects on endometrium
HRT	↓ LDL, ↑ HDL	Agonist	+++	+++
Raloxifene	↓ LDL, ↑ HDL	Antagonist	++	+/–
Tamoxifen	↓ LDL	Antagonist	+	++
Toremifene	↓ LDL, ↑ HDL	Antagonist	+	++
Idoxifene[a]	↓ LDL	Antagonist	+	++
Ospemifene[a]	↓ LDL, ↑ HDL	Antagonist	++	+/–
'Ideal SERM'	↓ LDL, ↑HDL	Antagonist	+++	–

[a]under development.
+++, clinically significant; ++, moderate; +, slight; +/–, slight-to-neutral; –, neutral.
HDL, high density lipoprotein; LDL, low density lipoprotein.

[a]K_d, equilibrium dissociation constant.

- downregulate the number of osteoclasts and increase proliferation of osteoblasts in bone marrow cultures isolated from neonatal mice[10]
- prevent bone loss at the distal metaphysic of the femur, proximal tibia and vertebrae of the ovariectomised rat[11]
- display antioestrogenic activity in several *in vivo* and *in vitro* mammary tumour models.[12,13]

Pharmacokinetics

The pharmacokinetics of a drug are of interest to healthcare professionals because it is important for them to understand the action of a drug on the body over a period of time.

The pharmacokinetic properties of raloxifene are summarised in Table 2.[1,3,14] Raloxifene displays linear pharmacokinetics with high interindividual variability, and can be administered to postmenopausal women regardless of food intake, age, body weight, cigarette smoking, ethnic origin or decreased renal functioning.[14] Absorbed rapidly following oral administration, raloxifene is distributed extensively throughout the body.[3] Raloxifene undergoes extensive first-pass glucuronidation to the glucuronide conjugates, raloxifene-4′-glucuronide (the primary metabolite), raloxifene-6-glucuronide and raloxifene-6,4′-diglucuronide.[3] Levels of raloxifene within the body are maintained by enterohepatic recycling – a process of continuous biliary excretion and intestinal reabsorption – which may ultimately prolong its pharmacological effects.[1,15] The primary route of elimination of raloxifene is faecal, and the majority of a dose of raloxifene and its glucuronide metabolites are excreted within 5 days of administration.[3] Less than 6% of a raloxifene dose, eliminated as glucuronide conjugates, is recovered in the urine.[3]

Dosage schedule

Raloxifene can be taken at any time of the day, in contrast to the bisphosphonates, the absorption of which is significantly inhibited by food.

Raloxifene is indicated for the treatment and prevention of osteoporosis in postmenopausal women.[3] The recommended daily dose is 60 mg. Raloxifene can be taken at any time of the day regardless of meal times,

Table 2. The pharmacokinetic properties of raloxifene.[1,3,14]

Pharmacokinetic parameter	
Absolute bioavailability (%)	2
Plasma protein binding (%)	98–99
Volume of distribution (L/kg)	2348
t_{max} (hours)	6
C_{max} (μg/L per mg/kg)	1.36
AUC (μg•L/hour per mg/kg)	24.2
Clearance (L/kg/hour)	44.1
$t_{1/2}$ (hours)	27.7

AUC, area under the concentration–time curve; t_{max}, time to reach maximum drug plasma concentration (C_{max}); $t_{1/2}$, elimination half-life.

in contrast to the bisphosphonates, the absorption of which is significantly inhibited by food.[3] The concurrent administration of calcium and vitamin D supplements is also advised in women with a low dietary intake of these nutrients. No dosage adjustment is necessary for the elderly, although raloxifene is not recommended in patients with cirrhosis or mild hepatic impairment (Child-Pugh Class A).[3]

Drug interaction profile

Colestyramine or other anion-exchange resins, may significantly reduce the absorption and enterohepatic cycling of raloxifene.[3] Peak concentrations of raloxifene may be reduced by coadministration with ampicillin, although concurrent administration is permitted.[3] Coadministration of raloxifene with warfarin may temporally reduce prothrombin time, and therefore careful monitoring is recommended in those patients who are receiving both agents.[3]

To date, raloxifene has displayed no evidence of clinically relevant interaction with calcium carbonate, aluminium- and magnesium hydroxide-containing antacids, methylprednisolone, digoxin, paracetamol, non-steroidal anti-inflammatory drugs (NSAIDs), oral antibiotics, H1 and H2 antagonists or benzodiazepines.[3]

Clinical efficacy

Most clinical trials of antiresorptive therapies use vertebral fracture as an endpoint, predominantly because fractures of this type are the first to be associated with important morbidity and mortality in postmenopausal women.[16] Since studies of this nature can be lengthy and expensive to conduct, surrogate markers (i.e. changes in BMD and biochemical markers of bone turnover) are used as indicators of patient response to drug therapy.[17] BMD is sometimes used as a surrogate marker for antifracture efficacy, although the relationship between treatment-induced changes in BMD and reductions in fracture risk is not clear.[17]

> Surrogate markers (i.e. changes in BMD and biochemical markers of bone turnover) are used increasingly as indicators of patient response to drug therapy.

Dose-ranging studies

The controlled clinical trials assessing the clinical efficacy of raloxifene (30–150 mg/day) are summarised in Table 3.[18–21] In general, raloxifene therapy was associated with significant increases in the BMD of the lumbar spine and total hip, as illustrated by the 2-year data presented in Figure 2.[21] Furthermore, long-term raloxifene treatment significantly reduced serum levels of a number of markers of bone turnover, including osteocalcin and bone-specific alkaline phosphatase (BSAP). As is evident from the table, the clinical benefits associated with raloxifene treatment were generally most pronounced amongst those patients receiving daily doses of 60 or 120 mg. Since the improvements associated with the 120 mg dose of raloxifene were not appreciably superior, and were in some instances inferior to those offered by the lower dose, raloxifene 60 mg, was selected as the optimal dosage.

> ☛ Dose-ranging studies are particularly important to ensure that the optimum dose of a drug can be determined in order that benefit can be realised with the least risk of side-effects.

Table 3. Summary of dose-ranging clinical trials of raloxifene (30–150 mg/day) in postmenopausal women.[18–21]

Study	Dosage regimen	Main outcomes
Delmas et al., 1997[18] Double-blind Placebo-controlled 24 months n=601	Raloxifene, 30, 60 or 150 mg/day, or placebo	• All doses of raloxifene were associated with significant increases in BMD from baseline, compared with placebo (lumbar spine: –0.8, 1.3, 1.6 and 2.2%, for placebo and raloxifene, 30, 60 and 150 mg, respectively; $p<0.03$ all doses vs placebo). • The increases from baseline in total hip BMD were –0.8, 1.0, 1.6 and 1.5% for placebo and raloxifene, 30, 60 and 150 mg, respectively ($p<0.03$ all doses vs placebo). • Increases in BMD in lumbar spine and total hip were independent of initial BMD, baseline serum osteocalcin, age and BMI. • Total cholesterol levels were reduced significantly across all raloxifene treatment groups compared with placebo (–1.2, –5.2, –6.4 and –9.7% for placebo and raloxifene, 30, 60 and 150 mg, respectively; $p<0.05$ all doses vs placebo).
Jolly et al., 2003[19] Double-blind Placebo-controlled Pooled data from two identical trials[18] 5 years n=328	Raloxifene, 60 mg/day, or placebo	• Over 5 years, raloxifene treatment significantly increased lumbar spine (2.8%; $p<0.001$) and total hip BMD (2.6%; $p<0.001$) compared with placebo. • Women taking raloxifene were less likely to develop osteoporosis (RR 0.13; $p=0.001$) or osteopenia (RR 0.23; $p=0.038$) at the lumbar spine than those patients taking placebo. • Raloxifene-treated patients were significantly more likely than placebo patients to convert to normal BMD status at the lumbar spine (RR 4.01; $p=0.043$) and total hip (RR 3.92; $p=0.011$) after 5 years of treatment. • At 5 years, markers of bone turnover were significantly reduced following raloxifene treatment compared with placebo (osteocalcin: –10.9%, $p<0.001$; BSAP: –7.2%, $p=0.042$; urinary C-telopeptide: –11.1%, $p=0.034$). • Compared with placebo, raloxifene treatment significantly reduced total cholesterol (–5.5%; $p<0.001$) and LDL-C (–8.7%; $p<0.001$). • The incidence of hot flushes was significantly higher amongst raloxifene-treated patients (28.8 vs 16.8%, respectively; $p=0.017$).

BMD, bone mineral density; BMI, body mass index; BSAP, bone-specific alkaline phosphatase; HDL-C, high density lipoprotein cholesterol; LDL-C, low density lipoprotein cholesterol; RR, relative risk.

Table 3. Continued

Study	Dosage regimen	Main outcomes
Lufkin et al., 1998[20] Double-blind 12 months n=143	Raloxifene, 60 or 120 mg/day, or control group receiving calcium, 750 mg/day, and vitamin D, 400 IU/day	• Over 12 months, the mean percentage changes in total hip BMD were greatest in the raloxifene, 60 mg group (−0.71, 0.95 and 0.47% for control and raloxifene, 60 and 120 mg, respectively; $p=0.027$ for raloxifene, 60 mg, vs control). • The change in anteroposterior and lateral lumbar spine BMD was not significantly different between treatment groups. • The percentage changes in serum osteocalcin and BSAP were most pronounced in the raloxifene treatment groups (osteocalcin: −12.4, −33.1 and −29.4% for control, and raloxifene, 60 and 120 mg, respectively; $p\leq0.005$ both doses vs control; BSAP: −21.1, −36.0 and −30.0%, respectively; $p\leq0.03$ both doses vs control). • Over 12 months, the LDL-C/HDL-C ratio decreased significantly following raloxifene therapy (−3.18, −13.2 and −8.34% for control and raloxifene, 60 and 120 mg, respectively; $p=0.001$ and $p=0.032$ for raloxifene 60 and 120 mg vs control).
Meunier et al., 1999[21] Double-blind Placebo-controlled 24 months n=129	Raloxifene, 60 or 150 mg/day, or placebo	• After 24 months, lumbar spine, total hip and femoral neck BMD increased significantly following both doses of raloxifene compared with placebo ($p<0.05$; Figure 2). • Serum osteocalcin levels declined significantly from baseline following raloxifene treatment, compared with placebo (−0.4, −28.4 and −25.2% for placebo and raloxifene, 60 and 150 mg, respectively; $p<0.001$ both doses vs placebo). • Serum BSAP levels declined significantly from baseline following raloxifene treatment compared with placebo (4.1, −13.7 and −15.8% for placebo and raloxifene, 60 and 150 mg, respectively; $p<0.001$, for raloxifene 150 mg, vs placebo; and $p<0.01$ for raloxifene 60 mg, vs placebo). • Serum LDL-C levels were significantly reduced from baseline following raloxifene treatment (2.93, −11.36 and −13.90%, respectively; $p<0.001$ vs placebo).

BMD, bone mineral density; BMI, body mass index; BSAP, bone-specific alkaline phosphatase; HDL-C, high density lipoprotein cholesterol; LDL-C, low density lipoprotein cholesterol; RR, relative risk.

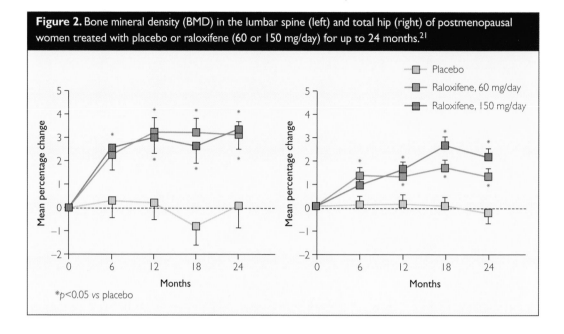

Figure 2. Bone mineral density (BMD) in the lumbar spine (left) and total hip (right) of postmenopausal women treated with placebo or raloxifene (60 or 150 mg/day) for up to 24 months.[21]

MORE study

Undertaken in 1994, the MORE study was a large-scale placebo-controlled study of 7,705 women with osteoporosis (defined as low BMD of the lumbar spine or femoral neck, or radiographical vertebral fractures) who had been postmenopausal for at least 2 years. Participants were randomly allocated to placebo or raloxifene, 60 or 120 mg/day, for a period of 4 years, and all women received daily calcium (500 mg) and vitamin D (400–600 IU) supplements. Both 36- and 48-month data have been published to date.[22,23] It should be noted that the concomitant use of other bone-sparing agents was permitted in the fourth year, in line with changes in therapeutic guidelines.

After 36 months of treatment, the percentage of patients discontinuing treatment was similar between treatment groups (22.5 *vs* 24.4% for raloxifene and placebo, respectively; *p*-value not reported). The proportion of patients continuing past 36 months of treatment was 78 and 72%, respectively (*p*-value not reported). At 36 months, radiographic data, available from 6828 women (89% of the study population), showed that 7.4% of participants had experienced at least one new vertebral fracture, including 10.1% of women receiving placebo, 6.6% of those receiving raloxifene, 60 mg, and 5.4% of those patients receiving raloxifene, 120 mg.[22] The reduction in vertebral fracture risk associated with raloxifene treatment is shown in Figure 3. However, raloxifene was not associated with a significant reduction in the risk of non-vertebral fracture (occurring in the wrist, hip or ankle), with 8.5% of raloxifene-treated patients reporting at least one fracture, compared with 9.3% of placebo patients (relative risk [RR] 0.9 for both raloxifene treatment groups combined; *p*=0.24). Compared with placebo, raloxifene treatment elicited significant increases in femoral

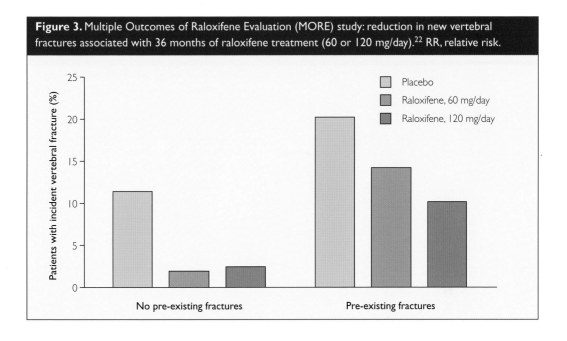

Figure 3. Multiple Outcomes of Raloxifene Evaluation (MORE) study: reduction in new vertebral fractures associated with 36 months of raloxifene treatment (60 or 120 mg/day).[22] RR, relative risk.

neck and lumbar spine BMD (2.1 and 2.6%, and 2.4 and 2.7%, for raloxifene, 60 and 120 mg, respectively; $p<0.001$ for all comparisons *vs* placebo). It is perhaps difficult to reconcile the positive changes in femoral hip BMD with the lack of fracture prevention reported in this region, although it should be acknowledged that the MORE study was not sufficiently powered to detect effects upon hip fracture. Overall, 3.6% of women assigned to placebo withdrew from the study as a result of multiple fractures or excessive BMD loss, compared with 1.1 and 0.9% of patients treated with raloxifene, 60 mg and 120 mg, respectively ($p<0.001$ for both doses *vs* placebo). The median reductions in serum osteocalcin concentrations over 36 months were 8.6, 26.3 and 31.1% for placebo, and raloxifene, 60 and 120 mg, respectively ($p<0.001$ *vs* placebo), whilst the excretion of urinary C-telopeptide, a marker of bone turnover, declined by 8.1, 34.0 and 31.5%, respectively ($p<0.001$ *vs* placebo). The adverse event rate was similar in the two raloxifene groups, with influenza-like illness, hot flushes, leg cramps, peripheral oedema and endometrial cavity fluid amongst the most commonly reported ($p\leq0.05$ *vs* placebo). The risk of experiencing a venous thromboembolic event, including deep vein thrombophlebitis and pulmonary embolism, was also heightened during raloxifene treatment (0.3, 1.0 and 1.0% for placebo, and raloxifene, 60 mg and 120 mg, respectively; RR 3.1 for both raloxifene treatment groups combined). Raloxifene was not associated with vaginal bleeding or breast pain, and was associated with a lower incidence of breast cancer (see later section).

Post hoc analysis of these data has shown that the risk reduction in vertebral fracture associated with raloxifene treatment was positively affected by baseline serum triglycerides ($p=0.03$), age ($p=0.04$) and lumbar spine BMD ($p=0.08$).[24]

Compared with placebo, raloxifene treatment elicited significant increases in femoral neck and lumbar spine BMD.

Forty-eight-month data have shown that the effects of raloxifene on vertebral fracture risk, BMD and bone turnover are sustained in the longer term.[23] Of those patients originally randomised to the three treatment groups, 72% of placebo- and 75% of raloxifene-treated patients underwent a 4-year follow-up visit (*p*-value not reported). The cumulative proportion of participants with at least one incident vertebral fracture at 4 years is shown in Figure 4. The RR for one or more new vertebral fractures after 4 years of raloxifene treatment was 0.64 for the 60 mg daily dose and 0.57 for the 120 mg dose. Consistent with the 3-year data, raloxifene treatment did not significantly alter the risk of non-vertebral fracture risk, with 11.5 and 10.7% of placebo- and raloxifene-treated patients reporting at least one new non-vertebral fracture (RR 0.93 for both raloxifene treatment groups combined). Compared with placebo, raloxifene treatment elicited significant increases in femoral neck and lumbar spine BMD at 4 years (2.5 and 2.3%, and 2.6 and 2.1%, for raloxifene, 60 and 120 mg, respectively; *p*<0.001 for all comparisons *vs* placebo). Again, the lack of positive correlation between the observed increase in femoral neck BMD and non-vertebral fracture risk does not lend great credibility to the use of BMD as a surrogate marker. The median baseline reductions in serum osteocalcin concentrations over 48 months were 8.6, 26.2 and 31.1% for placebo, and raloxifene, 60 mg and 120 mg, respectively (*p*<0.001 *vs* placebo), whilst BSAP declined by 19.9, 35.2 and 35.6%, respectively (*p*<0.001 *vs* placebo). These values remained in the premenopausal range throughout the 4-year study. The safety profile of raloxifene at 4 years was similar to that at 3 years, and this is covered more extensively in the Safety and Tolerability section of this review.

> The RR for one or more new vertebral fractures after 4 years of raloxifene treatment was 0.64 for the 60 mg daily dose and 0.57 for the 120 mg dose.

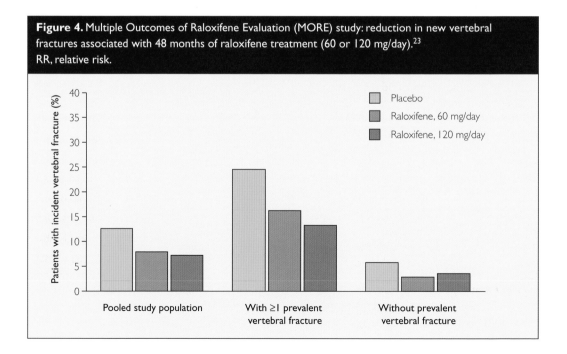

Figure 4. Multiple Outcomes of Raloxifene Evaluation (MORE) study: reduction in new vertebral fractures associated with 48 months of raloxifene treatment (60 or 120 mg/day).[23] RR, relative risk.

Fracture severity

Data from the MORE study were further examined in order to ascertain whether fracture severity at baseline predicted the patient's risk of sustaining a new vertebral or non-vertebral fracture.[25] In addition, the relative risk of fracture was determined in a subgroup of 614 women with severe prevalent vertebral fractures at baseline. Regardless of treatment, of those women who were free from fracture at baseline, 4.3 and 5.5% had sustained a new vertebral and non-vertebral fracture at 3 years. Of those women with mild, moderate and severe prevalent vertebral fractures at baseline (depending on the visually apparent degree of vertebral height loss), 10.5, 23.6 and 38.1% had new vertebral fractures and 7.2, 7.7 and 13.8% experienced new non-vertebral fractures after 3 years. The incidence of new non-vertebral fractures was significantly greater in women with severe prevalent vertebral fractures at baseline ($p<0.05$). To prevent one new fracture at 3 years in women with severe baseline vertebral fractures with raloxifene, 60 mg/day, the number needed to treat (NNT) was 10 for vertebral and 18 for non-vertebral fractures. The effect of raloxifene treatment was determined in the 614 women considered to be at high risk of fracture. New vertebral fractures occurred in 38.1, 28.1 and 25.1% of women in the placebo, and raloxifene, 60 and 120 mg, treatment groups, respectively. Raloxifene (60 mg) significantly decreased the risk of new vertebral (RR 0.74; $p=0.048$) and non-vertebral fracture (RR 0.53; $p=0.046$) at 3 years in this patient population. Therefore, this analysis showed that baseline vertebral fracture severity was the best independent predictor for new vertebral and non-vertebral fracture risk, and also identified women with severe vertebral fractures at baseline as being particularly responsive to raloxifene therapy.

> Raloxifene significantly decreased the risk of new vertebral and non-vertebral fracture at 3 years in women with severe vertebral fractures at baseline.

Are biochemical markers predictive of vertebral fracture risk?

Levels of N-terminal propeptide of type 1 procollagen (P1NP), a marker of bone turnover, were available for a subset of women (n=967) from the MORE cohort.[26] Treatment with raloxifene was associated with a significant reduction from baseline in P1NP levels (–40.8% [pooled data from both raloxifene doses]) compared with placebo (–11.0%; $p<0.001$). Serum osteocalcin levels were decreased by medians of 31.8 and 8.5% for pooled raloxifene and placebo groups, respectively ($p<0.001$ vs placebo) and BSAP concentrations were decreased by medians of 34.6 and 15.8%, respectively ($p<0.001$ vs placebo). The logistic regression relationship between 3-year vertebral fracture risk and the 1-year change for each biochemical marker was analysed and was found to be significant with P1NP (slope estimate 0.0085; $p=0.009$), osteocalcin (slope estimate 0.0068; $p=0.035$) and BSAP (slope estimate 0.0056; $p=0.039$). Thus, 1-year changes in P1NP, osteocalcin and BSAP, as biochemical markers of bone turnover, may predict the 3-year vertebral fracture risk reduction associated with raloxifene treatment.

However, it is generally accepted that markers of bone turnover are useful in population-based studies but lack precision, specificity and sensitivity to predict fracture risk in individuals.

Risk of breast cancer

The incidence of breast cancer was a secondary endpoint of the MORE study. Subsequent analysis of data from the MORE study has shown that long-term raloxifene therapy was associated with a significant reduction in invasive breast cancer.[27,28] Over the first 3 years of the study, the rate of breast cancer was significantly lower amongst raloxifene-treated patients (1.05 *vs* 0.25% for placebo and raloxifene [pooled], respectively; *p*<0.001).[27] Raloxifene decreased the risk of oestrogen receptor-positive breast cancer by 90% (RR 0.10), but not oestrogen receptor-negative invasive breast cancer (RR 0.88).[27] Four-year data, which included an additional 3,004 woman years of follow-up (23,315 woman years in total), reported a relative risk reduction in invasive breast cancer of 72% following raloxifene treatment.[28] The cumulative incidence of all confirmed breast cancer cases amongst MORE study participants is shown in Figure 5.[28]

Subsequent analysis of these data has shown that women with high estradiol levels (≥12 pmol/L) had a 2.07-fold higher risk of invasive breast cancer compared with women with lower levels.[29] For placebo-treated patients, the risk associated with high levels of estradiol was significant (RR 2.56; *p*<0.01), whilst raloxifene therapy appeared to protect these patients against breast cancer (RR 1.48; *p*>0.05).[29] In addition, patients with a family history of breast cancer experienced a

> Four-year data reported a relative risk reduction in invasive breast cancer of 72% following raloxifene treatment.

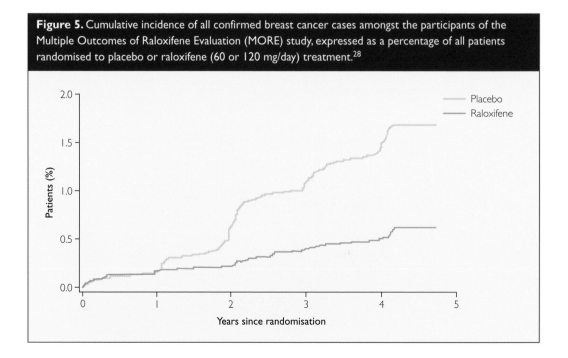

Figure 5. Cumulative incidence of all confirmed breast cancer cases amongst the participants of the Multiple Outcomes of Raloxifene Evaluation (MORE) study, expressed as a percentage of all patients randomised to placebo or raloxifene (60 or 120 mg/day) treatment.[28]

significantly greater breast cancer risk reduction with raloxifene treatment (*p*=0.015).[29] Previous hormone therapy use had no bearing on the incidence of breast cancer following raloxifene therapy (*p*=0.60).[30]

Whilst these data are encouraging, the role of raloxifene in the treatment of established breast cancer is still unclear, and the manufacturer currently advises against the use of raloxifene during the treatment of breast cancer.[3] The Study of Tamoxifen and Raloxifene (STAR), which was designed to assess the effects of both drugs on the incidence of invasive breast cancer (primary endpoint) and non-invasive breast cancer and endometrial cancer (secondary endpoints), is scheduled for completion during 2005. However, this study does not contain a placebo group so will not provide any information regarding the effect of raloxifene in osteoporotic women who are otherwise healthy.

The Continuing Outcomes Relevant to Evista (CORE) study examined the effect of an additional 4 years' raloxifene treatment on the incidence of invasive breast cancer in 5,213 women originally enrolled in the MORE study.[31] Overall, the 4-year rates of overall and oestrogen receptor positive invasive breast cancer were reduced by 59 and 66%, respectively, in the raloxifene treatment group compared with placebo. The incidence of oestrogen receptor negative breast cancer was unaffected by raloxifene treatment (*p*=0.86). Thus, over 8 years, the rates of overall and oestrogen receptor positive invasive breast cancer were reduced by 66 and 76%, respectively, following treatment with raloxifene compared with placebo.

Over 8 years, the rates of overall and oestrogen receptor positive invasive breast cancer were reduced by 66 and 76%, respectively, following treatment with raloxifene.

Cardiovascular risk

During the 4 years of the MORE study, the incidence of combined coronary and cerebrovascular events was not significantly affected by raloxifene treatment (3.7, 3.2 and 3.7% for placebo, and raloxifene 60 and 120 mg, respectively; RR 0.86 and 0.98 for raloxifene, 60 and 120 mg, respectively).[32] Raloxifene treatment did, however, significantly reduce the risk of cardiovascular events amongst those women with increased cardiovascular risk at baseline, as a result of prior coronary events or revascularisation procedures (n=1035; RR 0.60 for both raloxifene groups).

The effect of long-term raloxifene treatment on low density lipoprotein cholesterol (LDL-C) and other serum lipids was examined in an analysis of the 2413 women enrolled in the MORE study who did not take lipid-lowering medications at any point over the course of the trial.[33] At baseline, the percentage of women with LDL-C levels less than 4.1 mmol/L was comparable between the different treatment groups (57.5, 56.4 and 56.8% for placebo, raloxifene, 60 and 120 mg, respectively; *p*-value not reported). At 3 years, the proportion of women whose LDL-C had increased to above 4.1 mmol/L was significantly lower amongst the raloxifene than placebo groups (14.1, 5.0 and 5.1%, respectively; RR 0.35 and 0.36 compared with placebo). The proportion of women with LDL-C above 4.1 mmol/L at baseline (42.4, 43.6 and 43.2%, respectively; *p*-value not reported), in whom LDL-C decreased to less than 4.1 mmol/L after 3 years, was significantly higher amongst raloxifene patients (25.5, 49.7 and 55.6%, respectively; $p<0.0001$ *vs* placebo). Furthermore, a significantly higher proportion of these women achieved LDL-C levels of below 3.4 mmol/L following 3 years of raloxifene treatment (5.6, 13.5 and 17.4% for placebo and raloxifene, 60 and 120 mg, respectively; $p<0.0001$ *vs* placebo). The proportion of women initiating lipid-lowering therapy during the study was also significantly lower in the raloxifene treatment groups (5.7, 3.4 and 2.8%, respectively; $p<0.001$ *vs* placebo).

In summary, raloxifene therapy did not significantly affect the risk of cardiovascular events in the overall cohort, but significantly lowered risk amongst patients predisposed to cardiovascular complications at baseline. Previous hormone therapy use had no bearing on the incidence of cardiovascular events in this population ($p=0.56$).[30] Further analysis has shown that the long-term use of raloxifene did not compromise glycaemic control amongst patients with type 2 diabetes mellitus (3.9% of the study population).[34] The Raloxifene Use for The Heart (RUTH) trial, which has enrolled more than 10,000 patients, was specifically designed to determine whether raloxifene (60 mg/day) lowers the risk of coronary events. The findings of the study, which commenced in 2001 and will take 5 years to complete, are keenly anticipated.[35]

If a global index of clinical outcomes (defined as the earliest occurrence of coronary heart disease, stroke, pulmonary embolism, invasive breast cancer, endometrial cancer, colorectal cancer, hip fracture or death because of other causes) is applied to the MORE data, then raloxifene is associated with a hazard ratio of 0.75 compared with placebo (annual rates of 1.83 and 1.39% for placebo and raloxifene [combined doses], respectively).[36] Interestingly, this global risk reduction appeared to be more pronounced in obese compared with non-obese women ($p=0.03$).

Comparative studies

The efficacy of raloxifene has been compared with that of other antiresorptive therapies – predominantly the bisphosphonate, alendronate – in a relatively limited number of clinical trials, summarised in Table 4.[37–41] In general, the treatment-induced improvements in lumbar spine and total hip BMD were significantly greater amongst alendronate- than raloxifene-treated patients. Alendronate was also associated with more pronounced changes in BSAP and a significantly lower incidence of vasomotor events. It is envisaged that the upcoming Evista® Alendronate Comparison (EVA) trial, in which approximately 3,000 postmenopausal women with osteoporosis received either raloxifene (60 mg/day) or alendronate (10 mg/day) for a period of 5 years, will clarify the relative fracture risk reduction efficacy and safety profiles of these agents further.[17]

The additive effects of raloxifene and alendronate, when given in combination, have been investigated in a double-blind, placebo-controlled, year-long study in 331 postmenopausal women with osteoporosis.[42] Participants received either raloxifene (60 mg/day), alendronate (10 mg/day), or the same doses of each agent in

Table 4. Summary of clinical trials comparing the efficacy of raloxifene with that of other treatments for postmenopausal osteoporosis.[37–41]

Study	Dosage regimen	Main outcomes
Raloxifene *vs* alendronate		
Sambrook *et al.*, 2004[37] Double-blind 12 months n=487	Raloxifene, 60 mg/day, or alendronate, 70 mg/week	• Study completion rates were 86 and 88% for raloxifene and alendronate treatment groups, respectively (p-value not reported). • Lumbar spine BMD increased by 2.2 and 4.8% from baseline following raloxifene and alendronate treatment, respectively ($p<0.001$). • At 12 months, more patients in the alendronate than in the raloxifene group had maintained or increased lumbar spine BMD (87.2 *vs* 73.1% respectively; $p<0.001$). • Total hip BMD increased by 0.8 and 2.3% from baseline following raloxifene and alendronate, respectively ($p<0.001$). • At 12 months, the geometric mean change in BSAP was highest in the alendronate treatment group (50.6 *vs* 11.9%, respectively; $p<0.001$). • The proportion of patients reporting vasomotor events was highest in the raloxifene group (9.5 *vs* 3.7% for raloxifene and alendronate, respectively; $p=0.01$).
Luckey *et al.*, 2004[38] Double-blind 12 months n=456	Raloxifene, 60 mg/day, or alendronate, 70 mg/week	• Study completion rates were 82.8 and 80.3% for raloxifene and alendronate treatment groups, respectively (p-value not reported). • Lumbar spine BMD increased by 1.9 and 4.4% from baseline following raloxifene and alendronate, respectively ($p<0.001$). • At 12 months, more patients in the alendronate than in the raloxifene group had maintained or increased lumbar spine BMD (94 *vs* 75%, respectively; $p<0.001$). • Total hip BMD increased by 1.0 and 2.0% from baseline following raloxifene and alendronate, respectively ($p<0.001$). • At 12 months, the mean change in BSAP was highest in the alendronate treatment group (41 *vs* 22%, respectively; $p<0.001$). • The overall incidence of adverse events was similar between treatment groups (75.2 *vs* 74.2% for raloxifene and alendronate, respectively; $p=0.83$).
Turbi *et al.*, 2004[39] Open-label 12 months n=902	Raloxifene, 60 mg/day, or alendronate, 10 mg/day	• Compliance was significantly better amongst raloxifene-treated patients (68.7 *vs* 54.0% for raloxifene and alendronate, respectively; $p<0.001$). • Premature treatment discontinuation was significantly higher amongst alendronate-treated patients (25.8 *vs* 16.4%, respectively; $p<0.001$). • Adverse events represented the most common cause of premature withdrawal in both treatment groups (4.8 *vs* 11.0% for raloxifene and alendronate, respectively; $p<0.001$). • The proportion of patients who were satisfied or very satisfied with treatment was significantly higher amongst raloxifene- than alendronate-treated patients (95.7 *vs* 85.4%, respectively; $p<0.001$).

BMD, bone mineral density; BSAP, serum bone-specific alkaline phosphatase.

Table 4. Continued

Study	Dosage regimen	Main outcomes
Raloxifene vs monofluorophosphate (MFP)		
Reginster et al., 2003[40] Double-blind 18 months n=596	Raloxifene, 60 mg/day, plus MFP, 20 mg/day, or MFP, 20 mg/day, plus placebo	• The increase in BMD in the femoral neck was significantly greater in the raloxifene/MFP combination group (1.37 vs 0.33% for raloxifene/MFP and MFP, respectively; p=0.004). • The increase in BMD in the lumbar spine was significantly greater in the raloxifene/MFP combination group (8.80 vs 5.47% for raloxifene/MFP and MFP, respectively; p<0.001). • One patient in the combination group sustained multiple osteoporotic fractures, compared with 8 patients in the MFP group (p=0.02). • Hot flushes were significantly more common in the raloxifene/MFP combination group (9.7 vs 3.7%, respectively; p=0.005).
Raloxifene vs conjugated equine oestrogen (CEE)		
Reid et al., 2004[41] Double-blind Placebo-controlled 36 months n=619	Raloxifene, 60 or 150 mg/day, or CEE, 0.625 mg/day	• Over 3 years, BMD in the lumbar spine decreased by 2.0% from baseline in the placebo group, was maintained near baseline in the raloxifene treatment groups and increased by 4.6% in the CEE (p<0.001 raloxifene vs placebo and CEE). • Over the same period, BMD in the total hip decreased by 1.3% from baseline in the placebo group, was maintained near baseline in the raloxifene treatment groups and increased by 3.0% in the CEE (p<0.001 raloxifene vs placebo and CEE). • The mean reduction from baseline in serum osteocalcin at 3 years was 15, 27, 28.4 and 47.1% for placebo, raloxifene 60 and 150 mg, and CEE, respectively (p<0.001 for all active treatments vs placebo). • There were no significant differences between treatments in terms of the overall proportion of patients reporting adverse events.

BMD, bone mineral density; BSAP, serum bone-specific alkaline phosphatase.

> The positive effects of raloxifene and alendronate on BMD were independent and additive.

combination, and changes in BMD were evaluated after 12 months. Lumbar spine BMD increased by 2.1, 4.3 and 5.3% from baseline following treatment with raloxifene, alendronate and the raloxifene–alendronate combination, compared with a 0.004% decrease following placebo (p<0.05 vs placebo; p<0.05 raloxifene vs alendronate and raloxifene–alendronate). Femoral neck BMD was similarly affected, with increases of 1.7, 2.7 and 3.7% from baseline values, compared with 0.2% following placebo (p=0.02 alendronate vs raloxifene–alendronate; p<0.001 raloxifene vs raloxifene–alendronate). Further analysis of these data suggested that the positive effects of raloxifene and alendronate on BMD were independent and additive. The interaction effects for lumbar spine and femoral neck BMD were 0.153 and 0.654, respectively (the interaction effect was judged not to be significant if p>0.10).

This study highlights the potential advantages of combining raloxifene with a bisphosphonate, although the effect of such a treatment approach on clinical fracture risk has not been investigated to date. Currently unlicensed, the safety and financial implications of combination therapy must be resolved before such an approach becomes common clinical practice.

Meta-analysis

An analysis of data pooled from seven clinical trials, four of which have been published to date,[20–22,43] examined the changes in BMD following at least 1 year of raloxifene treatment.[44] Owing to its sheer size, the aforementioned MORE study dominates this analysis, and this should be borne in mind. All patients (n=10,199) received similar calcium and vitamin D supplementation over the course of each trial. Following raloxifene treatment, total body BMD (assessed in two of the trials) was increased by 1.33% over placebo (p=0.01). The increase in lumbar spine BMD associated with 1 year of raloxifene therapy, examined across all seven trials, was 1.82% over placebo (p<0.01), increasing to 2.51% after 2–3 years (in four trials; p<0.01). Improvements in combined hip BMD following raloxifene treatment followed a similar trend, measuring 1.47% after 1 year and increasing to 2.11% after 2–3 years (p<0.01 for both time points). Raloxifene-treated patients were more likely than placebo patients to discontinue treatment as a result of an adverse event (RR 1.15; p=0.05), and hot flushes were significantly more frequent amongst raloxifene-treated patients (RR 1.46; p<0.01).

Safety and tolerability

The majority of adverse events associated with raloxifene therapy do not necessitate the premature discontinuation of treatment.[3] The adverse events reported most frequently during randomised controlled trials, the MORE study and prescription-event monitoring, are summarised in Table 5.[45] Hot flushes, leg cramps, a 'flu-like' syndrome and peripheral oedema are amongst the most common side-effects associated with raloxifene therapy.[3]

Raloxifene treatment (60 or 120 mg/day for 12 months) was not associated with any significant deterioration in cognitive function, as assessed using the Memory Assessment Clinics (MAC) battery and Walter Reed Performance Assessment Battery (PAB), or mood, as assessed with the Geriatric Depression Scale (GDS), in a group of 143 postmenopausal women.[46]

The incidence of venous thromboembolic events following long-term treatment with raloxifene was thoroughly examined during the MORE study. Over a mean follow-up of 3.3 years, raloxifene-treated patients (60 and 120 mg daily dose groups pooled) were at an increased risk of venous thrombosis (RR 2.1; p=0.01 [Figure 6]).[47] Treatment with raloxifene was associated with an increased risk of deep vein thrombosis (RR 3.1; p<0.01) and pulmonary embolism (RR 4.5; p=0.05) compared with placebo treatment. Risk was highest in the raloxifene treatment

You are strongly urged to consult your doctor before taking, stopping or changing any of the products reviewed or referred to in BESTMEDICINE or any other medication that has been prescribed or recommended by your doctor.

Table 5. The incidence of selected adverse events reported during treatment with raloxifene in a prescription-event monitoring (PEM) study, during randomised clinical trials (RCTs) and in the Multiple Outcomes of Raloxifene Evaluation (MORE) study.[45]

Adverse event	Percentage of patients affected		
	PEM (n=13,987; 60 mg/day)	Pooled RCTs (n=1075; 60 mg/day)	MORE (n=5129; 60–120 mg/day)
Flatulence	0.2	3.0	–
Abdominal pain	0.6	6.5	–
Breast pain	0.8	4.7	2.6
CVA and TIA	0.4	–	0.5
Bradycardia	<0.1	–	0.6
DVT	<0.1	–	0.7
Hypertension	1.1	–	7.2
Coronary events (including IHD)	0.5	–	2.0
Oedema	1.9	–	5.9
Pulmonary embolus	0.1	–	0.3
Flushing/hot flushes/vasodilation	6.5	26.5	10.7
Urogenital bleeding	0.9	3.4	2.4
Diabetes/hyperglycaemia	0.3	–	1.2
Sweating	1.6	3.0	–
Leg cramps	3.4	5.4	6.9
Breast carcinoma	0.2	–	0.2
RTI/influenza-like illness	3.0	–	13.5
Haematuria	0.1	–	1.3

CVA, cardiovascular accident; DVT, deep vein thrombosis; IHD, ischaemic heart disease; RTI, respiratory tract infection; TIA, transient ischaemic attack.

Figure 6. Cumulative incidence of venous thromboembolic events amongst women in the Multiple Outcomes of Raloxifene Evaluation (MORE) study.[47] The difference between raloxifene (60 and 120 mg/day) and placebo treatment groups is significant (*p*=0.01).

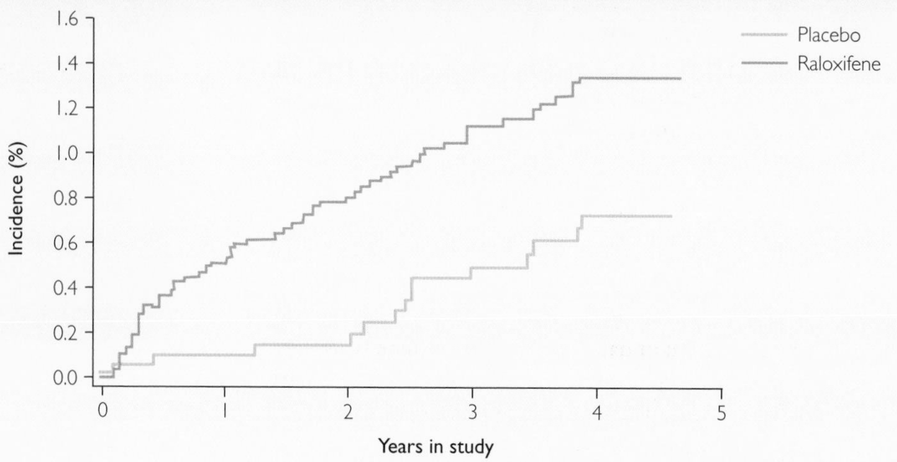

groups during the first 2 years of treatment but normalised to placebo levels thereafter. This safety analysis of the MORE study also determined that raloxifene had no impact on the incidence of cataracts or gallbladder disease, uterine bleeding (3.7% in placebo and raloxifene treatment groups; p=1.0) or endometrial cancer (0.25 vs 0.23% for placebo and raloxifene, respectively).

Hot flushes

The majority of clinical trials have identified an increased incidence of hot flushes associated with raloxifene therapy.[22,23] Although these vasomotor symptoms are unlikely to be severe enough to precipitate complete treatment discontinuation, they may interfere significantly with patient compliance and, therefore, may ultimately impede a positive clinical outcome.

A double-blind, placebo-controlled trial was conducted in order to evaluate the propensity for different raloxifene treatment regimens to elicit hot flushes over an 8-month treatment period.[48] A group of 487 postmenopausal women were randomly allocated to placebo, conventional (60 mg/day) or slow-dose escalation (60 mg every other day for 2 months and 60 mg/day thereafter) raloxifene treatment schedules. Throughout the study, the frequency, duration, intensity, severity and impact of hot flushes was measured. The rate of study completion was similar between treatment groups (87.4, 89.2 and 88.8% for placebo, conventional and slow-dose escalation raloxifene groups, respectively; p-values not reported). Amongst those patients who reported hot flushes over the course of the study, the mean number per week at study endpoint was 8.3, 11.6 and 11.9 for placebo, conventional and slow-dose escalation raloxifene groups, such that conventional, but not slow-dose escalation raloxifene, was associated with significantly more hot flushes per week than placebo (p=0.035 conventional vs placebo). The proportion of patients experiencing an increase of at least 14 hot flushes per week was 2.7, 9.7 and 7.7% for placebo, conventional and slow-dose escalation raloxifene groups, respectively (p=0.047 conventional raloxifene vs placebo).

Subsequent analysis of these data identified more recent menopause and surgical menopause as important predictors of hot flushes both before and during treatment with raloxifene.[49] Slow-dose escalation of raloxifene may represent a suitable therapeutic strategy for the reduction of the risk of hot flushes in women with early menopause.[49]

> More recent menopause and surgical menopause are important predictors of hot flushes both before and during treatment with raloxifene.

Contraindications and special precautions

Raloxifene is contraindicated in women of child-bearing potential, or in women with an active or past history of venous thromboembolic events, including deep vein thrombosis, pulmonary embolism and retinal vein thrombosis.[3] Owing to a lack of data, the use of raloxifene is also prohibited in women with hepatic impairment (including cholestasis), severe renal impairment, unexplained uterine bleeding, or signs or symptoms of endometrial cancer.[3]

Caution is advocated when prescribing raloxifene to women with:
- increased risk of venous thromboembolic events (e.g. a condition leading to a prolonged period of immobilisation)
- a history of oral oestrogen-induced hypertriglyceridaemia (>5.6 mmol/L)
- breast cancer (raloxifene treatment should only be initiated once treatment for breast cancer has ceased).[3]

Socioeconomic impact

The social and economic burden of osteoporosis is immense and in 2000, the condition was estimated to cost the UK £1.7 billion.[50] The annual incidence of fractures is set to increase dramatically over coming years in line with the increasingly ageing population.[51] Thus, the prevention of fractures is paramount to reduce the morbidity and mortality, healthcare and social care costs associated with osteoporosis.[52]

In a UK cost-effectiveness analysis of raloxifene, based on data derived from the MORE study, the costs per quality adjusted life year (QALY) gained from treating women without prior vertebral fractures were £18,000, £23,000, £18,000 and £21,000 at 50, 60, 70 and 80 years of age, respectively.[53] For women with prior vertebral fractures, the corresponding costs were £10,000, £24,000, £18,000 and £20,000 for these age groups, respectively. Take together with the emerging evidence regarding the positive effects of raloxifene on breast cancer, these data suggest that raloxifene is a cost-effective treatment option in postmenopausal women at high risk of vertebral fractures. However, general opinion surrounding the cost-effectiveness of raloxifene has been guided by its lack of demonstrated effect on hip fracture, the most costly fracture in health economic terms and in the morbidity and mortality associated with fracture outcome.

Raloxifene is a cost-effective treatment option in postmenopausal women at high risk of vertebral fractures.

Key points

- Raloxifene is licensed for the prevention and treatment of osteoporosis in postmenopausal women.

- As a SERM, raloxifene mimics the effects of oestrogen on bone and lipid metabolism but acts as an oestrogen antagonist in the uterine and breast tissues.

- By binding to the oestrogen receptor, raloxifene influences gene transcription and ultimately affects the proliferation and activity of osteoclasts and osteoblasts in bone.

- The MORE study demonstrated a significant reduction in the incidence of vertebral fracture following up to 4 years treatment with raloxifene in postmenopausal women.

- BMD was increased significantly following raloxifene therapy, together with concomitant alterations in biochemical markers of bone turnover (e.g. PINP, BSAP, osteocalcin), which may be predictive of long-term vertebral fracture risk.

- Long-term raloxifene treatment significantly reduced serum levels of LDL-C and reduced the incidence of cardiovascular events in at-risk patients.

- Aside from its effects in bone, raloxifene has also been shown to reduce the risk of invasive breast cancer significantly in postmenopausal women.

- Combining raloxifene with the bisphosphonate, alendronate, may represent a viable treatment option in the future. Although large-scale head-to-head comparative trials of these agents are currently ongoing, studies conducted to date tend to favour the bisphosphonate.

- Although generally well tolerated in clinical trials, raloxifene has been linked with an increased risk of venous thromboembolism. Leg cramps and hot flushes are commonly associated with long-term treatment.

References

A list of the published evidence which has been reviewed in compiling the preceding section of *BESTMEDICINE*.

1 Goldstein S, Siddhanti S, Ciaccia A, Plouffe L. A pharmacological review of selective oestrogen receptor modulators. *Hum Reprod Update* 2000; **6**: 212–24.

2 Silfen S, Ciaccia A, Bryant H. Selective estrogen receptor modulators: tissue selectivity and differential uterine effects. *Climacteric* 1999; **2**: 268–83.

3 Eli Lilly and Company Limited. Evista® 60 mg film-coated tablets. *Summary of product characteristics.* Basingstoke, 2004.

4 Grese T, Sluka J, Bryant H *et al.* Molecular determinants of tissue selectivity in estrogen receptor modulators. *Proc Natl Acad Sci USA* 1997; **94**: 14105–10.

5 Morello K, Wurz G, DeGregorio M. SERMs: current status and future trends. *Crit Rev Oncol Hematol* 2002; **43**: 63–76.

6 Buelke-Sam J, Bryant H, Francis P. The selective estrogen receptor modulator, raloxifene: an overview of nonclinical pharmacology and reproductive and developmental testing. *Reprod Toxicol* 1998; **12**: 217–21.

7 Yang N, Venugopalan M, Hardikar S, Glasebrook A. Identification of an estrogen response element activated by metabolites of 17beta-estradiol and raloxifene. *Science* 1996; **273**: 1222–5.

8 Vidal O, Kindblom L, Ohlsson C. Expression and localization of estrogen receptor-beta in murine and human bone. *J Bone Min Res* 1999; **14**: 923–9.

9 Yang N, Bryant H, Hardikar S *et al.* Estrogen and raloxifene stimulate transforming growth factor-beta 3 gene expression in rat bone: a potential mechanism for estrogen- or raloxifene-mediated bone maintenance. *Endocrinology* 1996; **137**: 2075–84.

10 Taranta A, Brama M, Teti A *et al.* The selective estrogen receptor modulator raloxifene regulates osteoclast and osteoblast activity *in vitro*. *Bone* 2002; **30**: 368–76.

11 Black L, Sato M, Rowley E *et al.* Raloxifene (LY139481 HCl) prevents bone loss and reduces serum cholesterol without causing uterine hypertrophy in ovariectomised rats. *J Clin Invest* 1994; **93**: 63–9.

12 Clemens J, Bennett D, Black L, Jones C. Effects of a new antiestrogen, keoxifene (LY156758), on growth of carcinogen-induced mammary tumors and on LH and prolactin levels. *Life Sci* 1983; **32**: 2869–75.

13 Wakeling A, Valcaccia B, Newboult E, Green L. Non-steroidal antioestrogens – receptor binding and biological response in rat uterus, rat mammary carcinoma and human breast cancer cells. *J Steroid Biochem* 1984; **20**: 111–20.

14 Hochner-Celnikier D. Pharmacokinetics of raloxifene and its clinical application. *Eur J Obstet Gynecol Reprod Biol* 1999; **85**: 23–9.

15 Roberts M, Magnusson B, Burczynski F, Weiss M. Enterohepatic circulation: physiological, pharmacokinetic and clinical implications. *Clin Pharmacokinet* 2002; **41**: 751–90.

16 Marcus R, Wong M, Heath H, Stock J. Antiresorptive treatment of postmenopausal osteoporosis: comparison of study designs and outcomes in large clinical trials with fracture as an endpoint. *Endocr Rev* 2002; **23**: 16–37.

17 Lufkin E, Sarkar S, Kulkarni P *et al.* Antiresorptive treatment of postmenopausal osteoporosis: review of randomized clinical studies and rationale for the Evista alendronate comparison (EVA) trial. *Curr Med Res Opin* 2004; **20**: 351–7.

18 Delmas P, Bjarnason N, Mitlak B *et al.* Effects of raloxifene on bone mineral density, serum cholesterol concentrations, and uterine endometrium in postmenopausal women. *N Engl J Med* 1997; **337**: 1641–7.

19 Jolly E, Bjarnason N, Neven P *et al.* Prevention of osteoporosis and uterine effects in postmenopausal women taking raloxifene for 5 years. *Menopause* 2003; **10**: 337–44.

20 Lufkin E, Whitaker M, Nickelsen T *et al.* Treatment of established postmenopausal osteoporosis with raloxifene: a randomized trial. *J Bone Min Res* 1998; **13**: 1747–54.

21 Meunier P, Vignot E, Garnero P *et al.* Treatment of postmenopausal women with osteoporosis or low bone density with raloxifene. Raloxifene Study Group. *Osteoporos Int* 1999; **10**: 330–6.

22 Ettinger B, Black D, Mitlak B *et al.* Reduction of vertebral fracture risk in postmenopausal women with osteoporosis treated with raloxifene: results from a 3-year randomized clinical trial. Multiple Outcomes of Raloxifene Evaluation (MORE) Investigators. *JAMA* 1999; **282**: 637–45.

23 Delmas P, Ensrud K, Adachi J *et al.* Efficacy of raloxifene on vertebral fracture risk reduction in postmenopausal women with osteoporosis: four-year results from a randomized clinical trial. *J Clin Endocrinol Metab* 2002; **87**: 3609–17.

24 Johnell O, Kanis J, Black D *et al.* Associations between baseline risk factors and vertebral fracture risk in the Multiple Outcomes of Raloxifene Evaluation (MORE) Study. *J Bone Min Res* 2004; **19**: 764–72.

25 Delmas P, Genant H, Crans G *et al.* Severity of prevalent vertebral fractures and the risk of subsequent vertebral and nonvertebral fractures: results from the MORE trial. *Bone* 2003; **33**: 522–32.

26 Reginster J, Sarkar S, Zegels B *et al.* Reduction in PINP, a marker of bone metabolism, with raloxifene treatment and its relationship with vertebral fracture risk. *Bone* 2004; **34**: 344–51.

27 Cummings S, Eckert S, Krueger K *et al.* The effect of raloxifene on risk of breast cancer in postmenopausal women: results from the MORE randomized trial. Multiple Outcomes of Raloxifene Evaluation. *JAMA* 1999; **281**: 2189–97.

28 Cauley J, Norton L, Lippman M *et al.* Continued breast cancer risk reduction in postmenopausal women treated with raloxifene: 4-year results from the MORE trial. Multiple outcomes of raloxifene evaluation. *Breast Cancer Res Treat* 2001; **65**: 125–34.

29 Lippman M, Krueger K, Eckert S *et al.* Indicators of lifetime estrogen exposure: effect on breast cancer incidence and interaction with raloxifene therapy in the multiple outcomes of raloxifene evaluation study participants. *J Clin Oncol* 2001; **19**: 3111–16.

30 Johnell O, Cauley J, Kulkarni P, Wong M, Stock J. Raloxifene reduces risk of vertebral fractures and breast cancer in postmenopausal women regardless of prior hormone therapy. *J Fam Pract* 2004; **53**: 789–96.

31 Martino S, Cauley J, Barrett-Connor E *et al.* Continuing outcomes relevant to Evista: breast cancer incidence in postmenopausal osteoporotic women in a randomized trial of raloxifene. *J Natl Cancer Inst* 2004; **96**: 1751–61.

32 Barrett-Connor E, Grady D, Sashegyi A *et al.* Raloxifene and cardiovascular events in osteoporotic postmenopausal women: four-year results from the MORE (Multiple Outcomes of Raloxifene Evaluation) randomized trial. *JAMA* 2002; **287**: 847–57.

33 Cox D, Sarkar S, Harper K, Barrett-Connor E. Effect of raloxifene on the incidence of elevated low density lipoprotein (LDL) and achievement of LDL target goals in postmenopausal women. *Curr Med Res Opin* 2004; **20**: 1049–55.

34 Barrett-Connor E, Ensrud K, Harper K *et al. Post hoc* analysis of data from the Multiple Outcomes of Raloxifene Evaluation (MORE) trial on the effects of three years of raloxifene treatment on glycemic control and cardiovascular disease risk factors in women with and without type 2 diabetes. *Clin Ther* 2003; **25**: 919–30.

35 Wenger N, Barrett-Connor E, Collins P *et al.* Baseline characteristics of participants in the Raloxifene Use for The Heart (RUTH) trial. *Am J Cardiol* 2002; **90**: 1204–10.

36 Barrett-Connor E, Cauley J. Risk-benefit profile for raloxifene: 4-year data from the Multiple Outcomes of Raloxifene Evaluation (MORE) randomised trial. *J Bone Min Res* 2004; **19**: 1270–5.

37 Sambrook P, Geusens P, Ribot C *et al.* Alendronate produces greater effects than raloxifene on bone density and bone turnover in postmenopausal women with low bone density: results of EFFECT (Efficacy of FOSAMAX versus EVISTA Comparison Trial) International. *J Intern Med* 2004; **255**: 503–11.

38 Luckey M, Kagan R, Greenspan S *et al.* Once-weekly alendronate 70 mg and raloxifene 60 mg daily in the treatment of postmenopausal osteoporosis. *Menopause* 2004; **11**: 405–15.

39 Turbi C, Herrero-Beaumont G, Acebes J *et al.* Compliance and satisfaction with raloxifene versus alendronate for the treatment of postmenopausal osteoporosis in clinical practice: An open-label, prospective, nonrandomized, observational study. *Clin Ther* 2004; **26**: 245–56.

40 Reginster J, Felsenberg D, Pavo I *et al.* Effect of raloxifene combined with monofluorophosphate as compared with monofluorophosphate alone in postmenopausal women with low bone mass: a randomized, controlled trial. *Osteoporos Int* 2003; **14**: 741–9.

41 Reid I, Eastell R, Fogelman I *et al.* A comparison of the effects of raloxifene and conjugated equine estrogen on bone and lipids in healthy postmenopausal women. *Arch Intern Med* 2004; **164**: 871–9.

42 Johnell O, Scheele W, Lu Y *et al.* Additive effects of raloxifene and alendronate on bone density and biochemical markers of bone remodeling in postmenopausal women with osteoporosis. *J Clin Endocrinol Metab* 2002; **87**: 985–92.

43 Johnston C, Bjarnason N, Cohen F *et al.* Long-term effects of raloxifene on bone mineral density, bone turnover, and serum lipid levels in early postmenopausal women: three-year data from 2 double-blind, randomized, placebo-controlled trials. *Arch Intern Med* 2000; **160**: 3444–50.

44 Cranney A, Tugwell P, Zytaruk N *et al.* Meta-analyses of therapies for postmenopausal osteoporosis. IV. Meta-analysis of raloxifene for the prevention and treatment of postmenopausal osteoporosis. *Endocr Rev* 2002; **23**: 524–8.

45 Layton D, Clarke A, Wilton L, Shakir S. Safety profile of raloxifene as used in general practice in England: results of a prescription-event monitoring study. *Osteoporos Int* 2004; **15**.

46 Nickelsen T, Lufkin E, Riggs B, Cox D, Crook T. Raloxifene hydrochloride, a selective estrogen receptor modulator: safety assessment of effects on cognitive function and mood in postmenopausal women. *Psychoneuroendocrinology* 1999; **24**: 115–28.

47 Grady D, Ettinger B, Moscarelli E *et al.* Safety and adverse effects associated with raloxifene: multiple outcomes of raloxifene evaluation. *Obstet Gynecol* 2004; **104**: 837–44.

48 Palacios S, Farias M, Luebbert H *et al.* Raloxifene is not associated with biologically relevant changes in hot flushes in postmenopausal women for whom therapy is appropriate. *Am J Obstet Gynecol* 2004; **191**: 121–31.

49 Aldrighi J, Quail D, Levy-Frebault J *et al.* Predictors of hot flushes in postmenopausal women who receive raloxifene therapy. *Am J Obstet Gynecol* 2004; **191**: 1979–88.

50 Seagger R, Howell J, David H, Gregg-Smith S. Prevention of secondary osteoporotic fractures – why are we ignoring the evidence? *Injury* 2004; **35**: 986–8.

51 Davenport G, Committee. PCRSS. Rheumatology and musculoskeletal medicine. *Br J Gen Pract* 2004; **54**: 457–64.

52 Dolan P, Torgerson D. The cost of treating osteoporotic fractures in the United Kingdom female population. *Osteoporos Int* 1998; **8**: 611–7.

53 Kanis J, Borgstrom F, Johnell O *et al.* Cost-effectiveness of raloxifene in the UK: an economic evaluation based on the MORE study. *Osteoporos Int* 2005; **16**: 15–25.

Acknowledgements

Figure 2 is adapted from Meunier *et al.,* 1999.[21]
Figure 3 is adapted from Ettinger *et al.,* 1999.[22]
Figure 4 is adapted from Delmas *et al.,* 2002.[23]
Figure 5 is adapted from Cauley *et al.,* 2001.[28]
Figure 6 is adapted from Grady *et al.,* 2004.[47]

5. Drug review – Risedronate (Actonel®)

Dr Eleanor Bull
CSF Medical Communications Ltd

Summary

Risedronate, a nitrogen-containing bisphosphonate, is indicated for the treatment and prevention of osteoporosis in postmenopausal women and in patients undergoing systemic glucocorticoid treatment for chronic inflammatory diseases. Localised to the bone following administration, risedronate targets the osteoclasts responsible for bone resorption and thereby normalises the bone remodelling process which is disrupted in osteoporosis. Consequently, risedronate increases or maintains bone mineral density (BMD) and reduces the incidence of vertebral and non-vertebral fractures in a clinical setting. In order to maximise bioavailability following oral administration, risedronate should be administered before food and following a period of fasting, with patients remaining upright for up to 30 minutes post-dosing. Failure to comply with dosage instructions may result in limited efficacy and an increased risk of side-effects. Risedronate is generally well tolerated with an adverse event profile resembling that of placebo. In contrast to some bisphosphonates, risedronate has a low propensity for causing gastrointestinal irritation, which, coupled with its minimal drug interaction profile, may further promote patient concordance.

Introduction

Since hormone replacement therapy (HRT) for osteoporosis is no longer recommended as a result of its association with an increased risk of heart disease and breast cancer, the bisphosphonates have become the first-line treatment option for this debilitating condition. In contrast to HRT, the bisphosphonates (e.g. cyclic etidronate, alendronate, ibandronate, pamidronate, risedronate, zolendronate) have a bone-specific mechanism of action – the inhibition of osteoclast-mediated bone resorption – and minimal associated side-effects.[1]

In contrast
to HRT, the
bisphosphonates
have a
bone-specific
mechanism of
action – the
inhibition of
osteoclast-
mediated bone
resorption –
and minimal
associated
side-effects.

The bisphosphonates were first developed as stable analogues of pyrophosphate, an endogenous inorganic compound with a strong affinity for hydroxyapatite crystals in bone.[2] Unlike pyrophosphate, bisphosphonates are resistant to hydrolysis and can thus be administered orally. Etidronate – the first bisphosphonate to be developed for the treatment of osteoporosis – was found to interfere with bone mineralisation at clinical doses and was therefore administered cyclically. The second-generation agents, alendronate and pamidronate, were 10–100-fold more potent than etidronate and exerted no detrimental effects on mineralisation. Potency was further enhanced through the incorporation of a tertiary nitrogen atom within the heterocyclic ring, a structure on which ibandronate, zolendronate and risedronate are based.[3] Risedronate is indicated for the prevention and treatment of postmenopausal and glucocorticoid-induced osteoporosis and may reduce the incidence of vertebral, non-vertebral and hip fracture.[3] This article reviews the pharmacological properties of risedronate and its efficacy in controlled clinical trials in the context of other available treatments for osteoporosis.

Pharmacology

Chemistry

The chemistry of
risedronate is of
essentially academic
interest and most
healthcare
professionals will, like
you, skip this section.

The chemical structure of risedronate, a nitrogen-containing bisphosphonate, is illustrated in Figure 1.[4] The P–C–P structure of the bisphosphonate group confers a high affinity for bone.[2] The antiresorptive potency of risedronate is thought to derive from the nitrogen-containing cyclic functional group attached to the main carbon atom of the bisphosphonate molecule.[5] Risedronate is available as 5, 30 and 35 mg film-coated tablets.[4] The recommended dosage regimen for the treatment of osteoporosis is a daily 5 mg or a weekly 35 mg tablet.[4]

Figure 1. The chemical structure of risedronate sodium ($C_7H_{10}NO_7P_2Na.2.5\ H_2O$).[4]

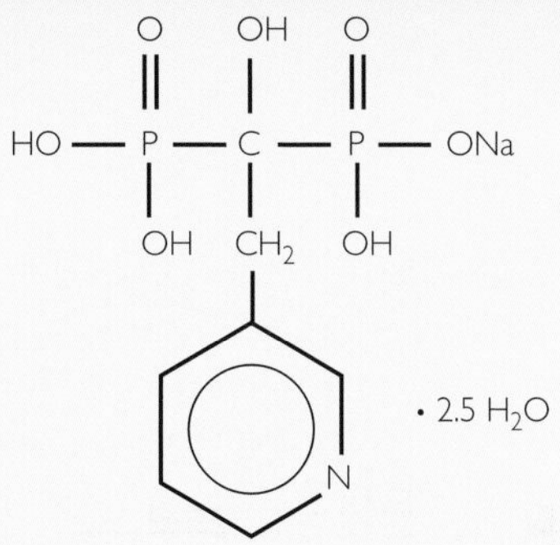

Mechanism of action

Localised to the bone following administration, risedronate targets the osteoclast directly either by increasing apoptosis or by affecting metabolic activity.[2] Following risedronate intervention, osteoclasts adhere normally to the bone surface but show reduced active resorption, evidenced by a lack of a ruffled border.

The farnesyl pyrophosphate synthase enzyme – implicated in the mevalonate pathway responsible for producing cholesterol and isoprenoid lipids – has been proposed as the intracellular target of risedronate and other nitrogen-containing bisphosphonates (e.g. alendronate, olpadronate and ibandronate).[6] The bisphosphonates inhibit this enzyme with an order of potency of zoledronic acid≈ minodronate> risedronate> ibandronate> incadronate> alendronate> pamidronate.[7] Subtle differences in the structure of the R^2 side chain are thought to account for the differing potencies of these compounds.[7]

> Localised to the bone following administration, risedronate targets the osteoclast directly either by increasing apoptosis or by affecting metabolic activity.

In vitro activity

The apoptotic effect of risedronate has been demonstrated *in vitro* using murine osteoclasts.[8] Risedronate, pamidronate and clodronate induced a 4–24-fold dose-dependent increase in the proportion of osteoclasts displaying the characteristic morphology of apoptosis, with risedronate showing the greatest potency (Figure 2).[8] This effect has been confirmed *in vivo* in normal mice, mice with increased bone resorption and in nude mice with osteolytic cancer metastases.[8]

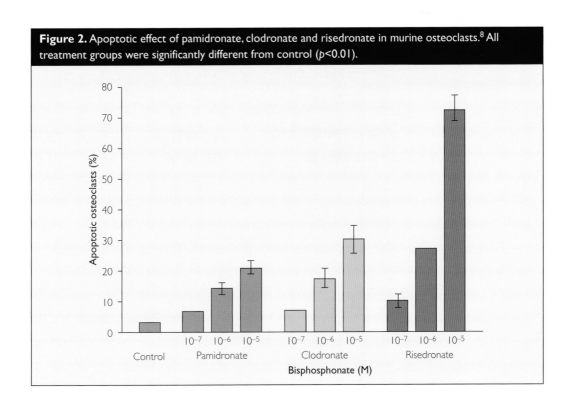

Figure 2. Apoptotic effect of pamidronate, clodronate and risedronate in murine osteoclasts.[8] All treatment groups were significantly different from control ($p<0.01$).

More recent evidence has suggested that risedronate may suppress bone resorption independently of its apoptotic effects, after dose–response studies showed that bone resorption was inhibited at doses 10-fold lower than those required to reduce the number of osteoclasts.[9]

In vivo *activity*

Risedronate treatment preserves trabecular architecture in ovariectomised rats and minipigs, common animal models used to study postmenopausal states.

The three-dimensional connectivity of vertebral cancellous bone from ovariectomised rats was significantly increased following risedronate treatment, 5 μg/kg daily – 1 week on, 3 weeks off – for a period of 1 year, compared with sham-operated and ovariectomised control rats.[10] Oestrogen, 10 μg/kg for 5 days of every week, maintained connectivity and cancellous bone volume at the level of the sham-operated rat. The authors proposed that the increase in connectivity following risedronate treatment reflected a combination of altered resorptive cell recruitment and function in the growing rat skeleton.

The effect of risedronate on trabecular architecture and bone mass was determined in ovariectomised minipigs given 18 months' risedronate treatment, 0.5 or 2.5 mg/kg/day.[11] Vertebral bone volume was higher following both doses of risedronate compared with control animals ($p<0.05$). These changes were most significant in the 2.5 mg group and more prevalent in the cranial-caudal ends compared with the midsection of the bone. Additionally, trabecular thickness, trabecular number and connectivity were greater with the higher dosage of risedronate ($p<0.05$).

Potential for gastric damage

Gastrointestinal disturbances are the most common adverse events associated with the bisphosphonates as a drug class. Rarely, ulcers of the oesophagus, stomach and small intestine may occur. The propensity for risedronate to elicit gastric damage has been evaluated in a number of rat models.[12–14]

Fasted, indometacin-treated rats received an oral dose of risedronate, pamidronate or alendronate at 150 or 300 mg/kg.[12] The gastric damage elicited by these compounds was in the order of pamidronate> alendronate> risedronate, which was in agreement with a separate study.[13] The degree of gastric damage was highly correlated with the pH of the dosing solution and was more pronounced at higher pH values.[12] When administered to rats at 5–150-times the recommended clinical dosage, risedronate, alendronate and etidronate elicited equivalent levels of gastric irritation as evaluated from gross and microscopic examination of multiple sections of the stomach. However, the gastric irritation potential was evident only at doses much higher than the clinical dose.[14]

The gastric irritation potential of risedronate was evident only at doses much higher than the clinical dose.

Pharmacokinetics

The pharmacokinetic properties of risedronate are presented in Table 1.[4,5,15] The absorption of risedronate is relatively rapid (t_{max} ~1 hour) and occurs throughout the upper gastrointestinal tract. Over the dose range 2.5–30 mg, the rate and extent of absorption is linear and independent of the site and rate of administration.[15,16] The absolute bioavailability of orally administered risedronate is ~0.6%, a value comparable with that of the other bisphosphonates, and is independent of formulation.[17] Risedronate is excreted unchanged primarily via the kidney.[4] Since it is not metabolised, risedronate does not induce or inhibit hepatic cytochrome P450 (CYP) enzymes.[4,18] Consequently, the potential for clinically significant drug–drug interactions is low (although no formal drug interaction studies have been performed), and risedronate can be administered with a large number of concomitant medications, with the exception of those containing polyvalent cations, which may otherwise interfere with absorption.

The pharmacokinetic profile of risedronate is not significantly altered in patients with mild-to-moderate renal impairment (creatinine clearance >20 mL/min) and no dosage adjustment is necessary in this patient population.[19] Risedronate is not recommended in patients with severe renal impairment (creatinine clearance <30 mL/min) owing to a lack of clinical experience in this population.[4] However, one study based on phase 3 clinical trial experience has suggested that renal function-related adverse events and creatinine clearance is unaffected by risedronate in patients with mild-to-severe renal impairment.[20] Dosage adjustment is not necessary in patients with hepatic impairment or in the elderly.[4] Risedronate has not been studied in patients under 18 years of age.[4]

☛ *The pharmacokinetics of a drug are of interest to healthcare professionals because it is important for them to understand the action of a drug on the body over a period of time.*

Table 1. The pharmacokinetic properties of risedronate administered as a single oral dose (2.5–30 mg).[4,5,15]

Pharmacokinetic parameter	
Absolute oral bioavailability (%)	0.63
t_{max} (hours)	~1
C_{max} (µg/L)	0.41–5.1
Plasma protein binding (%)	24
$t_{1/2}$ (hours)	480
Plasma clearance (mL/min)	122
Steady state volume of distribution (L/kg)	6.3
AUC (µg.L/hour)	1 hour before food – 10.44 4 hours before food – 15.28
Excretion	87% in urine

AUC, area under the concentration–time curve; t_{max}, time to reach maximum drug plasma concentration (C_{max}); $t_{1/2}$, elimination half-life.

Effect of food on absorption

As a drug class, the bisphosphonates exhibit characteristically low bioavailability following oral administration.[21] Absorption is significantly inhibited by food and so dosing instructions recommend that dosing should take place at least 30 minutes before food and following an overnight fast, or at another time during the day at the midpoint of a 4-hour fast.[4] Patients should take risedronate with a glass of plain water and remain upright for at least 30 minutes after dosing.[4]

In a dose-timing study, risedronate, 30 mg, was administered to volunteers at varying time points either preceding or following a meal.[21] The rate of absorption of risedronate was greater before than after a meal. When administered 1 or 4 hours in advance of a meal, absorption was increased by up to 2.3-fold. In general, the administration profile of risedronate permits a certain degree of flexibility and may help patients to achieve efficacy whilst maintaining their daily routine.[21] The once-weekly dosage also provides further flexibility.

Clinical efficacy

Placebo-controlled trials

The placebo-controlled trials assessing the effectiveness of risedronate in postmenopausal women with, or at risk of, osteoporosis are summarised in Table 2.[22–30] Clinical trials focused on the effect of risedronate on BMD and/or the incidence or risk of vertebral and non-vertebral (e.g. hip) fractures. Risedronate was taken with plain water, at least 30–60 minutes before the first meal of the day or 2 hours before going to bed and at least 2 hours after the last meal of the day. Patients were instructed to remain upright for up to 30 minutes after administration. Unless stated otherwise, patients received calcium and/or vitamin D supplements in addition to risedronate treatment.

The Vertebral Efficacy with Risedronate Therapy (VERT) trials, conducted both in North America and internationally, examined the effect of risedronate on the risk of fracture in postmenopausal women (Table 2).[25,26] The North American arm of the study incorporated 2,458 ambulatory postmenopausal women younger than 85 years with at least one vertebral fracture at baseline.[25] Patients received a daily dose of 2.5 or 5 mg risedronate or placebo for a period of 3 years, although the 2.5 mg treatment group was discontinued after 1 year as the 5 mg dose produced a more consistent effect on BMD whilst exhibiting a similar tolerability profile. Supplementary calcium and vitamin D were available if baseline levels were low. Over a 3-year period, a daily dose of 5 mg risedronate reduced the cumulative incidence of new vertebral fractures by 41% (p=0.003 vs placebo). The vertebral fracture reduction over the first year was 65% (p<0.001 vs placebo). The incidence of non-vertebral fractures was reduced by 39% following the 5 mg dose of risedronate (p=0.02 vs placebo). After 3 years of risedronate treatment, BMD was increased at the lumbar spine (5.4 vs 1.1% following placebo), femoral neck (1.6 vs –1.2%), femoral trochanter (3.3 vs

The rate of absorption of risedronate is greater before than after a meal.

Over a 3-year period, a daily dose of 5 mg risedronate reduced the cumulative incidence of new vertebral fractures by 41%. The fracture reduction over the first year was 65%.

Table 2. Summary of placebo-controlled trials with risedronate.[22–30]

Study	Design	Patient group	Dosage regimen	Main outcomes
Clemmesen et al., 1997[22]	Double-blind Multicentre 2 years' treatment 1-year follow-up	Postmenopausal women n=132	Continuous (2.5 mg daily) or cyclic (2.5 mg daily) for 2 weeks then 10 weeks' placebo Calcium supplements	• Lumbar spine BMD increased by 1.7% (NS) and 2.3% ($p<0.05$) after 2 and 3 years of cyclic risedronate, respectively. • After 3 years, differences in BMD between groups were significant ($p<0.01$). • Minor changes in markers of bone turnover. • No difference in fracture risk between groups.
Mortensen et al., 1998[23]	Double-blind Multicentre 2 years' treatment 1-year follow-up	Postmenopausal women n=111	Continuous, 5 mg daily, or cyclic, 5 mg daily, for 2 weeks then 2 weeks' placebo	• After 2 years, lumbar spine BMD altered by +1.4, –1.6 and –4.3% for daily, cyclic and placebo groups, respectively ($p<0.05$ vs placebo for both risedronate groups). • After 2 years, trochanter bone mass at hip increased by 5.4 and 3.3% for daily and cyclic groups vs placebo. • During follow-up, bone turnover increased towards baseline for both risedronate groups.
Fogelman et al., 2000[24]	Double-blind Multicentre 24 months	Postmenopausal women n=543	2.5 or 5 mg daily Calcium supplements	• At 24 months, lumbar spine BMD increased from baseline by 4 and 1.4% for 5 and 2.5 mg risedronate. No change following placebo ($p<0.001$ for risedronate, 5 mg, vs placebo). • Femoral neck and trochanter BMD increased following 5 mg risedronate and decreased in placebo group after 24 months. • BMD increases observed after 6 months following 5 mg risedronate. • Adverse event profile similar to placebo.

BMD, bone mineral density; BSAP, bone-specific alkaline phosphatase; MS/BS, mineralising surface as a percentage of bone surface; NS, non-significant; OS/BS, osteoid surface as a percentage of bone surface; VERT–MN, Vertebral Efficacy with Risedronate Therapy–Multinational; VERT–NA, Vertebral Efficacy with Risedronate Therapy–North America.

Table 2. Continued

Study	Design	Patient group	Dosage regimen	Main outcomes
Harris et al., 1999[25] VERT-NA	Double-blind Multicentre 3 years	Ambulatory postmenopausal women n=2,458	2.5[a] or 5 mg daily Calcium and vitamin D supplements	• Risk of new vertebral fractures reduced by 41% over 3 years (5 mg; p=0.003). • Vertebral fracture reduction 65% over 1 year (5 mg; p<0.001). • Non-vertebral fracture risk reduced by 39% over 3 years (5 mg; p=0.02). • BMD increased vs placebo at lumbar spine (5.4 vs 1.1%; p<0.05) and femoral trochanter (3.3 vs –0.7%; p<0.05). • Adverse event profile similar to placebo.
Reginster et al., 2000[26] VERT-MN	Double-blind Multicentre 3 years	Postmenopausal women n=1,226	2.5[b] or 5 mg daily Calcium and vitamin D supplements	• Risk of new vertebral fractures reduced by 49% over 3 years (5 mg; p<0.001). • Vertebral fracture reduction 61% over 1 year (5 mg; p=0.001). • Non-vertebral fracture risk reduced by 33% over 3 years (5 mg; p=0.06). • BMD increased at spine and hip within 6 months vs placebo (p<0.001). • Adverse event profile similar to placebo.
Sorensen et al., 2003[27] VERT-MN	2-year extension of VERT-MN	Postmenopausal women n=265	5 mg daily Calcium and vitamin D	• Risk of new vertebral fracture reduced by 59% in years 4 and 5 (p=0.01). • Mean increase in BMD over 5 years of supplements 9.3% (p<0.001 vs placebo).

[a]Treatment group discontinued after 1 year by protocol amendment.
[b]Treatment group discontinued after 2 years by protocol amendment.
BMD, bone mineral density; BSAP, bone-specific alkaline phosphatase; MS/BS, mineralising surface as a percentage of bone surface; NS, non-significant; OS/BS, osteoid surface as a percentage of bone surface; VERT–MN, Vertebral Efficacy with Risedronate Therapy–Multinational; VERT–NA, Vertebral Efficacy with Risedronate Therapy–North America.

Table 2. Continued

Study	Design	Patient group	Dosage regimen	Main outcomes
Ste-Marie et al., 2004[28] VERT-NA	2-year extension of Harris et al., 1999[25]	Postmenopausal women n=86	5 mg daily Calcium and vitamin D supplements	• OS/BS and MS/BS[c] were reduced from baseline by the greatest extent in placebo-treated patients (–5.4 vs –2.8% and –5.1 vs –2.8% for placebo and risedronate, respectively; $p=0.03$ and $p=0.01$). • Lumbar spine BMD increased by 9.2% following risedronate treatment compared with a 0.26% decrease in the placebo group ($p<0.05$).
Mellstrom et al., 2004[29] VERT-MN	4-year extension of Reginster et al., 2000[26]	Postmenopausal women n=164	5 mg daily Calcium and vitamin D supplements	• The incidence of new vertebral fracture during years 6–7 did not change significantly from that reported during years 4–5 (3.8 vs 5.2%, respectively; p-value not reported). • Lumbar spine BMD increased from baseline by 11.5% following 7 years of risedronate treatment ($p<0.05$ vs placebo).
McClung et al., 2001[30]	Double-blind Multinational 3 years	Postmenopausal women with osteoporosis (n=5,445) or at risk of hip fracture (n=3,886)	2.5 or 5 mg daily Calcium and vitamin D supplements	• Overall incidence of hip fracture 2.9% following risedronate vs 3.9% following placebo ($p=0.02$). • Incidence of vertebral fracture 8.4% following risedronate vs 10.7% following placebo in osteoporotic women ($p=0.03$).

[c]Bone formation parameters.
BMD, bone mineral density; BSAP, bone-specific alkaline phosphatase; MS/BS, mineralising surface as a percentage of bone surface; NS, non-significant; OS/BS, osteoid surface as a percentage of bone surface; VERT–MN, Vertebral Efficacy with Risedronate Therapy–Multinational; VERT–NA, Vertebral Efficacy with Risedronate Therapy–North America.

–0.7%), and the midshaft of the radius (0.2 vs –1.4%). The adverse event profile of risedronate was similar to that of placebo.

The multinational study adopted an identical treatment regimen, although the 2.5 mg risedronate group was discontinued after 2 years.[26] The patient population included 1,226 postmenopausal women with two or more prevalent vertebral fractures. Similar to the North American study, after 3 years of risedronate, 5 mg daily, the risk of new vertebral fractures was reduced by 49% ($p<0.001$; Figure 3). Over the first year

Figure 3. Incidence of new vertebral (top) and non-vertebral (bottom) osteoporosis-related fractures in patients receiving risedronate (2.5 or 5 mg) or placebo.[26]

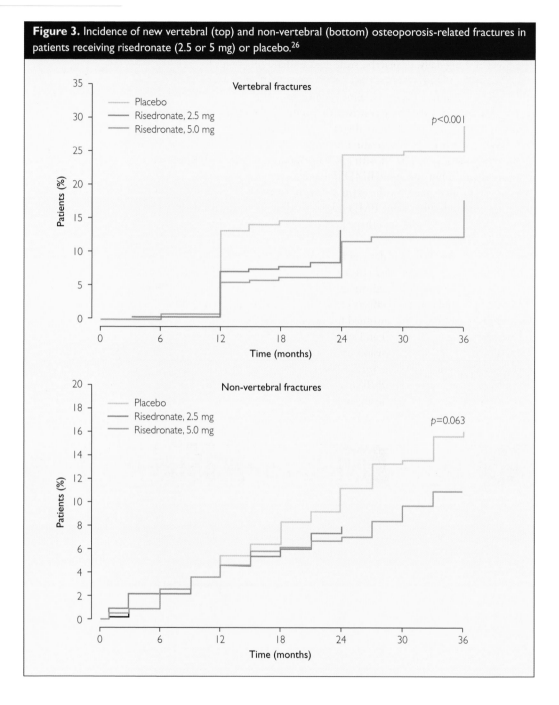

the fracture reduction was 61% (*p*=0.001). The 2.5 mg dosage of risedronate elicited a similar fracture reduction to the 5 mg dosage over 2 years. The risk of non-vertebral fractures was reduced by 33% over 3 years (*p*=0.06; Figure 3) and BMD at the spine and hip was significantly increased within 6 months of treatment initiation. Again, the side-effects associated with risedronate treatment resembled those encountered with placebo.

In a 2-year extension of the multinational VERT study, 265 women from the original study were selected to receive an additional 2 years of risedronate, 5 mg daily, or placebo treatment under double-blind conditions.[26,27] Patients were at least 5 years postmenopausal with at least two vertebral fractures at baseline. The fracture results obtained after 5 years of treatment were consistent with those obtained from the original 3-year study. Risedronate therapy was associated with a reduction in the risk of new vertebral fractures of 59% in years 4 and 5 ($p=0.01$ vs placebo), compared with a 49% reduction in years 1–3. The improvements in hip and spine BMD initiated over years 1–3 were maintained or increased over the extra 2 years of treatment. Overall, the mean increase in lumbar spine BMD due to risedronate treatment over 5 years was 9.3% ($p<0.001$), perhaps justifying long-term risedronate treatment (Figure 4).

Further extension studies derived from the original VERT-NA and VERT-MN trials have provided efficacy data for up to 7 years of continuous treatment with risedronate.[28,29] Analysis of these data has confirmed that the beneficial effects of risedronate are maintained in the long-term, suggesting that continued treatment for up to 7 years leads to further improvement in BMD and sustained vertebral fracture risk reduction (Table 2). One extension used, amongst others, mineralising surface as a percentage of bone surface (MS/BS) and osteoid surface as a proportion of bone surface (OS/BS), as markers of bone formation.[28] It was revealed that the changes associated with long-term risedronate

> Risedronate therapy was associated with a reduction in the risk of new vertebral fractures of 59% in years 4 and 5, compared with a 49% reduction in years 1–3.

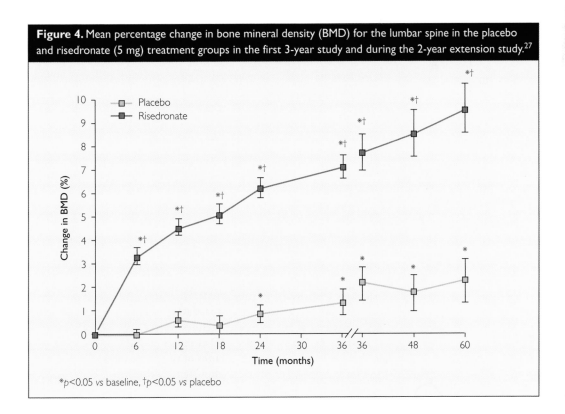

Figure 4. Mean percentage change in bone mineral density (BMD) for the lumbar spine in the placebo and risedronate (5 mg) treatment groups in the first 3-year study and during the 2-year extension study.[27]

*$p<0.05$ vs baseline, †$p<0.05$ vs placebo

treatment were consistent with the reduction in bone turnover observed at the bone-tissue level. No osteoid accumulation was found and mineralisation parameters remained within the normal range.[28]

Analyses are available relating to the short-term effects of risedronate on both vertebral and non-vertebral fracture risk over a 6-month period. Data derived from 2,442 postmenopausal women enrolled in the VERT trials, showed that within 6 months of initiating risedronate treatment, 5 mg daily, the relative risk of sustaining a vertebral fracture was 0.08.[31] By 9 months the relative risk was 0.16 (*p*=0.001 *vs* placebo). The risk of non-vertebral fracture was examined using data extrapolated from four clinical trials in 1172 women with postmenopausal osteoporosis.[24–26,30] Within 6 months, risedronate-treated patients experienced a 66% reduction in the risk of non-vertebral fracture compared with those patients receiving placebo (*p*=0.048).[32]

A further subset of patients from the VERT trials (n=693) was used to investigate the role of early decreases in bone resorption in the antifracture effects of risedronate.[33] Patients were screened for markers of bone resorption, including the urinary C- and N-telopeptides of type 1 collagen (CTX and NTX). The reductions in urinary CTX and NTX detected at 3–6 months of risedronate treatment (60 and 51%, respectively) correlated positively with the reduction in vertebral fracture risk (75% over 1 year and 50% over 3 years; *p*<0.05). This may signify that a large proportion of the reduction in fracture risk following risedronate is directly attributable to decreased bone resorption. The authors indicated that the relationship did not appear to be linear, as no contribution to fracture risk reduction was observed after a threshold of 40–60%.

The effect of risedronate on the risk of hip fracture was investigated in a large multinational study in 5,545 women with osteoporosis aged 70–79 years and 3,886 women aged over 80 years with at least one non-skeletal risk factor for hip fracture.[30] The entry criteria for the study was a T-score of –4 or –3 with a non-skeletal risk factor for hip fracture. All patients received risedronate, 2.5 or 5 mg daily, or placebo for 3 years, with supplemental calcium carbonate and vitamin D, if serum vitamin D levels at screening were below 16 ng/mL. Overall, the incidence of hip fracture in those women treated with risedronate was 2.9% compared with 3.9% in the placebo group (relative risk 0.7; *p*=0.02). In the 70–79 years age group, the incidence of fracture was 1.9% following risedronate, compared with 3.2% following placebo (relative risk 0.6; *p*=0.009). In the over 80 years age group, risedronate had no effect on the incidence of hip fracture (*p*=0.37). The rate of vertebral fracture was 8.4% in risedronate-treated patients compared with 10.7% in the placebo group (relative risk 0.8; *p*=0.03). These data suggest that risedronate reduces the risk of hip fracture in elderly women with osteoporosis but not in elderly women selected primarily on the basis of risk factors other than low BMD.

Meta-analyses

A meta-analysis of eight randomised, placebo-controlled trials in postmenopausal women receiving risedronate, examined the overall effect of the drug on the relative risk of vertebral and non-vertebral fractures.[22–26,30,34,35] The pooled relative risk of fracture in women receiving a daily dose of at least 2.5 mg risedronate was 0.64 and 0.73, for vertebral and non-vertebral fractures, respectively.[36] Additionally, risedronate exerted a positive effect on BMD changes in the lumbar spine and femoral neck, which was generally larger following a 5 mg dose than a 2.5 mg or cyclical dosage regimen. The percentage change in BMD between 5 mg risedronate and placebo after up to 3 years of treatment was 4.54% for the lumbar spine and 2.75% for the femoral neck.[36] These data show that risedronate is effective, in terms of reducing vertebral and non-vertebral fracture risk and increasing BMD, when administered to both early postmenopausal women and women with established bone loss.

The relationship between risedronate-induced changes in BMD and vertebral fracture risk was examined in a meta-analysis of data pooled from three double-blind, fracture endpoint trials of risedronate, of which two were the VERT-NA and VERT-MN studies described previously (Table 2).[25,26,37] In all studies, postmenopausal women (n=3,224) received up to 3 years of treatment with either risedronate (2.5 or 5 mg/day) or placebo. Overall, risedronate-treated patients whose lumbar spine BMD decreased over 3 years, were at a significantly increased risk of sustaining a vertebral fracture than those patients whose BMD increased (p=0.003). The risk of fracture was similar amongst risedronate-treated patients who experienced BMD increases of less than or more than 5% from baseline (relative risk 0.51 and 0.59; p=0.003 and p=0.008 for <5% and ≥5%, respectively), demonstrating that the magnitude of risedronate-induced increases in BMD has no significant bearing on the risk of vertebral fracture.

A recently published analysis looked at the effect of patients' age on the outcome of risedronate therapy.[38] Data derived from patients enrolled in three double-blind, fracture endpoint trials of risedronate, of which two were the VERT-NA and VERT-MN studies, were stratified according to age, creating a subgroup of 1,392 women aged 80 years or older.[38] After 1 year, the incidence of new vertebral fracture amongst these patients was 10.9 and 2.5% for placebo and risedronate, respectively, a risk reduction of 81% (p<0.001). At 3 years, the fracture risk reduction associated with risedronate treatment had decreased to 44%, but remained significant (p=0.003). Risedronate was well tolerated in this patient population and the proportion of patients withdrawing due to an adverse event was comparable between placebo and risedronate treatment groups (20.3 vs 20.6%, respectively; p=0.947). These data confirm that risedronate effectively reduced the risk of new vertebral fracture risk over 1 and 3 years in a subgroup of elderly women aged over 80 years.

Risedronate is effective, in terms of reducing fracture risk and increasing BMD, when administered to both early postmenopausal women and women with established bone loss.

Risedronate effectively reduced the risk of new vertebral fracture risk over 1 and 3 years in a subgroup of elderly women aged 80 years or older.

Once-weekly formulation

A 2-year, double-blind study in 1,456 postmenopausal women compared the once-daily and once-weekly risedronate treatment regimens.[39] All patients were aged over 50 years and had been postmenopausal for over
5 years with a lumbar spine or proximal femur T-score of –2.5 or lower. Risedronate was either administered as 5 mg daily, or as 35 or 50 mg weekly doses. All subjects also received 1 g calcium daily and supplemental vitamin D if baseline serum levels were low. After 12 months of treatment the percentage change in BMD at the lumbar spine was comparable between treatment groups (4.0, 3.9 and 4.2% for 5, 35 and 50 mg groups, respectively). Tolerability was again similar between groups, which lends credence to the weekly administration of 35 mg as the preferred treatment regimen.

Two-year data from this study concur with the 1-year results by demonstrating the clinical equivalence of the once-weekly and once-daily doses of risedronate.[40] Of the 1,456 women originally randomised to the various treatment groups, 77% completed the 2-year study, compared with the 83% of participants who completed 12 months. The incidence of new vertebral fractures was similar amongst all treatment groups (2.9, 1.5 and 1.7% for the 5 mg daily, 35 mg weekly and 50 mg weekly groups, respectively; $p=0.298$ between group comparison). After 24 months, the respective mean percentage changes in bone-specific alkaline phosphatase (BSAP) were 30.5, 29.9 and 37.5% for the 5 mg daily, 35 mg weekly and 50 mg weekly groups, respectively ($p>0.05$ between groups). In agreement with the 1-year data, which demonstrated non-inferiority of the weekly regimen compared with daily dosing, the mean percentage increases in lumbar spine BMD after 24 months were 5.17, 4.74 and 5.47%, respectively ($p>0.05$ between groups). The incidence of osteoporosis-related non-vertebral fractures reported as adverse events was comparable between treatment groups (5.0, 4.9 and 4.5%, respectively; $p=0.918$). The frequency of upper gastrointestinal adverse events was also similar between groups (22.7, 25.6 and 24.8%, respectively; $p=0.559$). Thus, these data confirm that the efficacy and safety of once-weekly risedronate are clinically equivalent to the once-daily treatment regimen.

The 35 mg weekly dose of risedronate was further examined in an analysis of the vertebral fracture risk over a 1-year period.[41] This study used matched historical controls to assess the relative efficacy of risedronate, which were generated by matching baseline characteristics of placebo-treated patients from the VERT trials to those of risedronate-treated patients in the current study. In those patients receiving the once-weekly 35 mg dose of risedronate (n=485), the risk of new vertebral fracture was reduced by 77% relative to the historical placebo group ($p=0.018$). This reduction was comparable with that reported following risedronate, 5 mg daily, in the VERT trials, which ranged between 61 and 65%. Over 2 years, the new vertebral fracture risk reduction following weekly administration of risedronate (n=403) was 87% compared with that reported in matched historical controls.[42]

The efficacy and safety of once-weekly risedronate are clinically equivalent to the once-daily treatment regimen.

Comparative trials

In order to make direct comparisons between antiresorptive agents and to evaluate relative antifracture efficacies, a well-designed randomised controlled clinical trial is needed. The first trial to compare the BMD-building and bone turnover marker (BTM)-reducing properties of risedronate with those of alendronate was conducted over 12 months in 549 postmenopausal women over 60 years of age.[43] The dosage regimens selected were judged to be the most convenient available at the time of the study. Risedronate was administered as 5 mg daily and was taken 2 hours after the main meal of the day in the upright position and at least 2 hours prior to the next food or beverage. In contrast, alendronate was administered as a 70 mg weekly dosage and was taken, in the upright position, in the fasted state upon rising for the day. The mean reduction in urine NTX corrected for creatinine level was greater in alendronate- than risedronate-treated patients (–52 vs –32%; p<0.001). After 6 months of treatment, alendronate elicited a greater increase in BMD than risedronate which was maintained at 12 months (4.8 vs 2.8% at the lumbar spine and 2.7 vs 0.9% at the hip for alendronate and risedronate, respectively; p<0.001). Both compounds were well tolerated and resembled placebo in terms of their adverse event profiles. However, in view of the between-meal dosage regimen employed for risedronate and not alendronate, it has been suggested that these data reflect differences in bioavailability rather than BMD build and BTM reduction. Additionally, as stated in the literature, caution is advocated when interpreting BMD-build and BTM-reduction data, which may not be linearly proportional to the fracture risk reduction.[33,44]

A recently published double-blind comparison of alendronate and risedronate has attempted to eliminate such bias by using the approved dose of each drug and employed standard morning oral dosing.[45] A group of 1,053 postmenopausal women with low BMD (≥2.0 SD below normal mean bone mass) received either risedronate (35 mg) or alendronate (50 mg) once weekly over a 12-month period. The rate of study completion was similar between treatment groups (85.2 vs 84.2% for risedronate and alendronate, respectively; p-value not reported). In general, treatment-associated increases in BMD were significantly greater amongst alendronate- than risedronate-treated patients. For example, the increases in BMD at the hip trochanter at 12 months were 3.4 and 2.1% for alendronate and risedronate, respectively (p<0.001). The increases in BMD at the total hip, femoral neck and lumbar spine followed a similar trend, with 12-month treatment differences of 1.1, 0.7 and 1.2%, respectively (p≤0.005), such that alendronate was associated with significantly greater gains in BMD than risedronate at all sites measured. The proportion of patients who showed at least a 3% increase in hip trochanter BMD at 12 months was significantly greater in the alendronate treatment group (51.1 vs 40.7%, respectively; p=0.002), a pattern also observed for lumbar spine BMD measurements. Urinary NTX was decreased by a greater extent in alendronate-treated patients over the course of the investigation (–52.8 vs –40.3%, respectively; p<0.001). Serum levels of NTX and BSAP were similarly affected at

> Alendronate was associated with significantly greater gains in BMD than risedronate at all sites measured.

12 months (–73.8 vs –54.7% and –40.6 *vs* –28.1% for alendronate and risedronate, respectively; $p<0.001$ for both comparisons). Both treatments were well tolerated, with upper gastrointestinal adverse events reported by 22.5 and 20.1% of alendronate- and risedronate-treated patients, respectively ($p=0.364$). Whether these treatment-related differences in markers of bone turnover and BMD translate into a reduced risk of fracture, remains to be confirmed in randomised controlled trials.

Glucocorticoid-induced osteoporosis

In light of the association between sustained glucocorticoid treatment and osteoporosis, the efficacy of risedronate has been extensively evaluated in this subgroup of patients.[46–48]

In a multicentre, double-blind study, 224 men and women who were initiating long-term glucocorticoid treatment, received risedronate, 2.5 or 5 mg daily, or placebo for 12 months.[46] Patients were receiving moderate-to-high doses of prednisolone or equivalent (>7.5 mg mean daily dose) for diseases which included rheumatoid arthritis, polymyalgia rheumatica, vasculitis and asthma. As shown in Figure 5, after 12 months, BMD at the lumbar spine was maintained in both risedronate groups but decreased from baseline in the placebo group (–0.1, 0.6 and –2.8% for 2.5, 5 mg and placebo, respectively; $p<0.05$ *vs* baseline). The differences in BMD between the 5 mg dose of risedronate and placebo were 3.8% at the lumbar spine ($p<0.001$), 4.1% at the femoral neck ($p<0.001$) and 4.6% at the femoral trochanter ($p<0.001$). There was a trend towards a decrease in the rate of vertebral fracture in the 5 mg risedronate group compared with placebo (5.7 *vs* 17.3%, a 71% reduction; $p=0.072$). The adverse event profile was comparable in all three treatment groups.

A group of men and women (n=290) having received high-dose oral glucocorticoid treatment for 6 months or more were selected for a year-long, placebo-controlled trial of risedronate, 2.5 or 5 mg daily.[47] All patients also received a daily dose of 1 g calcium and 400 IU of vitamin D. After 12 months of treatment, BMD in the lumbar spine (2.9%; $p<0.001$), femoral neck (1.8%; $p=0.004$) and trochanter (2.4%; $p=0.01$) were all significantly increased following risedronate treatment compared with placebo-treated patients, in whom BMD was maintained. Furthermore, up to a 70% reduction in the incidence of vertebral fractures was reported in the combined risedronate group relative to placebo ($p=0.042$).

The effect of risedronate, 2.5 or 5 mg daily, or placebo, was examined in a pooled analysis of the two previously mentioned studies, which included a total of 518 men and women who were receiving moderate-to-high doses of glucocorticoids for underlying diseases including rheumatoid arthritis and pulmonary conditions.[48] All patients received daily calcium supplementation, 500–1000 mg, and most received vitamin D, 400 IU. Following 12 months of treatment, BMD at the lumbar spine was increased by 1.9% from baseline in the 5 mg

Figure 5. Mean percentage change from baseline in bone mineral density (BMD) at the lumbar spine, femoral neck and femoral trochanter in patients treated with glucocorticoids and risedronate (2.5 or 5 mg) or placebo.[46]

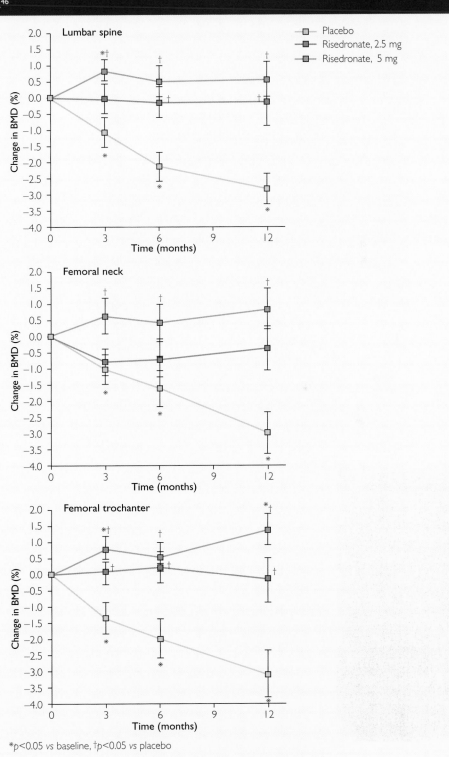

*p<0.05 vs baseline, †p<0.05 vs placebo

risedronate group ($p<0.001$) and decreased by 1% in the placebo group ($p=0.005$). BMD in the trochanter, femoral neck and radius was either maintained or increased following 5 mg risedronate but was reduced in the placebo group ($p<0.05$ at all skeletal sites). The 2.5 mg dose of risedronate had a positive effect on BMD although this was less pronounced than that observed with the 5 mg dose. There was a 70% reduction in the risk of vertebral fracture associated with risedronate (5 mg) after 12 months compared with placebo ($p=0.01$). Risedronate was equipotent in men and women irrespective of underlying disease status and duration of glucocorticoid therapy.

Glucocorticoid-treated patients with rheumatoid arthritis

The antiosteoporotic properties of risedronate were examined in a placebo-controlled study conducted in 120 postmenopausal women with rheumatoid arthritis, requiring long-term prednisolone treatment at a daily dose of at least 2.5 mg.[49] Patients received risedronate, 2.5 mg daily, or 15 mg cyclically for 2 weeks of every 12, for 96 weeks and were followed for a further year after treatment cessation. At 97 weeks, BMD was maintained in the daily risedronate group and reduced in the placebo group (1.4 *vs* –1.6% at the lumbar spine and 0.4 *vs* –4.0% at the trochanter for risedronate and placebo, respectively; $p=0.03$ and $p<0.005$). Overall, daily risedronate therapy was superior to placebo at the lumbar spine ($p=0.009$) and trochanter ($p=0.02$) but did not reach significance in the femoral neck. The overall effect of cyclical risedronate was similar to that of daily risedronate and was superior to placebo. The withdrawal of treatment led to significant bone loss at the lumbar spine in both risedronate groups. Adverse events were similar across all three treatment groups.

Safety and tolerability

Data derived from clinical trials show that, in general, risedronate is well tolerated and adverse events do not represent a significant factor governing treatment discontinuation. The most common side-effects associated with risedronate treatment are infection, back pain, gastrointestinal symptoms and arthralgia (Table 3).[4] The high-profile VERT clinical trials, which included a total of 3684 postmenopausal women, reported a similar incidence of side-effects between risedronate and placebo treatment groups. In addition, these trials did not exclude patients with a history of active gastrointestinal disease or concomitant use of non-steroidal anti-inflammatory drugs (NSAIDs).

Gastrointestinal effects

The bisphosphonates in general have attracted concerns related to their gastrointestinal effects, the most common of which is abdominal pain. Although the gastrointestinal disturbances associated with risedronate

Table 3. Adverse events reported during placebo-controlled clinical trials in at least 2% of patients receiving risedronate.[4]

Adverse event	Incidence of adverse event (%)	
	Placebo (n=1,914)	Risedronate (n=1,916)
Infection	29.7	29.9
Back pain	23.6	26.1
Pain	13.1	13.6
Abdominal pain	9.4	11.6
Hypertension	9.0	10.0
Nausea	10.7	10.9
Diarrhoea	9.6	10.6
Arthralgia	21.1	23.7
Joint disorder	5.4	6.8
Myalgia	6.3	6.6
Depression	6.2	6.8
Dizziness	5.4	6.4
Insomnia	4.5	4.7
Pharyngitis	5.0	5.8
Rash	7.2	7.7
Cataract	5.4	5.9
Urinary tract infection	9.7	10.9

appear to be minimal, adherence to the dosage instructions further limits adverse events.[50] The gastrointestinal toxicity potential of risedronate has been compared with that of alendronate and aspirin, which are strongly associated with gastrointestinal injury.[51,52]

A placebo-controlled study examined the extent of gastrointestinal toxicity following risedronate, alendronate and aspirin in 235 healthy volunteers.[52] Subjects, which included men and postmenopausal women aged 45–80 years in good general health with normal upper-gastrointestinal endoscopy, received a daily dose of risedronate, 30 mg, alendronate, 40 mg, or placebo for a period of 28 days, with aspirin administered at 650 mg four-times daily for the last 7 days. Risedronate and alendronate exhibited comparable mean gastric and duodenal erosion scores which were significantly lower than those for the aspirin group (0.73, 0.89, 3.07 and 0.31 for risedronate, alendronate, aspirin and placebo, respectively; $p<0.001$ for all groups *vs* aspirin [Figure 6]). Oesophageal erosion scores were similar for all treatment groups. The incidence of gastric ulcers and/or large numbers of gastric erosions was

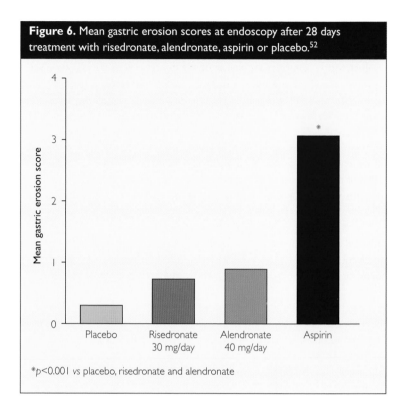

Figure 6. Mean gastric erosion scores at endoscopy after 28 days treatment with risedronate, alendronate, aspirin or placebo.[52]

*p<0.001 vs placebo, risedronate and alendronate

3% for both risedronate and alendronate compared with 60% in aspirin-treated subjects.

A similar trial conducted in 515 postmenopausal women in good general health with normal upper-gastrointestinal endoscopy, compared the gastrointestinal effects of risedronate, 5 mg, and alendronate, 10 mg, administered over a 2-week period.[51] Overall, gastric ulcers were detected in 4.1% of risedronate- and 13.2% of alendronate-treated subjects (p<0.001). At day 15, mean gastric endoscopy scores were significantly lower following risedronate than alendronate (0.91 vs 1.56; p<0.001), although mean oesophageal and duodenal scores were similar between groups.

A pooled analysis of gastrointestinal safety data accumulated from nine double-blind, placebo-controlled clinical trials of risedronate incorporated 10,068 men and women who had received either risedronate, 5 mg daily, or placebo for up to 3 years.[53] Of those patients having received risedronate, 29.8% experienced gastrointestinal disturbances, compared with 29.6% of placebo-treated patients. The concomitant use of NSAIDs or active pre-existing gastrointestinal tract disease had no effect on the frequency of upper-gastrointestinal tract adverse events in either risedronate- or placebo-treated patients.

> Of those patients having received risedronate, 29.8% experienced gastrointestinal disturbances, compared with 29.6% of placebo-treated patients.

Clinical practice

A UK-based questionnaire study of 219 patients receiving risedronate evaluated the adverse event profile of the drug.[54] Although patients were given detailed oral and written instruction on how to take risedronate, one-in-four patients were non-compliant with the dosage regimen. The study concluded that those patients who did not remain upright after taking risedronate were more likely to experience an adverse event. Adverse events were experienced by 38% of patients, the most common of which were gastrointestinal, occurring in 21% of patients. In total, 19% of patients stopped treatment due to adverse events. One-third of patients with an adverse event attempted a rechallenge with risedronate which was successful in 50% of patients.

A retrospective cohort analysis used women in a US-managed medical and pharmacy claims database (Protocare Sciences), to evaluate the frequency of gastrointestinal events following risedronate or alendronate treatment.[55] Of the 5,169 women assessed, 802 were receiving daily doses of risedronate and 4,367 were receiving either daily or weekly alendronate. The study found that alendronate-treated patients had a 42% higher risk of experiencing a gastrointestinal event during the first 4 months of therapy, compared with risedronate-treated patients (p=0.016). This figure takes into account adjustment for age and gastrointestinal-related events in the 6 months prior to initiating treatment.

> Those patients who did not remain upright after taking risedronate were more likely to experience an adverse event.

Pharmacoeconomics

The cost-effectiveness of risedronate for the treatment of osteoporosis has been analysed using a Markov simulation model.[56] The patients analysed were females aged approximately 75 years and at high risk of sustaining a hip fracture. Treating a cohort of 1,000 women with risedronate for the duration of their expected lifetimes resulted in net savings of £786,000. Over a period of 3 years, the net increment of quality-adjusted life-years (QALYs) was 16 per 1,000 women treated, with a cost per QALY of £8,625 per woman treated. In short, risedronate treatment resulted in an improvement in quality of life with possible cost savings when administered to elderly women at high risk of hip fracture.

A meta-analysis of a number of large double-blind trials examined the cost-effectiveness of risedronate in postmenopausal women, using a Markov model applied to a UK setting.[57] Over a period of 5 years, intervention with risedronate was shown to be cost-effective in women with established vertebral osteoporosis aged 60 years and over. The only group of women for whom treatment with risedronate was not cost-effective was those with no prior vertebral fractures and with a BMD T-score at the threshold for osteoporosis (–2.5 SD).

Key points

- Risedronate is a nitrogen-containing bisphosphonate currently indicated for the prevention and treatment of osteoporosis.

- An inhibitor of bone resorption, risedronate targets the osteoclast directly and either increases apoptosis or alters metabolic activity.

- In order to maximise bioavailability, risedronate should be administered before food and after a period of fasting, and patients should remain upright for up to 30 minutes following administration.

- Risedronate is not metabolised and thus can be administered in combination with a large number of other medications without complication.

- When administered to postmenopausal women with, or at risk of, osteoporosis, risedronate reduces the incidence of vertebral and non-vertebral hip fractures and increases or maintains bone mineral density.

- The clinical benefits associated with risedronate are first observed following 6 months of treatment initiation and are sustained over a 7-year treatment period.

- A once-weekly dosage regimen may represent a viable alternative to daily dosing and demonstrates similar clinical efficacy.

- Risedronate is well tolerated with an adverse event profile similar to placebo and has a low propensity for eliciting gastrointestinal side-effects.

References

A list of the published evidence which has been reviewed in compiling the preceding section of *BESTMEDICINE*.

1   Compston J, Rosen C. Fast Facts – Osteoporosis. 3rd ed. Oxford: Health Press, 2002.

2   Catterall J, Cawston T. Drugs in development: bisphosphonates and metalloproteinase inhibitors. *Arthritis Res Ther* 2003; **5**: 12–24.

3   Crandall C. Risedronate: a clinical review. *Arch Intern Med* 2001; **161**: 353–60.

4   Proctor and Gamble Pharmaceuticals UK Limited. Actonel® (risedronate sodium tablets). *Summary of product characteristics*. Egham, Surrey, 2003.

5   Dunn CJ, Goa KL. Risedronate: a review of its pharmacological properties and clinical use in resorptive bone disease. *Drugs* 2001; **61**: 685–712.

6   van Beek E, Pieterman E, Cohen L, Lowik C, Papapoulos S. Farnesyl pyrophosphate synthase is the molecular target of nitrogen-containing bisphosphonates. *Biochem Biophys Res Commun* 1999; **264**: 108–11.

7   Dunford J, Thompson K, Coxon F *et al.* Structure-activity relationships for inhibition of farnesyl diphosphate synthase *in vitro* and inhibition of bone resorption *in vivo* by nitrogen-containing bisphosphonates. *J Pharmacol Exp Ther* 2001; **296**: 235–42.

8   Hughes DE, Wright KR, Uy HL *et al.* Bisphosphonates promote apoptosis in murine osteoclasts *in vitro* and *in vivo*. *J Bone Miner Res* 1995; **10**: 1478–87.

9   Halasy-Nagy JM, Rodan GA, Reszka AA. Inhibition of bone resorption by alendronate and risedronate does not require osteoclast apoptosis. *Bone* 2001; **29**: 553–9.

10 Boyce RW, Wronski TJ, Ebert DC *et al.* Direct stereological estimation of three-dimensional connectivity in rat vertebrae: effect of estrogen, etidronate and risedronate following ovariectomy. *Bone* 1995; **16**: 209–13.

11 Borah B, Dufresne TE, Chmielewski PA *et al.* Risedronate preserves trabecular architecture and increases bone strength in vertebra of ovariectomized minipigs as measured by three-dimensional microcomputed tomography. *J Bone Miner Res* 2002; **17**: 1139–47.

12 Blank MA, Gibson GW, Myers WR *et al.* Gastric damage in the rat with nitrogen-containing bisphosphonates depends on pH. *Aliment Pharmacol Ther* 2000; **14**: 1215–23.

13 Lichtenberger LM, Romero JJ, Gibson GW, Blank MA. Effect of bisphosphonates on surface hydrophobicity and phosphatidylcholine concentration of rodent gastric mucosa. *Dig Dis Sci* 2000; **45**: 1792–801.

14 Peter CP, Kindt MV, Majka JA. Comparative study of potential for bisphosphonates to damage gastric mucosa of rats. *Dig Dis Sci* 1998; **43**: 1009–15.

15 Mitchell DY, Eusebio RA, Sacco-Gibson NA *et al.* Dose-proportional pharmacokinetics of risedronate on single-dose oral administration to healthy volunteers. *J Clin Pharmacol* 2000; **40**: 258–65.

16 Mitchell DY, Eusebio RA, Dunlap LE *et al.* Risedronate gastrointestinal absorption is independent of site and rate of administration. *Pharm Res* 1998; **15**: 228–32.

17 Mitchell DY, Barr WH, Eusebio RA *et al.* Risedronate pharmacokinetics and intra- and inter-subject variability upon single-dose intravenous and oral administration. *Pharm Res* 2001; **18**: 166–70.

18 Smith BJ, Hu JK, Schwecke WP. Evaluation of the effects of risedronate on hepatic microsomal drug metabolizing enzyme activities following administration to rats for 14 days: lack of an induction response. *Drug Chem Toxicol* 1998; **21**: 291–303.

19 Mitchell DY, St Peter JV, Eusebio RA *et al.* Effect of renal function on risedronate pharmacokinetics after a single oral dose. *Br J Clin Pharmacol* 2000; **49**: 215–22.

20 Miller P, Barton I, Dunlap L, Burgio D. Risedronate treated patients with reduced renal function show no significant increase in renal function-related AEs as compared to placebo. *J Bone Miner Res* 2003; **18**: S262–SU345.

21 Mitchell DY, Heise MA, Pallone KA *et al.* The effect of dosing regimen on the pharmacokinetics of risedronate. *Br J Clin Pharmacol* 1999; **48**: 536–42.

22 Clemmesen B, Ravn P, Zegels B *et al.* A 2-year phase II study with 1 year of follow-up of risedronate (NE-58095) in postmenopausal osteoporosis. *Osteoporos Int* 1997; **7**: 488–95.

23 Mortensen L, Charles P, Bekker PJ, Digennaro J, Johnston CC. Risedronate increases bone mass in an early postmenopausal population: two years of treatment plus one year of follow-up. *J Clin Endocrinol Metab* 1998; **83**: 396–402.

24 Fogelman I, Ribot C, Smith R *et al.* Risedronate reverses bone loss in postmenopausal women with low bone mass: results from a multinational, double-blind, placebo-controlled trial. BMD-MN Study Group. *J Clin Endocrinol Metab* 2000; **85**: 1895–900.

25 Harris ST, Watts NB, Genant HK *et al.* Effects of risedronate treatment on vertebral and nonvertebral fractures in women with postmenopausal osteoporosis: a randomized controlled trial. Vertebral Efficacy With Risedronate Therapy (VERT) Study Group. *JAMA* 1999; **282**: 1344–52.

26 Reginster J, Minne HW, Sorensen OH *et al.* Randomized trial of the effects of risedronate on vertebral fractures in women with established postmenopausal osteoporosis. Vertebral Efficacy with Risedronate Therapy (VERT) Study Group. *Osteoporos Int* 2000; **11**: 83–91.

27 Sorensen OH, Crawford GM, Mulder H *et al*. Long-term efficacy of risedronate: a 5-year placebo-controlled clinical experience. *Bone* 2003; **32**: 120–6.

28 Ste-Marie L, Sod E, Johnson T, Chines A. Five years of treatment with risedronate and its effects on bone safety in women with postmenopausal osteoporosis. *Calcif Tissue Int* 2004; **75**: 469–76.

29 Mellstrom D, Sorensen O, Goemaere S *et al*. Seven years of treatment with risedronate in women with postmenopausal osteoporosis. *Calcif Tissue Int* 2004; **75**: 462–8.

30 McClung MR, Geusens P, Miller PD *et al*. Effect of risedronate on the risk of hip fracture in elderly women. Hip Intervention Program Study Group. *N Engl J Med* 2001; **344**: 333–40.

31 Roux C, Seeman E, Eastell R *et al*. Efficacy of risedronate on clinical vertebral fractures within six months. *Curr Med Res Opin* 2004; **20**: 433–9.

32 Harrington JT, Ste-Marie LG, Brandi ML *et al*. Risedronate rapidly reduces the risk for nonvertebral fractures in women with postmenopausal osteoporosis. *Calcif Tissue Int* 2004; **74**: 129–35.

33 Eastell R, Barton I, Hannon RA *et al*. Relationship of early changes in bone resorption to the reduction in fracture risk with risedronate. *J Bone Miner Res* 2003; **18**: 1051–6.

34 McClung M, Bensen W, Bolognese M *et al*. Risedronate increases bone mineral density at the hip, spine and radius in postmenopausal women with low bone mass. *Osteoporos Int* 1998; **8**: 111 (Abstract).

35 Hooper M, Ebeling P, Roberts A *et al*. Risedronate prevents bone loss in early postmenopausal women. 26th European Symposium on Calcified Tissues 1999; Abstract.

36 Cranney A, Tugwell P, Adachi J *et al*. Meta-analyses of therapies for postmenopausal osteoporosis. III. Meta-analysis of risedronate for the treatment of postmenopausal osteoporosis. *Endocr Rev* 2002; **23**: 517–23.

37 Watts N, Cooper C, Lindsay R *et al*. Relationship between changes in bone mineral density and vertebral fracture risk associated with risedronate: greater increases in bone mineral density do not relate to greater decreases in fracture risk. *J Clin Densitom* 2004; **7**: 255–61.

38 Boonen S, McClung M, Eastell R *et al*. Safety and efficacy of risedronate in reducing fracture risk in osteoporotic women aged 80 and older: implications for the use of antiresorptive agents in the old and oldest old. *J Am Geriatr Soc* 2004; **52**: 1832–9.

39 Brown JP, Kendler DL, McClung MR *et al*. The efficacy and tolerability of risedronate once a week for the treatment of postmenopausal osteoporosis. *Calcif Tissue Int* 2002; **71**: 103–11.

40 Harris S, Watts N, Li Z *et al*. Two-year efficacy and tolerability of risedronate once a week for the treatment of women with postmenopausal osteoporosis. *Curr Med Res Opin* 2004; **20**: 757–64.

41 Watts NB, Lindsay R, Li Z, Kasibhatla C, Brown J. Use of matched historical controls to evaluate the anti-fracture efficacy of once-a-week risedronate. *Osteoporos Int* 2003; **14**: 437–41.

42 Watts N, Lindsay R, Li Z, Kasibhatla C, Brown J. Two year vertebral fracture risk reduction with risedronate 35 mg once-a-week. *Calcif Tissue Int* 2003; **72**: P193.

43 Hosking D, Adami S, Felsenberg D *et al*. Comparison of change in bone resorption and bone mineral density with once-weekly alendronate and daily risedronate: a randomised, placebo-controlled study. *Curr Med Res Opin* 2003; **19**: 383–94.

44 Delmas P, Li Z, Cooper C. Relationship between changes in bone mineral density and fracture risk reduction with antiresorptive drugs: some issues with meta-analyses. *J Bone Min Res* 2004; **19**: 330–7.

45 Rosen C, Hochberg M, Bonnick S *et al*. Treatment with once-weekly alendronate 70 mg compared with once-weekly risedronate 35 mg in women with postmenopausal osteoporosis: a randomized double-blind study. *J Bone Min Res* 2005; **20**: 141–51.

46 Cohen S, Levy RM, Keller M *et al*. Risedronate therapy prevents corticosteroid-induced bone loss: a twelve-month, multicenter, randomized, double-blind, placebo-controlled, parallel-group study. *Arthritis Rheum* 1999; **42**: 2309–18.

47 Reid DM, Hughes RA, Laan RF *et al*. Efficacy and safety of daily risedronate in the treatment of corticosteroid-induced osteoporosis in men and women: a randomized trial. European Corticosteroid-Induced Osteoporosis Treatment Study. *J Bone Miner Res* 2000; **15**: 1006–13.

48 Wallach S, Cohen S, Reid DM *et al*. Effects of risedronate treatment on bone density and vertebral fracture in patients on corticosteroid therapy. *Calcif Tissue Int* 2000; **67**: 277–85.

49 Eastell R, Devogelaer JP, Peel NF *et al*. Prevention of bone loss with risedronate in glucocorticoid-treated rheumatoid arthritis patients. *Osteoporos Int* 2000; **11**: 331–7.

50 Kherani RB, Papaioannou A, Adachi JD. Long-term tolerability of the bisphosphonates in postmenopausal osteoporosis: a comparative review. *Drug Saf* 2002; **25**: 781–90.

51 Lanza FL, Hunt RH, Thomson AB, Provenza JM, Blank MA. Endoscopic comparison of esophageal and gastroduodenal effects of risedronate and alendronate in postmenopausal women. *Gastroenterology* 2000; **119**: 631–8.

52 Lanza F, Schwartz H, Sahba B *et al*. An endoscopic comparison of the effects of alendronate and risedronate on upper gastrointestinal mucosae. *Am J Gastroenterol* 2000; **95**: 3112–17.

53 Taggart H, Bolognese MA, Lindsay R *et al*. Upper gastrointestinal tract safety of risedronate: a pooled analysis of 9 clinical trials. *Mayo Clin Proc* 2002; **77**: 262–70.

54 Hamilton B, McCoy K, Taggart H. Tolerability and compliance with risedronate in clinical practice. *Osteoporos Int* 2003; **14**: 259–62.

55 Worley K, Doyle J, Sheer R *et al*. Incidence of gastrointestinal events among women treated with bisphosphonates for osteoporosis. *Osteoporos Int* 2003; **14**: P293.

56 Iglesias CP, Torgerson DJ, Bearne A, Bose U. The cost utility of bisphosphonate treatment in established osteoporosis. *QJM* 2002; **95**: 305–11.

57 Kanis J, Borgstrom F, Johnell O, Jonsson B. Cost-effectiveness of risedronate for the treatment of osteoporosis and prevention of fractures in postmenopausal women. *Osteoporos Int* 2004; **15**: 862–71.

Acknowledgements

Figure 2 is adapted from Hughes *et al.*, 1995.[8]

Figure 3 is adapted from Reginster *et al.*, 2000.[26]

Figure 4 is adapted from Sorensen *et al.*, 2003.[27]

Figure 5 is adapted from Cohen *et al.*, 1999.[46]

Figure 6 is adapted from Lanza *et al.*, 2000.[52]

6. Drug review – Strontium ranelate (Protelos®)

Dr Eleanor Bull
CSF Medical Communications Ltd

Summary

Strontium ranelate is indicated for the treatment of osteoporosis in postmenopausal women to reduce the risk of vertebral and hip fractures. The effects of strontium ranelate on bone closely resemble those of calcium, with which it shares a chemical group. Unlike other agents commonly used in the management of osteoporosis, strontium ranelate stimulates the formation of new bone tissue, as well as reducing bone resorption. In this manner it redresses the bone remodelling process to favour bone formation. Formed by combining two stable strontium atoms with an organic moiety (ranelic acid), strontium ranelate localises almost exclusively to bone tissue following oral administration. Strontium ranelate prevents bone loss in ovariectomised rats, increases bone mass in osteopenic animals and increases bone strength in normal animals. Although relatively sparse, clinical studies conducted in postmenopausal women have revealed a dose-dependent increase in bone mineral density (BMD) of the lumbar spine and hip following up to 3 years of treatment. In women with osteoporosis, the risk of both vertebral and non-vertebral fracture was reduced by long-term treatment with strontium ranelate, with effects first evident after 1 year and sustained over 3 years. Data derived from clinical studies have shown strontium ranelate to be well tolerated, with an adverse event profile similar to that of placebo.

Introduction

Whilst effective in the treatment of postmenopausal osteoporosis, the antiresorptive therapies in common use today (e.g. alendronate, calcitonin, risedronate, raloxifene), alter the rate of bone remodelling and lower the risk of fracture, but do not address the reduction in bone formation that occurs within months of treatment initiation.[1] Ideally, an antiosteoporotic agent would have the ability both to decrease bone

Ideally, an anti-osteoporotic agent would have the ability both to decrease bone resorption and to maintain a relatively high rate of bone formation.

resorption and to maintain a relatively high rate of bone formation, uncoupling the bone remodelling process in a favourable manner. By directly stimulating bone formation, anabolic agents (e.g. growth hormone, insulin-like growth factor-I [IGF-I]), parathyroid hormone and strontium), may have greater potential than the antiresorptive compounds to increase bone mass and to decrease fractures.[2] It also follows that combinations of antiresorptive and anabolic agents have the potential to offer greater therapeutic benefits than those of either agent given alone.

Strontium ranelate, a compound consisting of two atoms of stable strontium and one molecule of ranelic acid, is emerging as a promising new drug for the treatment of postmenopausal osteoporosis.[3] Indeed, the beneficial effects of low-dose stable strontium in osteoporosis were first reported more than 50 years ago.[4] Strontium, an alkaline earth metal from the same chemical group as calcium, displays a great affinity for bone and following administration is almost exclusively deposited in the skeleton.[5] When used clinically, strontium ranelate exerts unique pharmacological effects on bone and bone cells, reducing bone resorption whilst maintaining or promoting bone formation.

Strontium ranelate is licensed for the treatment of postmenopausal osteoporosis to reduce the risk of vertebral and hip fractures. This current review discusses the pharmacological properties of strontium ranelate and its efficacy in controlled clinical trials in postmenopausal women with osteoporosis.

> Strontium displays a great affinity for bone and following administration is almost exclusively deposited in the skeleton.

Pharmacology

Mechanism of action

Strontium ranelate has a pharmacologically unique mechanism of action. In simple terms, it rebalances the bone turnover process in favour of bone formation. Experiments performed *in vitro* have shown strontium ranelate to increase bone formation by increasing osteoblast precursor replication and collagen synthesis, and to reduce bone resorption by decreasing osteoclast differentiation and resorbing activity (Figure 1).[3,6] Several of the actions of strontium on osteoclasts and osteoblasts closely resemble those of calcium, which are mediated by the extracellular calcium-sensing receptor.[7] This has prompted speculation that strontium ranelate may act as an agonist at the extracellular calcium-sensing receptor (or at an alternative cation-sensing receptor) in osteoblasts.[7]

> ☞ The chemistry of strontium ranelate is of essentially academic interest and most healthcare professionals will, like you, skip this section.

In vivo studies

A number of studies conducted in ovariectomised rats (which show an accelerated rate of bone resorption), immobilised rats (which show an increased rate of bone resorption in response to reduced bone formation) and intact rats, mice and monkeys, have further confirmed the antiresorptive and bone-stimulating actions of strontium ranelate, as summarised below.[8–12]

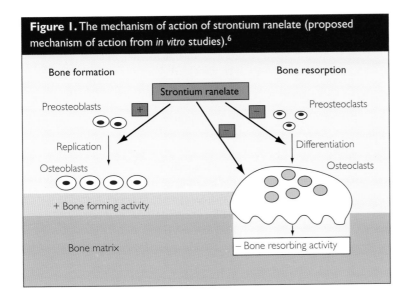

Figure 1. The mechanism of action of strontium ranelate (proposed mechanism of action from *in vitro* studies).[6]

- The treatment of ovariectomised rats with strontium ranelate (77, 154 or 308 mg/kg/day) for 8 weeks inhibited trabecular bone loss induced by oestrogen deficiency, without inhibiting bone formation.[8]

- In a rat model of osteopenia, induced by immobilising rats with a hind limb plaster cast, 10 days' treatment with strontium ranelate (50, 200 or 800 mg/kg/day) abolished the increased bone resorption and partially prevented trabecular bone loss in the immobilised limb.[9] Immobilised rats also showed increased serum alkaline phosphatase activity and decreased urinary hydroxyproline excretion, which suggests that bone resorption was reduced whilst bone formation was maintained.[9]

- Intact rats, having undergone long-term treatment with strontium ranelate (225–900 mg/kg/day) over a period of 2 years, showed increased bone mass in the lumbar vertebrae and femur, and increased trabecular bone volume in the tibial metaphysic.[10]

- In intact mice, exposed to strontium ranelate (200, 600 or 1800 mg/kg/day) for 2 years, vertebral bone mass was increased by 36 and 56% in male and female animals, respectively (*p*-value not reported).[11]

- Intact adult monkeys, aged 3–4 years, treated with strontium ranelate (100, 275 or 750 mg/kg/day) for 6 months, showed reductions in histomorphometric indices of bone resorption (i.e. osteoclast surface and number) with no adverse effects on bone mineralisation (as measured by mineral apposition rate and osteoid thickness).[12]

To summarise, strontium ranelate prevents bone loss in ovariectomised rats, increases bone mass in osteopenic animals and increases bone strength in normal animals. Consequently, strontium ranelate has been described as an uncoupling agent that separates bone

Strontium ranelate prevents bone loss in ovariectomised rats, increases bone mass in osteopenic animals and increases bone strength in normal animals.

resorption from bone formation, reducing bone resorption whilst maintaining bone formation. This results in net bone gain and may also improve bone microarchitecture and thus bone strength.[13]

Pharmacokinetics

The pharmacokinetics of a drug are of interest to healthcare professionals because it is important for them to understand the action of a drug on the body over a period of time.

The pharmacokinetic properties of strontium ranelate are summarised in Table 1.[3] Strontium ranelate shows characteristically low absorption, distribution and plasma protein binding following oral administration, and is rapidly eliminated via the kidneys and the gastrointestinal tract as the unchanged compound, with no evidence of metabolism in either animals or humans.[3] Steady-state concentrations are usually reached after 2 weeks of daily administration and strontium concentrations in bone tend to plateau after approximately 3 years of treatment.[3] Animal studies have shown that strontium levels in bone vary according to anatomical site, duration of treatment, dose and gender, although it is not clear to what extent these findings apply to humans.[14]

Dosing schedule

The bioavailability of strontium ranelate is reduced by up to 60–70% by coadministration with food or milk and its derivative products.

The recommended daily dose of strontium ranelate is 2 g, administered orally. The granules are taken as a suspension in a glass of water, and the manufacturer recommends that the suspension is consumed immediately and not stored for later use.[3] The bioavailability of strontium ranelate is reduced by up to 60–70% when coadministered with food or milk and other dairy products and hence, administration at bedtime, or at least 2 hours after eating, is advocated.[3] It is advisable that patients treated with strontium ranelate take vitamin D and calcium supplements, if their dietary intake is inadequate.[3] Since calcium-containing products may severely limit the bioavailability of strontium ranelate, it is also advisable that calcium supplements are taken at least 2 hours before or after the active drug.

Table 1. The pharmacokinetic properties of strontium ranelate after oral administration of a 2 g dose.[3]

Pharmacokinetic parameter	
Bioavailability (%)	25
t_{max} (hours)	3–5
Protein binding (%)	25
Volume of distribution (L/kg)	1
Plasma clearance (L/minute)	12
Renal clearance (L/minute)	7
$t_{1/2}$ (hours)	60

t_{max}, time to reach maximum drug plasma concentration (C_{max}); $t_{1/2}$, elimination half-life.

Strontium ranelate can be administered to the elderly and to patients with hepatic impairment or with mild-to-moderate renal impairment (30–70 mL/minute creatinine clearance), without the need for dosage adjustment.[3] However, strontium ranelate is not recommended for use by patients with severe renal impairment (below 30 mL/minute creatinine clearance), whilst a lack of efficacy and safety data prohibits its use in children and adolescents.[3]

Clinical efficacy

When assessing the efficacy of strontium ranelate in terms of changes in BMD, it is important to allow for the effect of strontium distribution in bone.[15] When performing dual-energy X-ray absorptiometry (DXA) to determine BMD, any metal with an atomic number greater than that of calcium (Z=20) will attenuate X-rays by a greater extent than calcium, which may in turn lead to an overestimation of BMD.[16] Strontium (Z=38) attenuates more X-rays than calcium and thus measurements of BMD should be adjusted to allow for this.[17] The adjustment factor for *in vivo* measurements in humans, providing the bone strontium content is known, is determined by the cube of the atomic number. A 1% strontium concentration *in vitro* induces a 10% increase in BMD at the iliac crest which is used as a proxy for the vertebral concentration. However, the relationship between bone strontium content at the iliac crest and the hip is unclear.[15]

Dose-ranging studies

The minimal effective dose of strontium ranelate was determined in a group of women with established postmenopausal vertebral osteoporosis. The Strontium Ranelate Treatment of Osteoporosis (STRATOS) study was designed for this purpose and recruited 353 osteoporotic women with at least one previous vertebral fracture and lumbar T-score of less than –2.4, who were at least 12 months postmenopausal.[17] Study participants were randomly allocated to 2 years' double-blind treatment with either placebo or strontium ranelate, 0.5, 1 or 2 g/day. All patients received supplementary calcium (500 mg/day) and vitamin D (800 IU/day) for the duration of the study.

The changes in lumbar spine BMD, before and after adjustment for bone strontium content, are illustrated in Figure 2. Over 2 years of treatment, strontium ranelate elicited dose-dependent increases in BMD in this region, such that the mean annual slopes of the percentage change in adjusted lumbar spine BMD were 0.5, 1.35, 1.65 and 2.97% for placebo, and strontium ranelate, 0.5 g, 1 g and 2 g, respectively ($p<0.01$ for strontium ranelate, 2 g, *vs* placebo). The corresponding mean annual slopes for the change in femoral neck BMD were –0.57, 0.24, 1.41 and 3.05%, respectively ($p<0.01$ for strontium ranelate, 2 g, *vs* placebo). During the second year of treatment, the proportion of strontium ranelate-treated patients who experienced a new vertebral deformity was significantly lower than placebo in both the 0.5 g and 2 g treatment groups (47.3 *vs* 24.2, 40.9 and 26.5% for placebo and

Dose-ranging studies are particularly important to ensure that the optimum dose of a drug can be determined in order that benefit can be realised with the least risk of side-effects.

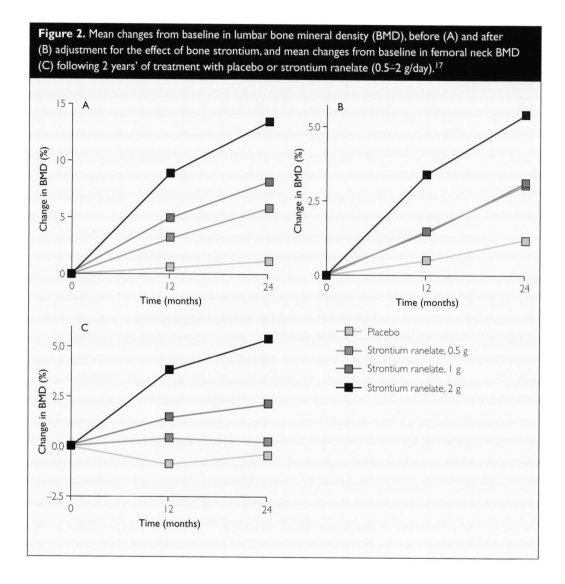

Figure 2. Mean changes from baseline in lumbar bone mineral density (BMD), before (A) and after (B) adjustment for the effect of bone strontium, and mean changes from baseline in femoral neck BMD (C) following 2 years' of treatment with placebo or strontium ranelate (0.5–2 g/day).[17]

strontium ranelate, 0.5 g, 1 g and 2 g, respectively; relative risks of 0.51 and 0.56 for strontium ranelate, 0.5 g and 2 g respectively). The authors reconcile a lack of a clear dose effect on fracture rate with the insufficient power of the study. Whilst the deformity rate in the 1 g strontium ranelate treatment group was maintained at the rate reported during the first year (39.7%), the rate of vertebral deformity increased by 13.6% in the placebo group over the same time period. The fracture rate during the first year of treatment was not affected by any dose of strontium ranelate compared with placebo (33.7, 36.6, 39.7, 29.7% for placebo, 0.5 g, 1 g and 2 g, respectively; $p=0.625$ group effect). The long cycle of bone remodelling may explain why it takes longer than 12 months for an antiosteoporotic effect to emerge, as suggested by the authors.

The urinary excretion of C-terminal telopeptide of type 1 collagen (CTX) decreased significantly relative to placebo over the first 6 months of treatment with strontium ranelate (group effect; $p=0.004$). The largest decreases in this marker of bone resorption occurred in the strontium ranelate, 1 and 2 g treatment groups, reaching 19.2 and 20.2%, respectively, compared with a 1.5% increase following placebo (p-values not reported). The incidence of treatment-emergent adverse events was similar across all treatment groups ($p=0.707$), with back pain, asthenia, nausea and headache amongst the most commonly reported side-effects (back pain was reported by 26.4, 17.6, 16.7 and 18.4% of patients for placebo, 0.5 g, 1 g and 2 g, respectively; p-value not reported).

Thus, in postmenopausal women with established osteoporosis, a 2 g daily dose of strontium ranelate was sufficient to increase vertebral BMD and reduce the incidence of vertebral deformities over a 2-year period.

Phase 3 studies

Two major studies, the Spinal Osteoporosis Therapeutic Intervention (SOTI) and the Treatment of Peripheral Osteoporosis (TROPOS) trials, further investigated the efficacy and tolerability of the 2 g daily dose of strontium ranelate in postmenopausal women with osteoporosis.[16,18] Both studies were carried out simultaneously in the same centres and all participants had previously undergone an open-label run-in period of calcium and vitamin D supplementation (of 2–24 weeks duration) – the Fracture International Run In for Strontium Ranelate Trials (FIRST) – in order to attempt to normalise their calcium and vitamin D status prior to treatment initiation.[19] Figure 3 demonstrates the rationale behind patient recruitment into either the SOTI or TROPOS studies.[19]

The main objective of the SOTI and TROPOS trials was to demonstrate a reduction in the number of postmenopausal women sustaining a new osteoporotic fracture, either vertebral (SOTI) or non-vertebral (TROPOS), following 3 years of continuous treatment with strontium ranelate.

The SOTI study

The SOTI study enrolled 1649 postmenopausal women with osteoporosis and at least one vertebral fracture.[18] Participants were randomised to receive either placebo or strontium ranelate, 2 g/day, over a period of 3 years. Daily calcium (up to 1 g) and vitamin D (400–800 IU) supplements were supplied for up to 24 weeks prior to randomisation, in accordance with the FIRST procedure mentioned previously, and also throughout the double-blind treatment phase. The proportion of patients completing the 3-year follow-up period was similar between the strontium ranelate and placebo treatment groups (87.3 vs 87.4%, respectively; p-value not reported). After 1 year of treatment, the new vertebral fracture rate was significantly lower in the strontium ranelate group than in the placebo group (6.4 vs 12.2%, respectively; relative risk 0.51, number needed to treat [NNT][a] 17; $p<0.001$). Over 3 years, the

In postmenopausal women with established osteoporosis, a 2 g daily dose of strontium ranelate was sufficient to increase vertebral BMD and reduce the incidence of vertebral deformities over a 2-year period.

After 1 year of treatment, the new vertebral fracture rate was significantly lower in the strontium ranelate group than the placebo group.

---

[a]The NNT represents the number of patients needed to be treated with study medication to prevent one vertebral fracture.

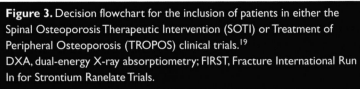

Figure 3. Decision flowchart for the inclusion of patients in either the Spinal Osteoporosis Therapeutic Intervention (SOTI) or Treatment of Peripheral Osteoporosis (TROPOS) clinical trials.[19]
DXA, dual-energy X-ray absorptiometry; FIRST, Fracture International Run In for Strontium Ranelate Trials.

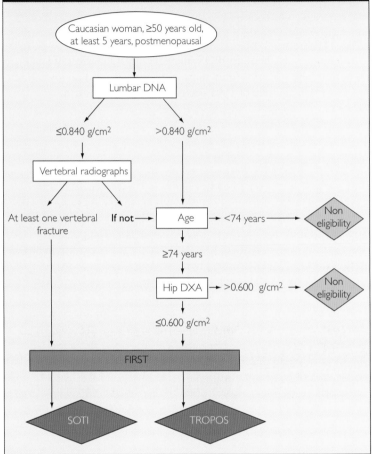

rate of new vertebral fracture was 20.9 and 32.8% for strontium ranelate and placebo, respectively, a risk reduction of 41% in favour of strontium ranelate (relative risk 0.59, NNT 9; $p<0.001$). At 3 years, non-adjusted BMD in the lumbar spine, femoral neck and total hip was increased significantly from baseline following treatment with strontium ranelate (increases of 12.7, 7.2 and 8.6%, respectively; $p<0.001$ *vs* baseline). The 3-year increase in BMD following active treatment was significantly greater than that reported in the placebo treatment group (differences of 14.4, 8.3 and 9.8% for lumbar spine, femoral neck and total hip, respectively; $p<0.001$ *vs* placebo). If lumbar spine BMD is adjusted for bone strontium content, then the difference between strontium ranelate and placebo remains significant (6.8 *vs* 1.3%, respectively; $p<0.001$ *vs* placebo). From 3 months onwards, serum concentrations of bone-specific alkaline phosphatase (BSAP) in the strontium ranelate group were significantly greater and serum CTX levels significantly lower than those recorded in the placebo group (Figure 4; $p \leq 0.05$). The rate and severity of adverse events were similar between treatment groups, although during the first 3 months, diarrhoea was reported significantly more frequently in the strontium ranelate group (6.1 *vs* 3.6% for strontium ranelate and placebo, respectively; $p=0.02$).

The TROPOS study

The recently published TROPOS study examined the effect of long-term treatment with strontium ranelate on vertebral and non-vertebral fracture risk in a group of 5091 postmenopausal women with osteoporosis, although non-vertebral fracture risk was the predetermined main evaluation criterion.[16] It should be noted however, that the study population was heterogeneous and 29.9% of women had a prevalent fragility fracture at baseline. In accordance with the FIRST procedure, participants completed between 2 weeks and 6 months of calcium (up to 1 g) and vitamin D (400–800 IU) supplementation prior to randomisation (which continued throughout the double-blind treatment period). Thereafter, patients were randomly allocated to treatment with either placebo or strontium ranelate, 2 g/day, for a double-blind period of 5 years, although the main findings presented here pertain to data from 3 years after randomisation. Over 3 years, treatment with strontium ranelate was associated with a 16% relative risk reduction in

> Over 3 years, treatment with strontium ranelate was associated with a 16% risk reduction in non-vertebral fractures relative to placebo.

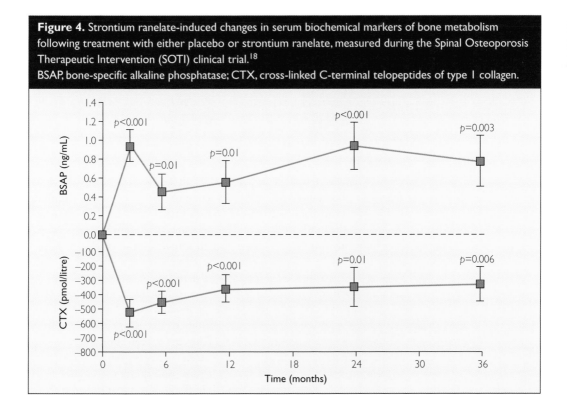

Figure 4. Strontium ranelate-induced changes in serum biochemical markers of bone metabolism following treatment with either placebo or strontium ranelate, measured during the Spinal Osteoporosis Therapeutic Intervention (SOTI) clinical trial.[18]
BSAP, bone-specific alkaline phosphatase; CTX, cross-linked C-terminal telopeptides of type I collagen.

non-vertebral fractures relative to placebo (Figure 5; NNT 55; *p*=0.04). The risk of sustaining a major non-vertebral fragility fracture (i.e. hip, wrist, pelvis, sacrum, ribs) was 19% lower in the strontium ranelate group than in the placebo group (NNT 56; *p*=0.031). In a subgroup of women who were designated as being at high risk of such fractures on account of their age (≥74 years) and femoral neck BMD (T-score: ≤–3 standard deviations from normal; the European reference range), the relative risk of hip fracture was reduced by 36% following treatment with strontium ranelate (NNT 48; *p*=0.046).

Of those patients undergoing annual spinal X-ray (n=3640), the risk of sustaining a new vertebral fracture with strontium ranelate relative to placebo, was reduced by 45% over 1 year and 39% over 3 years (*p*<0.001 for both comparisons). Of those patients with no previous vertebral fracture at baseline (n=2416), the risk of experiencing a first vertebral fracture was reduced by 45% following treatment with strontium ranelate (*p*<0.001).

Long-term treatment with strontium ranelate was associated with a significant increase from baseline in non-adjusted BMD at the femoral neck and total hip (3-year increases of 5.7 and 7.1%, respectively; *p*<0.001 *vs* baseline). At 3 years, the corresponding differences between the strontium ranelate and placebo groups were 8.2 and 9.8% for femoral neck and total hip, respectively (*p*<0.001 for both comparisons *vs* placebo).

The incidence of adverse events was comparable between treatment groups (87.9 *vs* 88.9% for strontium ranelate and placebo, respectively;

> The risk of sustaining a new vertebral fracture was reduced by 45% over 1 year and 39% over 3 years.

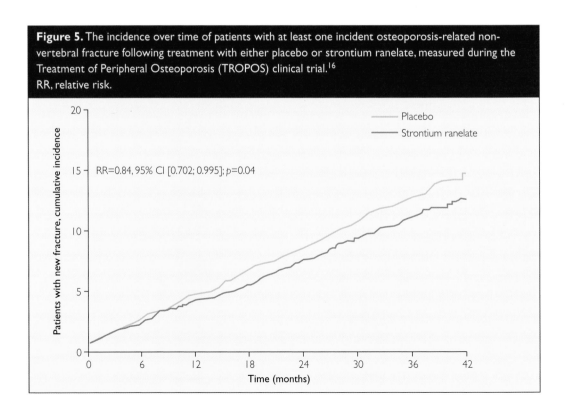

Figure 5. The incidence over time of patients with at least one incident osteoporosis-related non-vertebral fracture following treatment with either placebo or strontium ranelate, measured during the Treatment of Peripheral Osteoporosis (TROPOS) clinical trial.[16]
RR, relative risk.

RR=0.84, 95% CI [0.702; 0.995]; *p*=0.04

Placebo
Strontium ranelate

Patients with new fracture, cumulative incidence

Time (months)

p-value not reported). A similar proportion of strontium ranelate- and placebo-treated patients discontinued treatment as a result of adverse events (24.2 *vs* 21.6%, respectively; *p*-value not reported). The rate of diarrhoea was higher amongst strontium ranelate-treated patients during the first 3 months of treatment, although a lack of statistical analysis prevents comparison with the SOTI study (6.7 *vs* 5.0%, respectively; *p*-value not reported), but this resolved as treatment continued.

Safety and tolerability

Safety data derived from controlled clinical trials performed to date have shown strontium ranelate to be well tolerated, exhibiting a similar adverse event profile to that of placebo. Table 2 shows the adverse events reported most commonly during the phase 3 placebo-controlled clinical trials of strontium ranelate.[3] During the SOTI and TROPOS studies, diarrhoea, nausea, headache and eczema/dermatitis were reported more frequently in the strontium ranelate treatment groups than in placebo group over the first 3 months of administration, although such differences tended to resolve with continued treatment.[16,18]

The manufacturer recommends that strontium ranelate is not given to patients with severe renal impairment, and, in line with good clinical practice, advocates periodic assessment of renal function in patients with chronic renal impairment.[3] Strontium ranelate should be used with caution in patients at increased risk of venous thromboembolism, including patients with a past history of thromboembolic events.[3] The annual incidence of venous thromboembolism reported during phase 3 studies was 0.7% over 4 years, with a relative risk of 1.42 in strontium ranelate- compared with placebo-treated patients.

You are strongly urged to consult your doctor before taking, stopping or changing any of the products reviewed or referred to in *BESTMEDICINE* or any other medication that has been prescribed or recommended by your doctor.

Table 2. The most common[a] adverse events reported during phase 3 clinical trials of strontium ranelate (n=6669).[3]

Adverse event	Frequency (vs placebo)
Nervous system disorders	
Headache	3.0 *vs* 2.4%
Gastrointestinal	
Nausea	6.6 *vs* 4.3%
Diarrhoea	6.5 *vs* 4.6%
Loose stools	1.1 *vs* 0.2%
Skin and subcutaneous tissue disorders	
Dermatitis	2.1 *vs* 1.6%
Eczema	1.5 *vs* 1.2%

[a]Common, >1/100 and <1/10 patients.

Drug interactions

As a divalent cation, strontium ranelate is not metabolised and therefore, the likelihood of clinically relevant drug–drug interactions is limited. To date, no evidence of interaction has been detected with a number of commonly prescribed drugs (e.g. diuretics, non-steroidal anti-inflammatory drugs [NSAIDs], cardiac glycosides, calcium-channel blockers, β-blockers, angiotensin-converting enzyme [ACE] inhibitors and oral anticoagulants).[3]

The coadministration of strontium ranelate with aluminium and magnesium hydroxides decreases its absorption by 20–25%, and it is therefore recommended that these agents are given at least 2 hours after strontium ranelate administration.[3] Strontium ranelate may also form complexes with oral tetracycline and quinolone antibiotics, thereby reducing their absorption, and therefore concomitant administration is not recommended.[3]

Key points

- Strontium ranelate is an antiosteoporotic agent with a unique mechanism of action, and is indicated for the treatment of postmenopausal osteoporosis to reduce the risk of vertebral and hip fractures.

- By promoting bone formation and reducing bone resorption, strontium ranelate uncouples the bone remodelling process in a favourable manner.

- Administered orally, the absorption of strontium ranelate is impeded by coadministration with food and dairy products.

- Compared with placebo, strontium ranelate significantly increases BMD in postmenopausal women with osteoporosis.

- Postmenopausal women with osteoporosis showed reduced risk of vertebral and non-vertebral fracture following 3 years' of continuous treatment with strontium ranelate.

- Strontium ranelate is well tolerated, with an adverse event profile closely resembling that of placebo. Gastrointestinal effects, including diarrhoea, are mild-to-moderate in severity and tend to resolve during the first 3 months of treatment.

- As strontium ranelate is a divalent cation it is not metabolised. Therefore, it has limited potential for interaction with other commonly administered drugs.

References

A list of the published evidence which has been reviewed in compiling the preceding section of *BESTMEDICINE*.

1 Brandi M. New treatment strategies: ipriflavone, strontium, vitamin D metabolites and analogs. *Am J Med* 1993; **95**: S69–74.

2 Rubin M, Bilezikian J. New anabolic therapies in osteoporosis. *Curr Opin Rheumatol* 2002; **14**: 433–40.

3 Servier Laboratories Limited. Protelos®. *Summary of product characteristics.* Slough, 2004.

4 Shorr E, Carter A. The usefulness of strontium as an adjuvant to calcium in the remineralization of the skeleton in humans. *Bull Hosp Joint Dis* 1952; **16**: 59–66.

5 Pors Nielsen S. The biological role of strontium. *Bone* 2004; **35**: 583–8.

6 Marie P. Strontium ranelate: a novel mode of action optimizing bone formation and resorption. *Osteoporos Int* 2004; Epub ahead of print.

7 Brown E. Is the calcium receptor a molecular target for the actions of strontium on bone? *Osteoporos Int* 2003; **14**: S25–34.

8 Marie P, Hott M, Modrowski D *et al.* An uncoupling agent containing strontium prevents bone loss by depressing bone resorption and maintaining bone formation in estrogen-deficient rats. *J Bone Min Res* 1993; **8**: 607–15.

9 Hott M, Deloffre P, Tsouderos Y, Marie P. S12911–2 reduces bone loss induced by short-term immobilization in rats. *Bone* 2003; **33**: 115–23.

10 Ammann P, Shen V, Robin B *et al.* Strontium ranelate improves bone resistance by increasing bone mass and improving architecture in intact female rats. *J Bone Min Res* 2004; **19**: 2012–20.

11 Delannoy P, Bazot D, Marie P. Long-term treatment with strontium ranelate increases vertebral bone mass without deleterious effect in mice. *Metabolism* 2002; **51**: 906–11.

12 Buehler J, Chappuis P, Saffar J, Tsouderos Y, Vignery A. Strontium ranelate inhibits bone resorption while maintaining bone formation in alveolar bone in monkeys (*Macaca fascicularis*). *Bone* 2001; **29**: 176–9.

13 Ammann P. Strontium ranelate: A novel mode of action leading to renewed bone quality. *Osteoporos Int* 2004; Epub ahead of print.

14 Dahl S, Allain P, Marie P *et al.* Incorporation and distribution of strontium in bone. *Bone* 2001; **28**: 446–53.

15 Nielsen S, Slosman D, Sorensen O *et al.* Influence of strontium on bone mineral density and bone mineral content measurements by dual X-ray absorptiometry. *J Clin Densitom* 1999; **2**: 371–9.

16 Reginster J, Seeman E, Vernejoul M *et al.* Strontium ranelate reduces the risk of nonvertebral fractures in postmenopausal women with osteoporosis: TROPOS study. *J Clin Endocrinol Metab* 2005 Epub ahead of print.

17 Meunier P, Slosman D, Delmas P *et al.* Strontium ranelate: dose-dependent effects in established postmenopausal vertebral osteoporosis – a 2-year randomized placebo controlled trial. *J Clin Endocrinol Metab* 2002; **87**: 2060–6.

18 Meunier P, Roux C, Seeman E *et al.* The effects of strontium ranelate on the risk of vertebral fracture in women with postmenopausal osteoporosis. *N Engl J Med* 2004; **350**: 459–68.

19 Meunier P, Reginster J. Design and methodology of the phase 3 trials for the clinical development of strontium ranelate in the treatment of women with postmenopausal osteoporosis. *Osteoporos Int* 2003; **14**: S66–76.

Acknowledgements

Figure 1 is adapted from Marie, 2004.[6]
Figure 2 is adapted from Meunier *et al.*, 2002.[17]
Figure 3 is adapted from Meunier and Reginster, 2003.[19]
Figure 4 is adapted from Meunier *et al.*, 2004.[18]
Figure 5 is adapted from Reginster *et al.*, 2005.[16]

7. Drug review – Teriparatide (Forsteo®)

Dr Rebecca Fox-Spencer
CSF Medical Communications Ltd

Summary

Teriparatide, the biologically active fragment of human recombinant parathyroid hormone, is now commercially available in the UK as a treatment for postmenopausal osteoporosis. By extending the life span of bone-forming osteoblast cells, teriparatide exerts an anabolic effect, particularly on sites rich in trabecular bone. In this way, teriparatide promotes normalisation of bone mineral density (BMD) and reduces fracture risk, both at vertebral and non-vertebral sites. Teriparatide is effective in postmenopausal women on a background of hormone replacement therapy (HRT) and chronic corticosteroid treatment, though it is not licensed for treatment of corticosteroid-induced osteoporosis. It is also effective in men with osteoporosis, though again, it is not licensed in this patient population. Teriparatide is reported to be more effective than antiresorptive therapies such as alendronate. Whilst the mechanisms of action of teriparatide and the bisphosphonates are distinct, they are not synergistic, and a prior history of antiresorptive treatment may delay the anabolic actions of teriparatide. Clinical studies have demonstrated that teriparatide is a well-tolerated treatment option. Although animal studies have raised some safety concerns regarding osteosarcoma development after long-term treatment with teriparatide, these are considered to have little relevance to clinical practice in humans. However, as a consequence of these concerns, the recommended treatment duration of 18 months should not be exceeded when used clinically. Despite the clear clinical benefits of teriparatide in the treatment of osteoporosis, there are pharmacoeconomic barriers preventing its adoption as a first-line therapy.

Introduction

Antiresorptive therapies have long been the mainstay of treatment for osteoporosis. By reducing the rate of bone resorption (breakdown), these treatments stabilise or promote an increase in BMD. Thus, these treatments are effective in interrupting the progressive vertebral and hip fracture risk associated with postmenopausal osteoporosis. However, for those patients who already have significant bone loss, antiresorptive treatment may not afford sufficient protection against the risk of future fractures. Antiresorptive drugs do not restore the disordered bone architecture characteristic of osteoporosis or stimulate net bone formation. Ideally, treatment for osteoporosis should normalise bone mass and architecture, thereby reducing fracture risk. Therefore, an agent with anabolic properties is desirable.[1,2]

As the primary endogenous regulator of calcium and phosphate metabolism in bone and kidney, parathyroid hormone has been recognised for over 70 years to exert anabolic effects on bone.[3] When the hormone was first manufactured synthetically in 1974, the potential arose to exploit these anabolic properties in a clinical setting.

Intact human parathyroid hormone is composed of 84 amino acids, but the N-terminal 34-amino acid fragment of the human recombinant hormone constitutes the biologically active region.[4] As it has been suggested that the C-terminal fragment of the hormone may exert biological effects over and above those required therapeutically, the N-terminal 34-amino acid is likely to be associated with a reduced adverse event profile compared with the full-length hormone.[5] The recombinant human 34-amino acid fragment of parathyroid hormone is now commercially available as teriparatide.[6]

> Parathyroid hormone has been recognised for over 70 years to exert anabolic effects on bone.

In the UK, teriparatide is currently only licensed for the treatment of postmenopausal women.[7] In the USA, however, teriparatide is also approved for the treatment of severe osteoporosis in men, and a number of trials have demonstrated appreciable clinical efficacy in male patients. Consequently, this article will review data on the efficacy and safety of the 1–34 amino acid fragment of parathyroid hormone in both women and men, in the interests of completeness.

In some of the trials described in this review, a synthetic parathyroid hormone fragment has been used rather than the commercially available recombinant fragment, teriparatide. This synthetic form is expected to have identical properties to teriparatide, but is denoted in this review as 'synthetic parathyroid hormone (1–34)' for accuracy. These two forms of the parathyroid hormone fragment are further distinguished by the units used to describe the administered dose. Thus, teriparatide is administered as a microgram dose, whereas the dose of the synthetic form is measured in units (U), generally 400 U, which is considered to be equivalent to 25 μg of teriparatide.

Although the anabolic effects on bone induced by intact parathyroid hormone are understood to be equivalent to those of the 34-amino acid fragment of parathyroid hormone, the abundant data concerning the full-length hormone are beyond the scope of this review.

Pharmacology

Chemistry

The 34-amino acid sequence of teriparatide is shown in Figure 1.

Method of administration

In patients considered suitable for teriparatide treatment, therapy should be initiated by a specialist – either a hospital consultant or a GP with a special interest in osteoporosis. The recommended dose of teriparatide is 20 µg once daily, administered by subcutaneous injection into the thigh or abdomen. The drug is supplied in a pre-filled injection pen, with a total of 3 mL drug in solution. This volume contains 750 µg teriparatide, providing sufficient doses for a 28-day period.[6]

The recommended dose of teriparatide is 20 µg daily, administered by subcutaneous injection into the thigh or abdomen.

Pharmacokinetics

The principle pharmacokinetic parameters associated with the parathyroid hormone 1–34 fragment (data from synthetic parathyroid hormone [1–34]) are shown in Table 1.[1,8] The plasma clearance rate is particularly high and exceeds the rate of normal hepatic blood flow, indicating that clearance occurs both hepatically and extra-hepatically.[6] Serum concentrations are 20 to 30% lower in men than in women, whereas plasma clearance rates are approximately 50% higher.[1,6] When evaluated over an age range of 31 to 85 years, no effect of age has been observed on the pharmacokinetic properties of synthetic parathyroid hormone (1–34).[6] No specific data are available on the metabolism or excretion of teriparatide. However, by extrapolating from data relating to the full length parathyroid hormone, peripheral metabolism of teriparatide is predicted to occur via enzymatic mechanisms in the liver with excretion via the kidneys.[9]

The pharmacokinetics of a drug are of interest to healthcare professionals because it is important for them to understand the action of a drug on the body over a period of time.

Figure 1. The 34-amino acid sequence of teriparatide.

NH_2 – Ser – Val – Ser – Glu – Ile – Gin – Leu – Met – His – Asn
| Leu
| Gly
| Glu – Val – Arg – Glu – Met – Ser – Asn – Leu – His – Lys
| Trp
| Leu
| Arg – Lys – Lys – Leu – Gin – Asp – Val – His – Asn – Phe – COOH

Table 1. Pharmacokinetic properties of synthetic parathyroid hormone (1–34) following a subcutaneous dose (400 U) in women with postmenopausal osteoporosis.[1,8]

Pharmacokinetic parameter	
Bioavailability (%)	95
C_{max} (pmol/L)	58–181
t_{max} (minutes)	15–45
$t_{1/2}$ (minutes)	48–100
Apparent volume of distribution (L)	100[a]
Plasma clearance (mL/minute)	790

t_{max}, time to peak plasma concentration (C_{max}); $t_{1/2}$, plasma half-life.
[a]Substantially greater than total body water estimate – it is suggested that there may have been significant local degradation of the hormone fragment, leading to a reduction in its concentration and hence an over-estimation of the volume of distribution.

Data suggest that the pharmacokinetic profile of teriparatide is unaffected in patients with mild-to-moderate renal insufficiency (creatinine clearance 30–72 mL/minute) or heart failure (New York Heart Association class I–III).[9] The half-life of the drug was increased, however, in patients with severe renal insufficiency (creatinine clearance <30 mL/minute), and teriparatide is contraindicated in this patient population. No data are yet available from patients with hepatic impairment.[9]

Mode of action and preclinical data

☛ *These preclinical data sections describe the results of the earliest phases of a drug's development (see Readers Guide).*

Loss of bone strength caused by oestrogen deficiency is associated with a high rate of 'remodelling' or turnover. An increase in bone strength may be induced by improved mineralisation of existing bone, enhanced architectural organisation or increased bone volume. Traditionally, antiresorptive therapies have been used to prevent and treat osteoporosis by reducing the rate of bone turnover. The down regulation of both bone resorption and formation increases the time available for mineralisation of the remaining bone, thus improving its strength. However, these drugs do not restore bone architecture or volume.[10]

More recently, drugs with anabolic properties on bone have been developed. These have included sodium fluoride, growth hormone and insulin-like growth factor-1 (IGF-I), and more recently, teriparatide. Strontium ranelate is also reported, on the basis of animal data, to have anabolic properties, in addition to an antiresorptive action.[11] Teriparatide binds to the same parathyroid receptor on bone as the full-length hormone, and exerts its anabolic action through the second messenger, cyclic adenosine-3',5'-monophosphate (cAMP). In direct contrast to antiresorptive drugs, teriparatide increases both bone resorption and bone formation. The balance between these two processes following therapeutic administration of teriparatide is such that the increased rate of turnover is accompanied by a net increase in the amount of bone laid down. Thus, teriparatide mediates a replacement of lost bone. Although the increased rate of remodelling induced by teriparatide would be expected to impair bone strength to some extent, the anabolic effects more than compensate for this. Thus, although antiresorptive drugs are effective for both the treatment and the prevention of osteoporosis, teriparatide has the potential to mediate a greater reduction in fracture risk in patients with established disease, due its greater potential to normalise the strength of affected bone.[5]

A wealth of data exist which demonstrate the anabolic effects of parathyroid hormone (1–34) in animal models.[12–16] Intermittent treatment (generally by daily subcutaneous injections) with parathyroid hormone (1–34) has been shown to increase trabecular bone mass, though its effects on cortical bone are less pronounced.[17] Importantly, although pulsatile administration of parathyroid hormone (1–34) exerts an anabolic action, continuous infusion leads to bone loss.[18] This is because continuous administration alters the balance of bone resorption and formation in favour of the former.

Investigations in animals have also progressed our understanding of the mechanism by which the anabolic effect of intermittent parathyroid hormone (1–34) treatment is exerted. A study in mice has revealed that the prevention of programmed cell death (apoptosis) of osteoblasts is a major mechanism by which parathyroid hormone (1–34) increases bone mass.[19] The balance between bone-formation (osteoblast) and bone-resorption (osteoclast) cells dictates skeletal homeostasis, and disruption of this balance leads to bone diseases such as osteoporosis. Parathyroid hormone (1–34) appears to redress this balance by prolonging the life span of osteoblasts (normally approximately 8 days in mice, but a matter of months in humans). The increase in bone mass is most likely to be the cumulative result of repeated daily postponement of apoptosis over several generations of osteoblasts.[19] The antiapoptotic action of parathyroid hormone (1–34) is in direct opposition to the promotion of osteoblast apoptosis induced by oestrogen withdrawal or glucocorticoid treatment, both of which are known risk factors for the development of osteoporosis.[20,21]

In addition to its effect on osteoblasts, parathyroid hormone (1–34) also promotes bone strength indirectly by increasing intestinal absorption of calcium, tubular reabsorption of calcium, phosphate excretion at the kidney and renal synthesis of 1,25-dihydroxyvitamin D_3.[6,9]

Clinical efficacy

There are a number of outcome measures commonly used in clinical trials of osteoporosis treatments, ranging from measurements of biochemical markers of bone turnover, through qualitative and quantitative indications of bone composition and size, to the incidence of fractures. Serum levels of bone-specific alkaline phosphatase (BSAP), osteocalcin and C-terminal propeptide of type 1 procollagen (P1CP) are all markers of bone formation, whereas urinary N-telopeptide (NTX), urinary free deoxypyridinoline and 1,25-dihydroxyvitamin D_3 are markers of bone resorption. The most common measure of bone integrity is BMD, usually measured by dual-energy X-ray absorptiometry (DXA). BMD is derived from two independent measurements – bone mineral content and projected bone area – and is strongly predictive of fracture risk in the untreated population. BMD does not, however, reflect changes in the microarchitecture of bone. This can be evaluated qualitatively by two-dimensional or three-dimensional imaging. The number of incident fractures, particularly vertebral fractures, was the primary outcome in the 'Fracture Prevention Trial'. Vertebral fractures are often defined, quantitatively, by a reduction in height (for example a 20% reduction).[22] Non-vertebral fractures are generally diagnosed following examination of radiographs and radiological reports. Non-vertebral 'fragility fractures' are defined as those caused by a trauma, which would not be expected to result in a fracture of normal bone (e.g. a fall from standing height or less).[22]

BMD is the most frequently used method for diagnosing osteoporosis and is often used in a clinical trial setting to define the study population. The BMD T-score is the difference between the measured BMD and that established in a normal, young population of the same gender. A T-score of less than –2.5 (BMD at least 2.5 standard deviations below the predicted healthy average) is commonly used as the threshold for diagnosis of osteoporosis (see Table 2 in the Disease Overview of this edition of *BESTMEDICINE*).

The clinical trials described in this review generally excluded patients with comorbid disease, particularly those affecting bone or calcium metabolism. Patients with hepatic or renal dysfunction were generally excluded, as were those with secondary causes of osteoporosis, unless the trial design dictated otherwise.

The Fracture Prevention Trial

A major trial, conducted in postmenopausal osteoporotic women, has clearly demonstrated the anabolic effects of teriparatide.[22] Subsequently referred to as the 'Fracture Prevention Trial', this investigation was designed with a duration of 3 years, but was terminated early when new data from a study in rats indicated a risk of osteosarcomas following long-term treatment with a high dose of teriparatide.[23] It is now thought unlikely that these data are of clinical relevance in humans; this issue is discussed in more detail in the Safety and Tolerability section of this review. Women were eligible for entry into the Fracture Prevention Trial if they were ambulatory, were at least 5 years postmenopausal, and had suffered at least one moderate or two mild non-traumatic vertebral fractures on radiographs of the thoracic and lumbar spine. If fewer than two moderate fractures were present, an additional criterion for inclusion was a BMD T-score at the hip or lumbar spine of –1 or less.

A total of 1637 women were enrolled into the study and each received daily supplements of calcium (1000 mg) and vitamin D (400–1200 IU). After daily self-administration of a placebo injection for 2 weeks, each patient was randomised to receive a daily self-administered injection of placebo (n=544) or teriparatide at 20 µg (n=541) or 40 µg (n=552). The mean duration of treatment, prior to the premature termination of the trial, was 17–18 months, and was not significantly different between the three groups. In the 1326 patients for whom baseline and follow-up radiographs were available, teriparatide, 20 or 40 µg, reduced the risk of new vertebral fractures by 65 and 69%, respectively, compared with placebo. The corresponding reductions in risk for two or more new fractures were 77 and 86%, respectively, and 90 and 78%, respectively, for at least one new moderate or severe vertebral fracture. The total number of new vertebral fractures per 1000 patient years of treatment was 136 in the placebo group, compared with 49 and 30 in the 20 µg and 40 µg teriparatide groups, respectively. Amongst those patients who suffered at least one new vertebral fracture, the mean loss in height was greater in the placebo group (–1.1 cm) than in the 20 µg or 40 µg teriparatide groups (–0.2 and –0.3 cm, respectively; $p=0.002$ vs placebo). New or worsening back pain was reported by 23% of patients in the placebo group, compared with 17 and 16% in the low- and high-dose teriparatide groups, respectively ($p=0.007$ vs placebo).

Women treated with teriparatide (20 µg or 40 µg) were 35 and 40% less likely, respectively, to experience new non-vertebral fractures than those in the placebo group and 53 and 54% less likely, respectively, to have new non-vertebral fragility fractures. The absolute risks of non-vertebral fragility fractures were 6% in the placebo group compared with 3% in the teriparatide group (no differences were apparent between doses). Data reflecting the cumulative incidence of non-vertebral fractures indicated that the superiority of teriparatide over placebo did not emerge until 9–12 months after the initiation of treatment (Figure 2). This is an important consideration, given that, in the UK, teriperatide is currently licensed for a maximum treatment duration of only 18 months.[6]

At baseline, all three treatment groups demonstrated a mean BMD T-score of –2.6 at the spine. Teriparatide generated greater improvements in BMD than placebo at the lumbar spine, femoral neck, trochanter, intertrochanter and total hip ($p<0.001$). For BMD in the shaft of radius, only the higher dose of teriparatide afforded significantly greater benefits than placebo ($p<0.001$) whilst there was no treatment effect on BMD in the distal radius ($p>0.05$). Both doses of teriparatide generated greater improvements in total body BMD than placebo ($p<0.001$).

Treatment with teriparatide did not significantly increase the number of deaths, hospitalisations, or the incidence of cardiovascular disorders, urolithiasis or gout, in comparison with placebo. Despite the concerns arising from the teriparatide study in rats, no cases of osteosarcoma were reported in study participants. In fact, the incidence of cancer was higher in the placebo group (4%) than in the 20 µg or 40 µg teriparatide groups (2% in each; $p=0.02$ and $p=0.07$, respectively). Six per cent of

> Teriparatide, 20 or 40 µg, reduced the risk of new vertebral fractures by 65 and 69%, respectively, compared with placebo.

> Teriparatide generated greater improvements in BMD than placebo at the lumbar spine, femoral neck, trochanter, intertrochanter and total hip ($p<0.001$).

Figure 2. Cumulative proportion of women receiving placebo or teriparatide (20 or 40 µg/day) with at least one non-vertebral fracture (left) or at least one non-vertebral fragility fracture (right) occurring during the course of the study.[22]

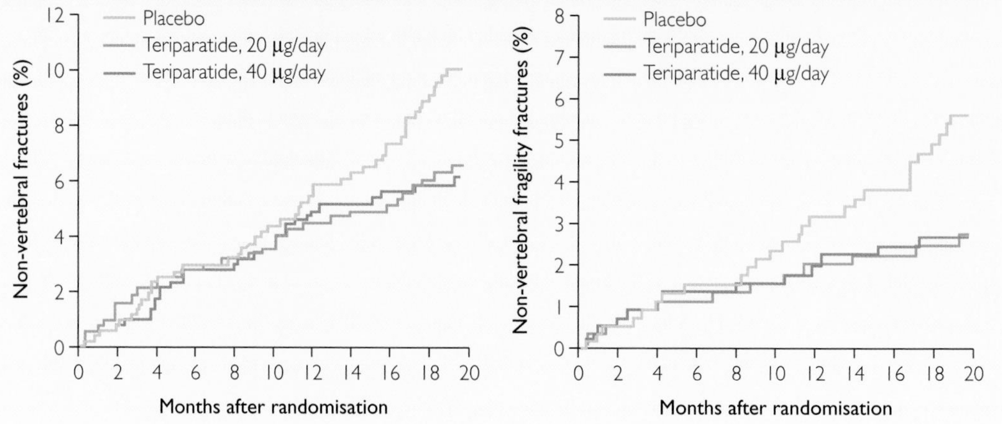

the placebo and the lower-dose teriparatide groups, and 11% of the higher-dose teriparatide group withdrew from the trial as a consequence of adverse events. Nausea and headache were more common in the teriparatide 40 µg (but not the 20 µg) group than in the placebo group ($p<0.001$ and $p=0.01$, for nausea and headache, respectively). In contrast, dizziness and leg cramps were more common in the teriparatide 20 µg group than in those receiving placebo ($p=0.05$ and $p=0.02$, respectively), but were similar in the 40 µg and placebo groups. Mild hypercalcaemia (4–6 hours after injection) occurred at least once in 2, 11 and 28% of patients receiving placebo, and 20 and 40 µg teriparatide, respectively. However, on retesting a few weeks later, only approximately one-third of these patients still had high serum calcium concentrations. In one patient in each of the placebo and 20 µg teriparatide groups, and in nine patients in the 40 µg teriparatide group, treatment was withdrawn due to repeatedly high serum calcium concentrations. Furthermore, serum calcitriol concentrations increased significantly in both teriparatide groups but remained stable with placebo. The incidence of hypercalciuria was not increased with active treatment. Serum uric acid levels increased in a dose-dependent manner with teriparatide but were not associated with clinical sequelae. Serum magnesium concentrations decreased slightly in both active treatment groups, whereas serum creatinine and creatinine clearance were unaffected. Circulating antibodies to teriparatide developed in under 1% of patients in the placebo group, 3% in the 20 µg teriparatide group and 8% of the 40 µg teriparatide group.

In conclusion, this trial demonstrated a clear effect of teriparatide in preventing both vertebral and non-vertebral fractures and in improving BMD. The data from this study do not indicate any increased risk of

> This trial demonstrated a clear effect of teriparatide in preventing both vertebral and non-vertebral fractures and in improving BMD.

serious adverse events as a result of teriparatide treatment. The tolerability profile was, however, inferior in the 40 μg group compared with the lower-dose teriparatide group, and these data are supportive, therefore, of the selection of the 20 μg dose as the appropriate choice for clinical use.[6]

Subgroup analyses of the Fracture Prevention Trial

The Fracture Prevention Trial has generated the core clinical data supporting the efficacy of teriparatide, and these data have been subject to a number of *post hoc* analyses. These analyses have evaluated the influence of baseline parameters on the effectiveness of teriparatide,[24,25] as well as addressing concerns regarding the 'cortical steal' hypothesis.[26,27]

Effect of age

In a *post hoc* analysis of the Fracture Prevention Trial data, patients were grouped according to age: under 65 years, 65–75 years and 75 years and older.[24] The percentage increase in vertebral BMD in patients treated with teriparatide was found to be greatest in older patients (treatment-by-age interaction, $p=0.037$). This age effect, however, was also observed in the placebo group and is therefore more likely to reflect the greater baseline calcium and vitamin D deficiencies of the older population. No treatment-by-age interaction was identified when the outcome considered was the relative risk reduction of vertebral fracture ($p=0.558$).

Effect on BMD

The effect of baseline vertebral BMD on treatment efficacy was evaluated by dividing the patients into groups with baseline T-scores of less than –3.3, between –3.3 and –2.1, or greater than –2.1.[24] In patients treated with teriparatide, the percentage increase in vertebral BMD was inversely related to the baseline value. However, the absolute increase in vertebral BMD was similar in all three baseline groups (treatment-by-BMD interaction, $p=0.615$). Furthermore, there was no significant difference between the three subgroups in terms of the relative risk for developing new vertebral fractures (treatment-by-BMD interaction, $p=0.817$).

The risk of new vertebral fractures was further evaluated by dividing patients into two groups with T-scores of either less than –2.5, or at least –2.5. Although the interaction remained non-significant ($p=0.203$), teriparatide reduced the risk of vertebral fracture in patients with more severe BMD impairment at baseline (T score <–2.5; $p<0.001$) but was ineffective in the less severe group (T score ≥–2.5; $p=0.130$).

Effect of number and severity of prevalent fractures

A *post hoc* analysis revealed that patients in the placebo group who had experienced at least two vertebral fractures at baseline were more likely to have new vertebral fractures during the trial than if they had one or

The effectiveness
of teriparatide
was largely
independent of
the baseline
prevalent
fracture status.

fewer at baseline ($p<0.001$).[24] However, in the two teriparatide groups, the number of new vertebral fractures was not related to the number of baseline fractures. Furthermore, the number of prevalent vertebral fractures (none, one or at least two) had no impact on the percentage increase in BMD in response to teriparatide. Thus, the effectiveness of teriparatide was largely independent of the baseline prevalent fracture status.

This has been demonstrated further in another *post hoc* analysis which evaluated the effect of baseline number and severity of fractures on the teriparatide-mediated reduction of new fracture risk.[25] This analysis was performed on a subset of the Fracture Prevention Trial population who received either placebo or the 20 µg dose of teriparatide and who had at least one vertebral fracture at baseline (n=931). The observations from this analysis are illustrated in Figure 3. In patients who received placebo, the number of prevalent vertebral fractures at baseline was significantly associated with the risk of any new vertebral fractures and of moderate or severe new vertebral fractures ($p<0.001$ in both cases). These risks were also significantly associated with the severity of the prevalent vertebral fractures at baseline ($p<0.001$). In addition, the number of non-vertebral fragility fractures at baseline was significantly associated with the risk of new non-vertebral fractures ($p=0.002$) and of new non-vertebral fragility fractures ($p<0.001$) in patients receiving placebo during the study. In contrast, in the patients who received teriparatide (20 µg), there was no significant association between the risk of new vertebral fractures (either total or moderate/severe only) and the number or severity of prevalent vertebral fractures at baseline. Neither was there a significant association in teriparatide-treated patients between the number of non-vertebral fragility fractures at baseline and the risk of new non-vertebral and non-vertebral fragility fractures during the treatment period.

Teriparatide
reduces fracture
risk by a similar
level regardless
of the baseline
prevalent
fracture burden.

In summary, this analysis demonstrates that the correlation between current fracture burden and increased risk of future fractures in postmenopausal osteoporotic women is abolished by treatment with teriparatide. Thus, teriparatide reduces fracture risk by a similar level regardless of the baseline prevalent fracture burden.

Effect of teriparatide on cortical bone

Several studies in which parathyroid hormone has been used in the treatment of osteoporosis have demonstrated maintenance or even loss of cortical bone at some sites, despite increased trabecular bone mass.[17,28] This trade-off would be unsatisfactory, as a reduction in the rate of vertebral fractures (due to increased trabecular bone mass) may be offset by an increase in the risk of hip fractures (due to reduced cortical bone mass), which are associated with higher mortality, morbidity and cost. The proposal of this so-called 'cortical steal' hypothesis has raised some concern about the use of parathyroid hormone or its fragments in the clinical management of osteoporosis.

Figure 3. Proportion of women with new vertebral (A and B) or non-vertebral (C) fractures in placebo and teriparatide 20 µg/day groups, by number (A) and severity (B) of prevalent vertebral fractures or number of prevalent non-vertebral fractures (C).[25]

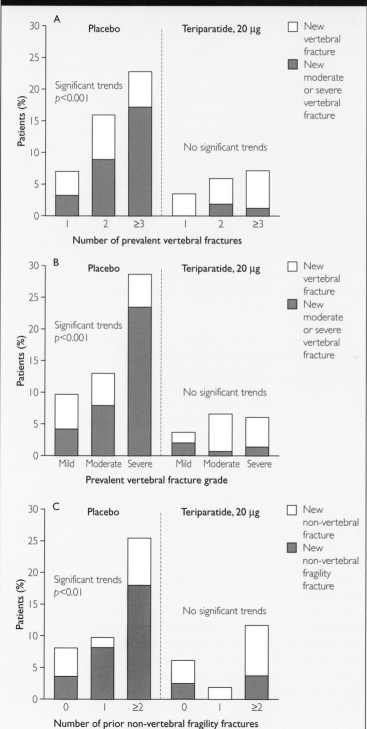

An analysis of the study population from the Fracture Prevention Trial has directly addressed the 'cortical steal' hypothesis.[26] A subset of the trial population underwent iliac crest biopsies before and after treatment with teriparatide, yielding a total of 51 paired specimens of sufficient quality for analysis. Bone structural characteristics were similar across all three treatment groups. For the purpose of this analysis, data from the two teriparatide treatment groups (20 and 40 µg) were pooled. Qualitative two-dimensional analysis of the biopsy specimens revealed increased trabecular and cortical thickness in most teriparatide-treated patients. However, patients receiving the higher dose also demonstrated some evidence of marrow fibrosis (in 14%) and tunnelling resorption (in 29%). Indices reflecting activity, turnover, erosion depth and wall thickness did not differ between treatment groups. Teriparatide mediated a 14% increase in trabecular bone volume compared with a 24% reduction in the placebo group ($p=0.001$). The increase in marrow star volume (a measure of porosity) was considerably smaller than that observed in the placebo group (16 *vs* 112%, respectively; $p=0.004$). Cortical thickness increased in teriparatide-treated patients (0.9%) and decreased in the placebo group (–10.8%), but this trend did not reach significance ($p=0.197$). There was no significant difference between the placebo and teriparatide groups in terms of cortical porosity ($p=0.094$).

The 'structural model index' quantifies the form of a three-dimensional structure in terms of the amount of plates and rods composing the structure. A numerical increase (between 0 and 3) in this index reflects a shift from plate to rod elements. It is well documented that the structure of trabecular bone changes radically from 'plate-like' to 'rod-like' during ageing, bone remodelling and osteoporosis. Three-dimensional analysis of the biopsy specimens from this analysis revealed that teriparatide decreased the structural model index relative to placebo (–12 *vs* +7%, respectively; $p=0.025$), reflecting a reversal in osteoporotic changes. Teriparatide also increased the connectivity density (+19 *vs* –14%; $p=0.034$) and cortical thickness (+22 *vs* +3%; $p=0.012$) compared with placebo. The teriparatide-mediated increase in three-dimensional trabecular bone volume fraction was not significantly different to the reduction recorded in the placebo group (+7 *vs* –5%, respectively, $p=0.098$). As in the two-dimensional analysis, there was no significant difference between the placebo and teriparatide groups in terms of cortical porosity ($p=0.457$).

In summary, these investigations demonstrate that teriparatide was able to improve both trabecular and cortical bone structure. Thus, contrary to speculation that the anabolic effects of teriparatide on trabecular bone may occur at the expense of cortical bone, teriparatide actually improved cortical bone structure, which was reflected in an increase of approximately 20% in cortical thickness. This was accompanied by an increase in trabecular bone volume, improved trabecular bone connectivity and a shift from 'rod-like' to 'plate-like' trabecular morphology. Teriparatide did not, however, induce any changes in indices of trabecular bone remodelling, bone resorption, or bone formation rates.

Qualitative two-dimensional analysis of the biopsy specimens revealed increased trabecular and cortical thickness in most teriparatide-treated patients.

These investigations demonstrate that teriparatide was able to improve both trabecular and cortical bone structure.

The issue of whether or not teriparatide-mediated anabolic effects on trabecular bone occur at the expense of cortical bone mass has been further addressed by an additional subgroup analysis of the Fracture Prevention Trial.[17,22,27] This investigation made use of peripheral quantitative computed tomography as a non-invasive method of assessing bone structure *in vivo*, which has the potential to evaluate trabecular and cortical bone effects separately. A study which focused on the effects of teriparatide on cortical bone took measurements at the distal radial diaphysis, as this area is known to contain only a very small proportion of trabecular bone (<10%). Of the 118 women tested, usable scans were obtained from 101 women. Both doses of teriparatide (20 and 40 µg) increased total bone mineral content ($p<0.05$) and total bone area ($p<0.01$) (but not total bone density) compared with placebo. Cortical bone area was increased by 5% ($p=0.005$) and 7% ($p<0.001$) compared with placebo in the 20 and 40 µg groups, respectively. Cortical bone mineral content was also higher in the 20 and 40 µg teriparatide groups than in the placebo group (by 6 and 4%, respectively), though this trend was not statistically significant ($p=0.054$). The thickness of cortical bone was statistically equivalent in all the treatment groups, though there was a non-significant trend for lower cortical bone density in the higher-dose teriparatide group compared with placebo. Calculations were made to determine the axial and polar cross-sectional moments of inertia, which serve as architectural indicators of the resistance of bone to bending and torsional loading, respectively. Both the 20 µg and 40 µg teriparatide groups had higher polar moments of inertia than the placebo group (by 9 and 21%, respectively; $p<0.001$). The higher dose teriparatide group also had a higher axial moment of inertia compared with placebo (16%; $p<0.0001$). These data indicate that teriparatide mediated improvements in bone geometry, which would be predicted to increase bone strength and resistance to fracture, as supported by data from the Fracture Prevention Trial.[22]

Teriparatide mediated improvements in bone geometry, which would be predicted to increase bone strength and resistance to fracture.

Effect of prior osteoporotic treatment

Given the predominance of antiresorptive treatment for osteoporosis, it is important to consider whether the clinical efficacy of teriparatide is altered by a history of long-term use of antiresorptive therapy. A prospective, open-label, non-randomised, 18-month trial has directly addressed this issue, by administering teriparatide treatment to women who had previously received alendronate (10 mg/day) or raloxifene (60 mg/day) for 18–36 months prior to study entry.[29] Raloxifene is a selective oestrogen receptor modulator (SERM), and like alendronate, has an antiresorptive mode of action.

Women entering this study were aged between 60 and 87 years, and were required to have a prior recorded lumbar spine or total hip BMD T-score of –2.5 or less, along with a score of –2.0 or less at study entry. Patients with a recent history of oestrogen or progestin treatment were excluded from this trial. A total of 59 eligible women were assigned to treatment with teriparatide (20 µg/day) and daily supplements of calcium (1000 mg) and vitamin D (400 IU). Of the 98.3% patients who completed the initial 12-month treatment period, 86.2% consented to partake in a 6-month extension, and 96% of these completed this additional phase.

The only statistically significant difference recorded between the prior alendronate and prior raloxifene groups at baseline was in the median levels of bone turnover markers, which were approximately twice as high in the raloxifene group. Following 1 month of treatment with teriparatide, all markers of bone turnover (BSAP, osteocalcin, C-terminal propeptide of type 1 procollagen [P1CP] and NTX) had increased significantly from baseline in both groups. The prior raloxifene group, however, demonstrated greater increases in markers of bone formation (osteocalcin, P1CP and BSAP) than the prior alendronate group after 1 month ($p<0.05$). At all later time points, there were non-significant trends towards a larger magnitude of effect in the prior raloxifene group than in the prior alendronate group. Between 6 and 12 months after the commencement of teriparatide treatment, levels of all bone turnover markers tended to plateau in both groups.

Measurements were made of lumbar spine and total hip BMD in this study. During the period between 3 and 6 months after the initiation of teriparatide treatment, lumbar spine BMD increased significantly from baseline in the prior raloxifene group but did not change in the prior alendronate group (Figure 4). From 6 months onwards, this parameter increased at a similar rate in the two groups, but the earlier onset of effect in the prior raloxifene group ensured a greater magnitude of overall effect (10.2 *vs* 4.1% respective increases over baseline at 18 months; $p<0.05$). The first 6 months of treatment were also responsible for the discrepancy between the two groups in total hip BMD measurements. Whereas this parameter remained close to baseline

> Lumbar spine BMD increased significantly from baseline in the prior raloxifene group but did not change in the prior alendronate group.

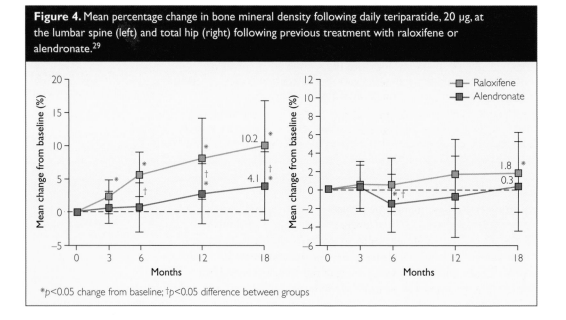

Figure 4. Mean percentage change in bone mineral density following daily teriparatide, 20 µg, at the lumbar spine (left) and total hip (right) following previous treatment with raloxifene or alendronate.[29]

*$p<0.05$ change from baseline; †$p<0.05$ difference between groups

in the prior raloxifene group, it decreased significantly in the prior alendronate group (Figure 4). Although the two groups demonstrated a similar rate of increase in total hip BMD from 6 months onwards, a non-significant superior effect for the prior raloxifene group was apparent throughout the study (mean change from baseline to 18 months: 1.8 *vs* 0.3%; $p>0.05$). Moreover, there were significant correlations between the 12-month spinal BMD change and markers of bone turnover in the prior raloxifene group, whereas such correlations were not apparent in the prior alendronate group.

Hypercalcaemia occurred in 9.1% of women in the prior raloxifene group and 12.1% of those who previously receiving alendronate. All of these cases normalised without any alteration to treatment. Serious adverse events occurred in 9.1 and 18.1% of the prior raloxifene and alendronate groups, respectively, but no additional details were reported. No adverse treatment effects were observed in terms of haematology or chemistry tests.

In summary, patients with a prior history of treatment with raloxifene or alendronate respond favourably to teriparatide, both in terms of markers of bone turnover and measurements of BMD. However, there was a less pronounced effect of teriparatide treatment upon markers of bone turnover in patients previously exposed to alendronate compared with prior raloxifene patients. This was suggested to be due to the lower bone turnover induced by alendronate treatment. For example, bone turnover has been shown to remain suppressed for at least 1 year after discontinuation of alendronate.[30] The low turnover at baseline in prior alendronate patients may have reduced the availability of target cells for the teriparatide-induced bone formation process to occur or, alternatively, reduced the effect of teriparatide in inducing bone resorption, thus preventing the stimulation of bone formation. Similarly, whereas prior raloxifene-treated patients demonstrated teriparatide-induced increases in BMD comparable with those observed in treatment-naïve patients,[22] the prior alendronate patients experienced a markedly inferior effect in the first 6 months. This impairment was suggested to be attributable to a reduction in remodelling and increased mineralisation in alendronate-treated bone. Thus, alendronate pre-treatment alters the usual time course of teriparatide-induced changes, as well as interfering with the relationships between bone turnover and changes in BMD. Although these effects may be expected to delay the teriparatide-mediated reductions in fracture risk, this has not yet been explicitly demonstrated.

Efficacy on a background of HRT

Although HRT has prophylactic properties on osteoporosis if started early in the menopause, it is no longer considered to be a first-line option for long-term prevention of osteoporosis, due to safety concerns relating to an increased incidence of breast cancer and adverse cardiovascular effects.[7] However, some of the available clinical data concerning the efficacy of parathyroid hormone (1–34) in postmenopausal osteoporosis have been obtained on a background of HRT (summarised in Table 2).[31–33] In one such trial, eligible patients had a bone mass T-score of –2.5 or less and/or non-traumatic fractures.[31] All patients had received HRT for at least 1 year. A total of 34 patients completed a 1-year observation period and were randomised to 3 years of treatment with either synthetic parathyroid hormone (1–34; 400 U/25 µg daily) plus oestrogen or oestrogen alone. Calcium supplementation was used to ensure a total daily intake of 1500 mg/day. Oestrogen was supplemented with a progestin in those patients who had not had a hysterectomy.

BMD at the lumbar spine increased throughout the trial in patients receiving synthetic parathyroid hormone (1–34) but did not change significantly in patients continuing on HRT alone (Figure 5). The effects of synthetic parathyroid hormone (1–34) were less pronounced in the total hip region and at the proximal forearm, but again there was no significant change associated with HRT alone. Total-body bone mineral content increased by a total of 7.8% in the synthetic parathyroid hormone (1–34) group, yet remained unchanged in the HRT alone group.

According to biochemical measurements, there were no significant changes in either group in serum calcium, phosphorus, parathyroid hormone, 25-hydroxyvitamin D, 1,25-dihydroxyvitamin D_3 or 24-hour urinary calcium. There were no cases of hypercalciuria or alterations in serum urea nitrogen, creatinine, electrolytes, complete blood cell count, hepatic function or evidence of development of antibodies to synthetic parathyroid hormone (1–34). Osteocalcin increased significantly within the first month of synthetic parathyroid hormone (1–34) treatment, whereas NTX did not increase until the sixth month of treatment. The levels of these markers of bone turnover then declined towards baseline. Following 3 years of treatment, osteocalcin and NTX levels were equivalent in the synthetic parathyroid hormone (1–34) and HRT-only groups.

Using a 15% reduction in vertebral height to indicate a vertebral fracture, 13 new vertebral fractures were identified over the course of the study. Of these, 77% occurred in the HRT-only group ($p<0.03$ *vs* synthetic parathyroid hormone [1–34] group). When a 20% reduction in vertebral height was used to indicate a vertebral fracture, the number of incident fractures was reduced to six, five of which occurred in the HRT-only group ($p=0.09$ *vs* synthetic parathyroid hormone [1–34] group).

Analysis of adverse events revealed that most patients experienced pain at the site of injection with synthetic parathyroid hormone (1–34) and many had macular redness at the injection site, which lasted between 15 minutes and 12 hours after injection. Discomfort and redness generally resolved as the study progressed. One case of urinary infection with possible renal stone occurred in the synthetic parathyroid hormone (1–34) group, but this patient continued the trial with no further complications. There were four withdrawals from the study, all in the synthetic parathyroid hormone (1–34) group. Only two of these,

Table 2. Summary of trials of synthetic parathyroid hormone (1–34)/teriparatide on a background of hormone-replacement therapy with or without corticosteroid treatment.[31–33]

Study	Study population	Treatment groups	Main outcomes
Lindsay et al., 1997[31]	Postmenopausal osteoporosis (T-score <–2.5 and/or non-traumatic fractures). HRT taken for at least a year previously. n=34	• Oestrogen + synthetic PTH (1–34; 400 U/25 μg/day) • Oestrogen ('control') 3 years In both cases, oestrogen was either conjugated equine, 0.625 mg/day, or transdermal, 50 μg/day. Patients prescribed a progestin if they had not had a hysterectomy. Calcium supplementation to give total intake of 1500 mg/day	• Bone mass at lumbar spine increased by 13% in PTH group after 3 years (p<0.02), with a non-significant decline in control group. • PTH-induced increases in bone mass were less pronounced at other sites. • No significant difference between groups after 3 years in indices of calcium homeostasis or bone turnover. • Most patients had pain at injection site, some with macular redness. • Two withdrawals due to PTH treatment (back pain and subcutaneous nodules).
Lane et al., 1998[32]	Postmenopausal (for ≥3 years) women, aged 50–82 years. T-score <–2.5. Chronic stable doses of both HRT and corticosteroids. n=51	• Oestrogen + corticosteroid + synthetic PTH (1–34; 400 U/25 μg/day) • Oestrogen + corticosteroid ('control') 1 year In both cases, oestrogen and corticosteroid maintained at individual regimen. Calcium supplementation to give total intake of 1500 mg/day; 800 IU vitamin D₃/day	• BMD at lumbar spine increased significantly in PTH group (p<0.001), no significant effect in control group. • PTH-induced increases in bone mass were less pronounced at other sites. • 96% classified as 'responders' in PTH group, 40% in control group. • New vertebral fractures in 0/1 of PTH/control groups, respectively. New non-vertebral fractures in two patients from each group. • Cases of hypercalciuria (one in each group) normalised on reduction of calcium intake. Three cases of hypercalcemia (all in PTH group) resolved with reduction in PTH dose and calcium intake. • Markers of bone formation increased significantly in PTH group. • Mild headaches and mild injection-site tenderness were the most common side-effects.

BMD, bone mineral density; HRT, hormone replacement therapy; PTH, parathyroid hormone.

Table 2. Continued

Study	Study population	Treatment groups	Main outcomes
Rehman et al., 2003[33]	As for Lane study.	• Oestrogen + corticosteroid + teriparatide (40 µg/day) • Oestrogen + corticosteroid ('control') 1 year In both cases, oestrogen and corticosteroid maintained at individual regimen.	• Vertebral cross-sectional area in the lumbar spine increased significantly after a year of teriparatide treatment. This increase remained significant a year after discontinuation of treatment. • However, there were no significant differences between groups in the vertebral cross-sectional area at 12 or 24 months. • Vertebral BMD increased by 35% after 1 year of teriparatide treatment, and a further 2.9% after 1 year of follow-up (compared with 1.3 and 0.3% in the control group). • Estimated vertebral compressive strength increased by nearly 200% after 1 year of teriparatide treatment, and was maintained throughout the year of follow-up. No change was reported in the control group.

BMD, bone mineral density; HRT, hormone replacement therapy; PTH, parathyroid hormone.

Figure 5. Changes in bone mineral density (BMD) at the total hip (left) and lumbar spine (right) in patients receiving hormone replacement therapy (HRT) with or without synthetic parathyroid hormone (1–34).[31]

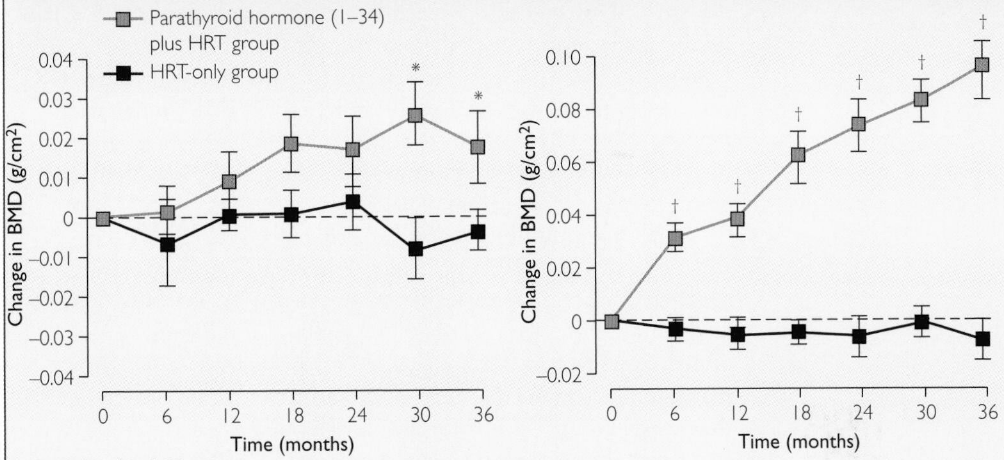

*p<0.001; †p<0.02

however, were considered to be related to study treatment (one case of back pain and one of subcutaneous nodules at the injection sites). The other two withdrawals were due to cases of breast cancer and otosclerosis.

To summarise, synthetic parathyroid hormone (1–34) generates considerable benefit to BMD in patients receiving concurrent HRT, particularly in vertebral bone. The anabolic effects of synthetic parathyroid hormone (1–34) were less pronounced in other regions such as the total hip and forearm (which are, in fact, not recommended sites for monitoring treatment efficacy), though there was no detrimental effect at these sites.

> Synthetic parathyroid hormone (1–34) generates considerable benefit to BMD in patients receiving concurrent HRT, particularly in vertebral bone.

Efficacy on a background of corticosteroid therapy

The most common cause of drug-related osteoporosis is chronic corticosteroid use.[34] Corticosteroids suppress bone formation, and so teriparatide, with its anabolic action, would appear particularly suitable for this patient population. Furthermore, trabecular bone is the most susceptible to corticosteroid-induced bone loss, due to its high turnover rate. As discussed previously, the anabolic effects of teriparatide are most prominent in the trabecular bone compartment, lending further support to this treatment strategy in patients with corticosteroid-induced osteoporosis. Although teriparatide is not currently licensed for use in patients with corticosteroid-induced osteoporosis, the efficacy of parathyroid hormone (1–34) on a background of corticosteroid (as well as HRT) treatment has been evaluated in a clinical trial setting.

Two such reports have been published, both evaluating data originating from apparently equivalent study populations, though one publication reports the use of synthetic parathyroid hormone (1–34) whilst the other describes the dose in terms of the recombinant hormone (data summarised in Table 2).[32,33] These populations comprised women aged between 50 and 82 years, with a variety of chronic non-infectious diseases and osteoporosis (defined by a bone mass T-score <–2.5 at the lumbar spine and/or femoral neck). These women were required to have been postmenopausal for at least 3 years and were receiving stable HRT and corticosteroid therapy. In each study, a total of 51 women were randomised to 12 months of treatment with the hormone fragment or no additional treatment, administered on the existing background of oestrogen and corticosteroid therapy.

In the first study, synthetic parathyroid hormone (1–34) was administered at 400 U/25 µg daily.[32] Patients also received calcium supplements to ensure a total dietary intake of 1500 mg per day, as well as vitamin D_3 supplements of 800 IU per day. In this study, BMD in the lumbar spine increased from baseline in patients receiving synthetic parathyroid hormone ([1–34]; 11.1%; $p<0.001$) but did not change in the control group.[32] The difference between the treatment groups was significant after 12 months at the lumbar spine ($p<0.001$), but there was no significant advantage of synthetic parathyroid hormone (1–34) over the control group in BMD at any other site tested. A positive response to treatment (defined as any positive change in spinal BMD between baseline and the 12-month treatment endpoint) was achieved in 96% of the synthetic parathyroid hormone (1–34) group compared with only 40–45% (depending on method of measurement) in the control group. There were similar and low rates of new vertebral and non-vertebral fractures in the synthetic parathyroid hormone (1–34) and control groups, though the study was not powered for the analysis of fracture rates.

Osteocalcin, BSAP and urinary excretion of deoxypyridinoline crosslinks were measured in patients receiving synthetic parathyroid hormone (1–34). Levels of all three of these markers of bone turnover increased by approximately 200% at 6 months. However, markers of bone formation were maximally increased within 1–3 months of treatment, whereas the marker of bone resorption did not reach its maximum level until 6 months. Small increases in serum calcium and 1,25-dihydroxyvitamin D_3, and small decreases in the levels of endogenous intact parathyroid hormone occurred in the group being administered synthetic parathyroid hormone (1–34; $p<0.05$ from baseline to 6 months), but these levels remained within the normal range. There were no significant changes in serum phosphorus, 25-hydroxyvitamin D or 24-hour urinary calcium in either group. There were two cases of hypercalciuria (one in each group) and three of hypercalcaemia (all in the synthetic parathyroid hormone [1–34] group), but all resolved spontaneously upon reduction of calcium and/or parathyroid hormone intake. In the few patients tested, there was no evidence of antibody development to synthetic parathyroid hormone (1–34) and it was well tolerated, with mild headaches during the early stages of treatment amongst the most common adverse events. Mild injection site tenderness was also reported, but these adverse events did not lead to any withdrawals from the trial.

The second study used teriparatide, 40 µg/day, and employed the change in vertebral cross-sectional area as the primary efficacy outcome.[33] This was based on the hypothesis that if bone formation increased at the periosteal surface, vertebral size would be expected to increase accordingly. After 1 year of teriparatide treatment, the vertebral cross-sectional area of the first and second lumbar vertebrae had increased by 4.8% from baseline ($p<0.001$). A 2.6% increase over baseline persisted after 12 months of follow-up without teriparatide treatment ($p<0.05$). No significant changes from baseline were observed in the group who remained on HRT and corticosteroids alone. Similarly, estimated vertebral compressive strength increased by nearly 200% in the teriparatide group over the 12-month treatment period ($p<0.01$), an effect which was maintained throughout the 12-month follow-up period ($p<0.01$). There was no change in the HRT and corticosteroid only group. Consistent with other reports, teriparatide increased vertebral BMD by nearly 35% after 1 year of treatment ($p<0.001$), whilst the density increased by an additional 2.9% during the 12-month follow-up period ($p<0.001$ *vs* baseline). The increases were non-significant in the group remaining on HRT and corticosteroids alone (1.3 and 0.3%, respectively). The increase in compressive strength was interpreted to be primarily a result of the increase in BMD, and, to a lesser extent, the increase in vertebral cross-sectional area. This is because compressive strength increases in proportion to the square of BMD.

In conclusion, these data indicate that teriparatide is able to override the suppressive effects of chronic corticosteroid treatment on osteoblast function and stimulate bone formation. This effect has also been demonstrated on a background of HRT treatment.

> Teriparatide is able to override the suppressive effects of chronic corticosteroid treatment on osteoblast function and stimulate bone formation.

Efficacy in men

Osteoporosis is primarily a problem in postmenopausal women. However, osteoporosis in men is also a significant health burden, and the aetiology of the disease appears to be more complex in male patients.[35,36] Osteoporosis may be secondary to other conditions, such as hypogonadism, but a considerable proportion of cases in men are idiopathic. These cases are characterised by a low rate of bone turnover, and this characteristic invites the use of anabolic therapies such as teriparatide. Furthermore, skeletal regions composed primarily of trabecular bone are the most severely affected in male patients with idiopathic osteoporosis. Given that the anabolic effects of teriparatide are most pronounced in trabecular bone, significant benefits might, again, be expected in this patient group. Although teriparatide is not currently licensed in the UK for use in male patients, trial data are available to suggest that it may be a useful treatment option in this population.

A large randomised, double-blind, placebo-controlled trial[37] has supplemented data from a number of small trials which have indicated that the 1–34 fragment of parathyroid hormone increases BMD in men with osteoporosis.[38] Male participants were eligible for the trial if they were aged between 30 and 85 years, ambulatory and with a lumbar spine or proximal femur T-score of at least –2. Those with secondary causes of metabolic bone disease such as glucocorticoid excess were excluded, but approximately half had low levels of serum free testosterone. The 437 study participants were randomised to receive placebo or teriparatide, 20 or 40 μg daily, each self-administered by the patient subcutaneously. As was the case in the Fracture Prevention Trial, this study was terminated prematurely due to the concerns arising from the detection of osteosarcomas in rats treated long-term with high doses of teriparatide.[22,23] As a result, the median duration of treatment exposure was 11 months (intended duration was 24 months), though the duration of treatment was significantly less in the teriparatide groups than in the placebo group (median of 313 and 302 days for 20 and 40 μg teriparatide, respectively, *vs* 328 days with placebo; p=0.046).

Teriparatide induced dose-dependent increases in lumbar spine and femoral neck BMD compared with placebo (p<0.001 and p<0.03, respectively) in this male population. At the end of the treatment period, there was a net decrease in lumbar spine BMD in approximately 40% of patients receiving placebo, compared with 7.1 and 6.2% in the 20 and 40 μg teriparatide groups, respectively. Both doses of teriparatide also increased whole body bone mineral content relative to placebo (20 μg, p=0.021; 40 μg, p=0.005), though no significant differences were apparent between the two doses. Teriparatide mediated significant increases in markers of bone formation (BSAP and P1CP) and resorption (NTX/creatinine ratio and free deoxypyridinoline [FDPD]/creatinine ratio) compared with placebo, though at 12 months, P1CP levels in the 20 μg teriparatide group had fallen below those in the placebo group (Figure 6). The effects on BMD and biochemical markers of bone remodelling were shown to be independent of baseline free testosterone or estradiol levels, as well as baseline measurements of body mass index (BMI), lumbar spine BMD, smoking and alcohol intake.

> Teriparatide induced dose-dependent increases in lumbar spine and femoral neck BMD compared with placebo amongst this male population.

Mean serum calcium concentrations (measured 4–6 hours after injection) were higher in teriparatide- than placebo-treated patients at all time points (p<0.001). These levels exceeded the upper limit of normal (2.64 mM) in 6.2% patients who received the lower dose (p=0.003 *vs* placebo) and in 16.8% receiving the higher dose of teriparatide (p<0.001 *vs* placebo). A reduction in calcium supplementation was permitted and indeed implemented in some patients. Nonetheless 2% of patients in the 20 μg teriparatide group and 4% in the 40 μg group withdrew from the trial due to elevated post-injection serum calcium levels.[a] Mean urinary calcium excretion increased in all groups, but this was shown to occur in response to calcium and vitamin D supplementation rather than teriparatide or placebo injections. Concentrations of serum 1,25-dihydroxyvitamin D_3 increased in both active treatment groups compared with placebo, though from 6 months onwards, the difference was only significant in the 40 μg group (p<0.05). At month 12, the mean serum concentration of intact parathyroid hormone was below the limit of quantification in approximately 90% of patients in all three

---

[a]Hypercalcaemic events are considered rare in clinical practice, and patients receiving teriparatide treatment are advised to maintain dietary calcium and vitamin D supplementation.

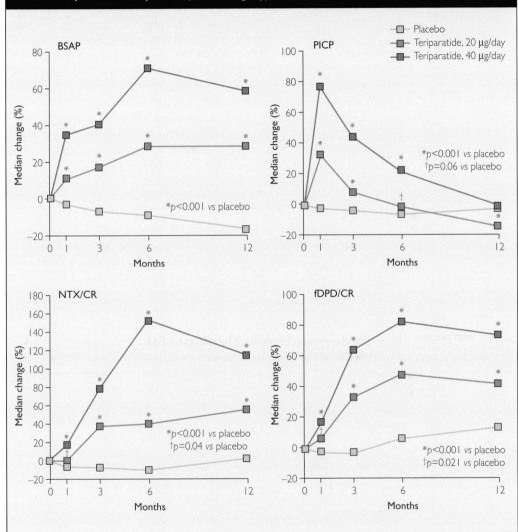

Figure 6. Median percentage changes in biochemical markers of bone formation (bone-specific alkaline phosphatase [BSAP]; procollagen I carboxy-terminal [PICP]) and bone resorption (urinary N-telopeptide/creatinine ratio [NTX/CR]; free deoxypyridinoline/creatinine ratio, [fDPD/CR]) in patients treated with placebo or teriparatide (20 or 40 µg/day).[37]

groups. The incidence of urolithiasis was statistically equivalent in all three groups. Small changes in levels of uric acid, serum chloride and serum magnesium were not associated with any adverse clinical events.

Adverse events occurred with a similar incidence in all three groups, and led to withdrawal from the trial in 4.8, 9.3 and 12.9% of patients in the placebo, and teriparatide, 20 µg and 40 µg, groups, respectively (p=0.052 for pooled teriparatide vs placebo). The rate of nausea was greater in the 40 µg teriparatide group than in the placebo group (18.7 vs 3.4%, respectively; p<0.001) but not in the 20 µg group (5.3%). There was a non-significant trend for an increased rate of headache in the 40 µg teriparatide group. The rate of non-vertebral fractures was low (≤2.0%) and was statistically equivalent in all three groups. Two deaths were reported, but neither was considered to be related to the study treatment or procedures. There were also six cases of cancer (three in placebo group and three in 20 µg teriparatide group) but none of these were osteosarcomas.

This trial demonstrated, therefore, that daily injections of teriparatide increased spinal and femoral BMD, as well as whole body bone mineral content in men with osteoporosis. The time course and magnitude of the change in lumbar spinal BMD were similar to those in postmenopausal women in the Fracture Prevention Trial.[22] The similarities of the observations made in a male osteoporotic population compared with the findings in female patients would suggest that the reduction in fracture risk identified in women would also apply to male patients, but this would need to be formally demonstrated in a trial setting.

<aside>Daily injections of teriparatide increased spinal and femoral BMD, as well as whole body bone mineral content in men with osteoporosis.</aside>

Efficacy compared with alendronate

A number of comparative trials have evaluated the relative efficacy of teriparatide and alendronate. As antiresorptive agents remain the most widely used treatments for osteoporosis in postmenopausal women, these comparisons are directly relevant to clinical practice. A multicentre, randomised, double-blind, double-dummy trial has compared the efficacy of teriparatide and alendronate in ambulatory women who were at least 5 years postmenopausal (n=146).[39] Eligible women were aged between 30 and 85 years and demonstrated a lumbar spine or femoral neck BMD T-score of –2.5 or less. Participants in this trial completed a screening and run-in phase of up to 2 months, during which time they received training in self-injection using placebo, as well as at least 1 month of daily supplements of calcium (1000 mg) and vitamin D (400–1200 IU). Participants were then randomised to 24 months' treatment with either teriparatide (40 µg once daily) plus oral placebo or alendronate sodium (10 mg orally) plus a once-daily placebo injection. The trial was, however, terminated prematurely after a median of 14 months of treatment (in both groups), due to the findings of the rat carcinogenicity study described previously.[23] There was no difference by treatment group in the number of women completing 6 and 12 months of testing. The median compliance during the treatment period was 67 and 71% for the teriparatide and alendronate groups, respectively.

In the lumbar spine, teriparatide increased BMD, bone mineral content and projected bone area by a greater extent than alendronate treatment. The difference in BMD between treatment groups at 3 months amounted to 2.7% in favour of teriparatide, which increased to 5.4% at 6 months and 8.3% at 12 months ($p<0.001$ *vs* alendronate at each time point). The change in bone mineral content from baseline to endpoint was 15.1% in the teriparatide group, compared with 6.6% in the alendronate group ($p<0.001$). Spinal bone area was increased by 1.29 cm^2 in the teriparatide group, compared with 0.49 cm^2 in the alendronate group ($p=0.002$).

Femoral neck and total hip BMD were also increased by a greater extent following treatment with teriparatide than with alendronate ($p \leq 0.01$). Teriparatide also increased total body bone mineral and decreased one-third distal radius by a greater extent than alendronate ($p \leq 0.05$ and $p \leq 0.001$, respectively).

The superiority of teriparatide compared with alendronate on bone translated to a significantly lower non-vertebral fracture frequency (4.1 vs 13.7%; $p = 0.042$). Mean height did not, however, change significantly from baseline in either treatment group. The anabolic effect of teriparatide was demonstrated by significant increases in markers of bone resorption (NTX corrected for creatinine) and of bone formation (serum BSAP).

The proportion of women withdrawing from the teriparatide and alendronate groups due to adverse events was not significantly different (19 vs 10%, respectively; $p = 0.099$). The rates of adverse events and serious adverse events were also statistically equivalent in the two groups. One patient in the teriparatide group died of a cardiac arrest, but this was not considered to be related to the study treatment. New or worsened back pain was more common in the teriparatide than in the alendronate group (19.2 vs 5.5%; $p = 0.012$), as were leg cramps (8.2 vs 0%; $p = 0.012$).

Median post-dose (within 4–6 hours) serum calcium levels with teriparatide peaked 6 months into the treatment period, and were higher than those recorded in the alendronate group (10.0 vs 9.2 mg/dL; $p < 0.001$). These elevations, however, were not associated with any clinically significant adverse outcomes. In addition, there was a significant increase in urinary calcium in the teriparatide group (by 38 mg/day) at the 1-month visit but not in the alendronate group ($p = 0.001$ between groups and between teriparatide and baseline). After this time point, however, there was no significant difference in urinary calcium excretion between treatment groups. Teriparatide increased total alkaline phosphatase, whereas alendronate reduced this parameter, consistent with the respective modes of action of the two drugs. Teriparatide also mediated a slight increase in serum uric acid at 12 months, as well as a significant increase in serum 1,25-dihydroxyvitamin D_3 and significant decreases in serum intact parathyroid hormone and in 25-hydroxyvitamin D compared with alendronate. Antiteriparatide antibodies developed in three women but were not associated with any adverse clinical events.

The superior efficacy of teriparatide compared with alendronate was further demonstrated in a trial which, in addition to comparing the individual monotherapies, investigated the hypothesis that the combination of an antiresorptive and an anabolic drug would provide a therapeutic advantage by virtue of their differing mechanisms of fracture risk reduction.[40] However, this trial used the full length parathyroid hormone (1–84) rather than the 1–34 fragment and as such will not be discussed in detail here. Nonetheless, it is worth considering the major conclusion of this trial – that there was no evidence of synergy between parathyroid hormone and alendronate. This finding was mirrored in a

> The superiority of teriparatide compared with alendronate on bone translated to a significantly lower non-vertebral fracture frequency.

There was no
evidence of
synergy between
parathyroid
hormone and
alendronate.

study which compared the efficacy of the 1–34 parathyroid fragment and alendronate when given alone or combination to an exclusively male population.[41] In order to be eligible, men were required to be between 46 and 85 years of age and to have a lumbar spine or femoral neck BMD T-score of –2 or less (n=83). Patients were randomised to treatment with alendronate alone (10 mg/day), teriparatide alone (40 μg/day once daily) or both drugs given concurrently. In addition to these, patients received 400 U of vitamin D daily and calcium intake was maintained at 1000–1200 mg daily.

This trial has generated useful data on the differing effects of the drug on BMD at various skeletal sites (Figure 7). However, it should be emphasised that teriparatide is not currently licensed for use by male patients in the UK. A further important consideration is that the maximum duration of treatment in this trial was 30 months, whereas the maximum recommended duration is 18 months.[6] Teriparatide increased BMD relative to either alendronate or combination therapy ($p<0.001$ in all cases) at the posteroanterior and lateral spine, as well as the femoral neck. In the posteroanterior and lateral spine, the combination therapy was more effective than alendronate alone ($p<0.001$ and $p=0.02$, respectively), whereas at the femoral neck, combination therapy and alendronate mediated equivalent increases in BMD ($p=0.08$). The BMD measurement for the total hip was greater in the teriparatide group than in the alendronate alone group ($p=0.005$), but was not significantly different from the group receiving combination therapy ($p=0.08$). Alendronate as a monotherapy was also equivalent in efficacy to the combination treatment on this parameter ($p=0.2$). At the radial shaft, BMD increased in the alendronate and combination groups, but decreased in the teriparatide group ($p=0.002$ *vs* alendronate; $p=0.009$ *vs* combination group). There were no significant differences between the three groups in total body BMD ($p=0.6$).

The trabecular BMD at the spine increased with teriparatide compared with either alendronate or the combination treatment ($p<0.001$), with the combination superior to alendronate alone ($p=0.005$). The peak serum alkaline phosphatase level was greater in the teriparatide group than in the combination or alendronate-only groups ($p<0.001$), which did not differ from each other in this parameter ($p=0.14$).

There were no significant differences in serum calcium levels measured either 4 or 24 hours after injection. Urinary calcium excretion exceeded 400 mg/day in more patients receiving the combination therapy than alendronate (10.5 *vs* 2.1%; $p=0.004$). Teriparatide treatment was associated with more headache ($p=0.05$), dizziness ($p=0.05$), joint pain ($p<0.001$), back pain ($p=0.003$), but less chest pain ($p=0.02$) than alendronate alone. Teriparatide was also associated with more joint pain ($p=0.01$), back pain ($p=0.03$), but less shortness of breath ($p=0.007$) than the combination therapy.

This trial has therefore shown that alendronate impairs the ability of teriparatide to stimulate new bone formation in male osteoporotic patients. The fact that a reduction in bone resorption (due to

Teriparatide
increased BMD
relative to either
alendronate or
combination
therapy at the
posteroanterior
and lateral spine,
as well as the
femoral neck.

Figure 7. Mean percentage change in bone mineral density at various skeletal sites with alendronate, teriparatide, or combination therapy.[41]

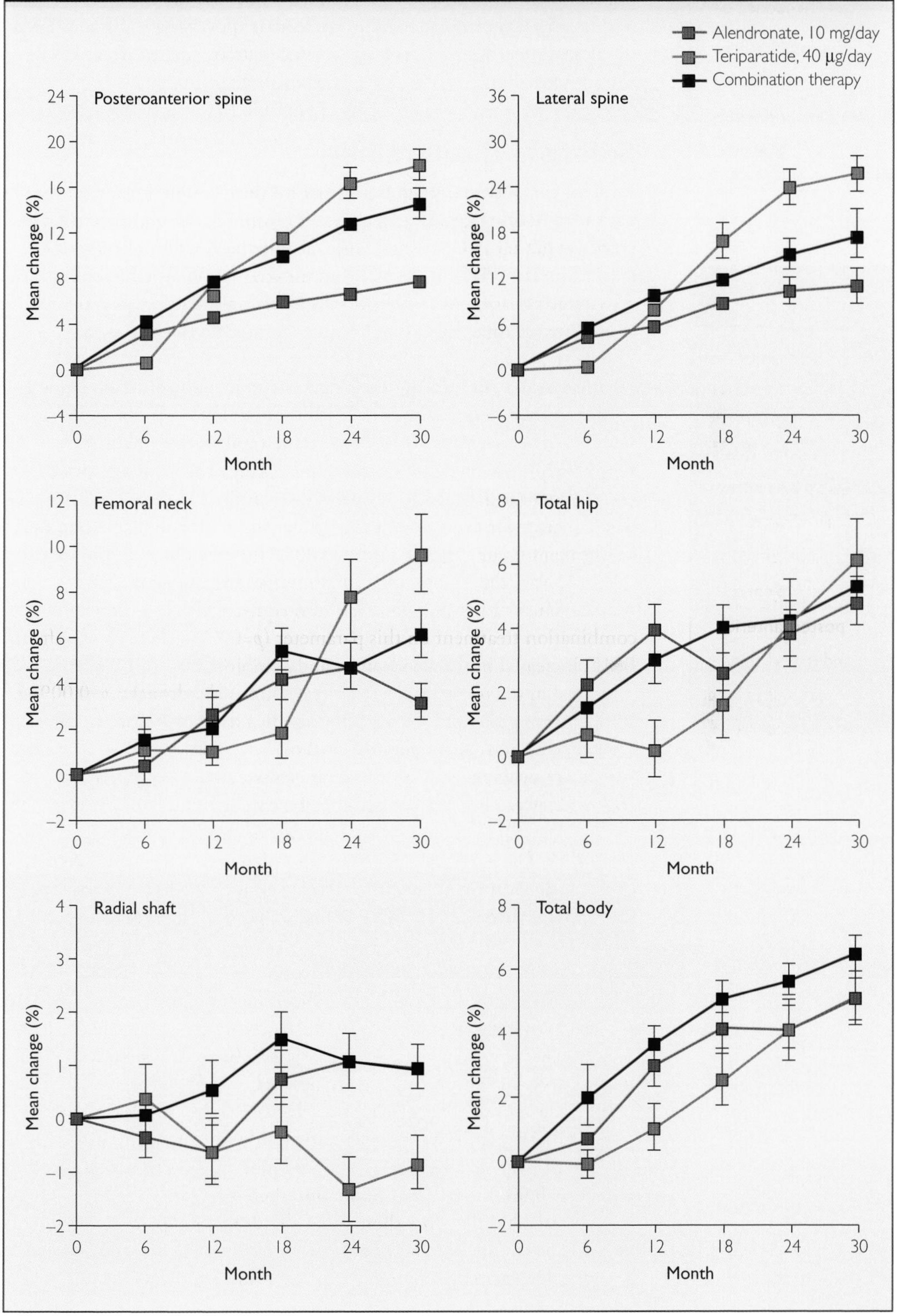

Alendronate impairs the ability of teriparatide to stimulate new bone formation in male osteoporotic patients.

You are strongly urged to consult your doctor before taking, stopping or changing any of the products reviewed or referred to in *BESTMEDICINE* or any other medication that has been prescribed or recommended by your doctor.

alendronate treatment, for example) mitigates the anabolic effects of teriparatide on bone was interpreted as evidence that the hormone acts indirectly, stimulating new bone formation by first increasing osteoclastic bone resorption. The addition of alendronate also prevented the teriparatide-induced decrease in BMD at the radial shaft, a skeletal site composed mainly of non-weight-bearing cortical bone.

Safety and tolerability

Although a considerable proportion of patients experience adverse events with teriparatide treatment in clinical trials, the same applies to patients receiving placebo.[6] Consistent with this, the most common adverse event is pain in the limb, which is most likely a non-specific result of the subcutaneous injection. Other common adverse events in patients treated with teriparatide include nausea, headache and dizziness (Table 3).[9]

Elevated serum calcium levels do not appear to be of major clinical concern as most cases of hypercalcaemia are mild.[22,37] Indeed, as mentioned earlier, patients receiving teriparatide are advised to supplement their diet with calcium and vitamin D.[6] Urinary calcium excretion was unaffected by teriparatide treatment in the majority of cases. Two trials have reported cases of hypercalciuria, but these resolved following reductions in calcium intake.[33,42] In one isolated trial, serum calcium levels and urinary calcium excretion decreased following teriparatide treatment.[43] There has been some evidence of development of antibodies which cross-react with teriparatide, but there have been no reports of hypersensitivity or allergic reactions.[6,22,39]

The major safety concern associated with teriparatide treatment arose from a routine preclinical safety trial conducted in male and female Fischer 344 rats.[23] These rats were treated with teriparatide at 75 µg/kg, which was predicted to be the maximum tolerated dose, but is also over 200-times greater than that used therapeutically in humans. As expected,

Table 3. Incidence of the most common adverse events following treatment with teriparatide, 20 µg/day, in clinical trials.[9,22,37]

Adverse event	Incidence (%)
Elevated serum calcium level[a]	6.2–11
Nausea	5.3–8
Headache	5.3–8
Leg cramps	0.7–3
Dizziness	9
Withdrawal due to adverse drug event	6–9.3

[a]Elevated level defined in this case as >10.6 mg/dL. In the UK, it is usually defined as >2.65 mmol/L.

teriparatide generated increases in bone mass. However, these increases were excessive in magnitude, and not only raised BMD, but also induced periosteal expansion and alterations in bone size and shape. Furthermore, these exaggerated changes were accompanied by a dose-dependent increase in the incidence of bone proliferative lesions, including osteosarcoma. As previously discussed, these findings have raised serious concerns over the safety of chronic treatment with parathyroid hormone or its fragments. A number of factors, however, were highlighted by the investigators at the time of this study, and have been upheld since, which suggest that these data are of little relevance to the clinical setting.[23,44] These discussions focus on three main aspects. First, the rats in this trial were treated daily for approximately 80–90% of their normal life span, whereas in humans, the recommended maximum duration of therapy (18 months) represents less than 2% of the average life span. Similarly, the treatment period in rats encompassed approximately 25–30 bone-turnover cycles, whereas only 1–3 cycles would be expected to occur in osteoporotic women during the course of treatment with teriparatide. Thirdly, the physiology of rat and human bone is fundamentally different. In rats, longitudinal skeletal growth occurs throughout life, whereas in humans, growth plates close and longitudinal growth ceases to occur by the age of approximately 30 years. The potential for teriparatide-induced changes in bone mass and development of proliferative lesions appears therefore to be much greater in rats.

In support of these considerations, there have been no reported cases of osteosarcoma in patients treated with teriparatide thus far. Furthermore, the drug was deemed neither mutagenic nor genotoxic in a series of standard *in vitro* and *in vivo* tests.[37] Although the osteosarcoma cases in rats are not considered to be clinically relevant in humans, precautionary measures with teriparatide treatment are advised. The maximum treatment period is currently set at 18 months, and the drug is contraindicated in patients who have received prior radiation therapy to the skeleton.[6]

Teriparatide is also contraindicated in patients with pre-existing hypercalcaemia, severe renal impairment, unexplained elevations of BSAP and in patients with metabolic bone diseases other than osteoporosis, including hyperparathyroidism and Paget's disease of the bone. Studies in rabbits have demonstrated some reproductive toxicity, hence teriparatide is not licensed in patients who are pregnant or breast-feeding.[6,7] No significant drug–drug interactions have been reported.[9]

Pharmacoeconomics

Despite the potential benefits of teriparatide treatment, it is an expensive option, with direct drug costs over ten-times those of alendronate.[7] Comprehensive pharmacoeconomic studies are yet to be conducted to assess to what extent the clinical efficacy of teriparatide reduces direct and indirect disease-associated costs. However, given the current discrepancy in drug costs, teriparatide is not considered a first-line

> Although the osteosarcoma cases in rats are not considered to be clinically relevant in humans, precautionary measures with teriparatide treatment are advised.

treatment option in the UK at present, and this is likely to remain the case for the foreseeable future. The treatment is most likely to be cost-effective in elderly post-menopausal women who have established osteoporosis, a very high fracture risk, and inadequate response to alternative therapies.[45]

Key points

- Teriparatide is the N-terminal 34-amino acid fragment of human recombinant parathyroid hormone and demonstrates the same effect on bone as the full-length (84-amino acid) hormone.

- Teriparatide exerts an anabolic effect on bone, which appears to be promoted by a postponement of apoptosis in osteoblasts, the cells responsible for bone formation.

- Teriparatide acts preferentially on trabecular-rich skeletal sites, such as the vertebrae. The efficacy at cortical-rich sites appears to be less pronounced, though the existing evidence is not generally supportive of the 'cortical steal' hypothesis.

- The major clinical trial of teriparatide – the Fracture Prevention Trial – has demonstrated that 20 and 40 µg/day doses are similarly effective at reducing the risk of vertebral and non-vertebral fractures, though the higher dose was less well tolerated. Only the 20 µg/day dose is licensed in the UK.

- Teriparatide appears to be equally effective over a range of baseline age, BMD or prevalent fracture burden.

- Teriparatide is effective in patients previously exposed to antiresorptive therapy, though persisting effects of prior alendronate, in particular, can affect the time course of teriparatide-induced changes. Concurrent use of teriparatide and bisphosphonates is not recommended.

- Teriparatide is effective on a background of HRT, with or without concurrent corticosteroid therapy, though it is not licensed for treatment of corticosteroid-induced osteoporosis.

- Although not licensed for use in men in the UK, teriparatide exerts similar benefits in men with osteoporosis as in women with postmenopausal osteoporosis. The effect on risk of incident fractures in teriparatide-treated men has yet to be reported.

- Teriparatide is generally well tolerated, and the risk of osteosarcoma identified in rats is considered to have little relevance to human patients.

References

A list of the published evidence which has been reviewed in compiling the preceding section of *BESTMEDICINE*.

1 Brixen KT, Christensen PM, Ejersted C, Langdahl BL. Teriparatide (biosynthetic human parathyroid hormone 1–34): a new paradigm in the treatment of osteoporosis. *Basic Clin Pharmacol Toxicol* 2004; **94**: 260–70.

2 McClung M. Parathyroid hormone for the treatment of osteoporosis. *Obstet Gynecol Surv* 2004; **59**: 826–32.

3 Selye H. On the stimulation of new bone formation with parathyroid extract and irradiated ergosterol. *Endocrinology* 1932; **16**: 547–58.

4 Dempster DW, Cosman F, Parisien M, Shen V, Lindsay R. Anabolic actions of parathyroid hormone on bone. *Endocr Rev* 1993; **14**: 690–709.

5 Hodsman AB, Bauer DC, Dempster D *et al.* Parathyroid hormone and teriparatide for the treatment of osteoporosis: a review of the evidence and suggested guidelines for its use. *Endocr Rev* 2005; E-pub ahead of print.

6 Eli Lilly and Company Ltd. Forsteo® (teriparatide). *Summary of product characteristics*. Basingstoke, July 2003.

7 *British National Formulary (BNF) 49*: London: the British Medical Association and the Royal Pharmaceutical Society of Great Britain. March 2005.

8 Lindsay R, Nieves J, Henneman E, Shen V, Cosman F. Subcutaneous administration of the amino-terminal fragment of human parathyroid hormone-(1–34): kinetics and biochemical response in estrogenized osteoporotic patients. *J Clin Endocrinol Metab* 1993; **77**: 1535–9.

9 Cappuzzo KA, Delafuente JC. Teriparatide for severe osteoporosis. *Ann Pharmacother* 2004; **38**: 294–302.

10 Sharpe M, Noble S, Spencer CM. Alendronate: an update of its use in osteoporosis. *Drugs* 2001; **61**: 999–1039.

11 Marie PJ. Strontium ranelate: a novel mode of action optimizing bone formation and resorption. *Osteoporos Int* 2005; **16(Suppl 1)**: S7–10.

12 Liu CC, Kalu DN. Human parathyroid hormone-(1–34) prevents bone loss and augments bone formation in sexually mature ovariectomized rats. *J Bone Miner Res* 1990; **5**: 973–82.

13 Ejersted C, Andreassen TT, Oxlund H *et al.* Human parathyroid hormone (1–34) and (1–84) increase the mechanical strength and thickness of cortical bone in rats. *J Bone Miner Res* 1993; **8**: 1097–101.

14 Oxlund H, Ejersted C, Andreassen TT, Torring O, Nilsson MH. Parathyroid hormone (1–34) and (1–84) stimulate cortical bone formation both from periosteum and endosteum. *Calcif Tissue Int* 1993; **53**: 394–9.

15 Podbesek R, Edouard C, Meunier PJ *et al.* Effects of two treatment regimes with synthetic human parathyroid hormone fragment on bone formation and the tissue balance of trabecular bone in greyhounds. *Endocrinology* 1983; **112**: 1000–6.

16 Hirano T, Burr DB, Turner CH *et al.* Anabolic effects of human biosynthetic parathyroid hormone fragment (1–34), LY333334, on remodeling and mechanical properties of cortical bone in rabbits. *J Bone Miner Res* 1999; **14**: 536–45.

17 Rubin MR, Cosman F, Lindsay R, Bilezikian JP. The anabolic effects of parathyroid hormone. *Osteoporos Int* 2002; **13**: 267–77.

18 Dobnig H, Turner RT. The effects of programmed administration of human parathyroid hormone fragment (1–34) on bone histomorphometry and serum chemistry in rats. *Endocrinology* 1997; **138**: 4607–12.

19 Jilka RL, Weinstein RS, Bellido T *et al.* Increased bone formation by prevention of osteoblast apoptosis with parathyroid hormone. *J Clin Invest* 1999; **104**: 439–46.

20 Tomkinson A, Gevers EF, Wit JM, Reeve J, Noble BS. The role of estrogen in the control of rat osteocyte apoptosis. *J Bone Miner Res* 1998; **13**: 1243–50.

21 Weinstein RS, Jilka RL, Parfitt AM, Manolagas SC. Inhibition of osteoblastogenesis and promotion of apoptosis of osteoblasts and osteocytes by glucocorticoids. Potential mechanisms of their deleterious effects on bone. *J Clin Invest* 1998; **102**: 274–82.

22 Neer RM, Arnaud CD, Zanchetta JR *et al.* Effect of parathyroid hormone (1–34) on fractures and bone mineral density in postmenopausal women with osteoporosis. *N Engl J Med* 2001; **344**: 1434–41.

23 Vahle JL, Sato M, Long GG *et al.* Skeletal changes in rats given daily subcutaneous injections of recombinant human parathyroid hormone (1-34) for 2 years and relevance to human safety. *Toxicol Pathol* 2002; **30**: 312–21.

24 Marcus R, Wang O, Satterwhite J, Mitlak B. The skeletal response to teriparatide is largely independent of age, initial bone mineral density, and prevalent vertebral fractures in postmenopausal women with osteoporosis. *J Bone Miner Res* 2003; **18**: 18–23.

25 Gallagher JC, Genant HK, Crans GG, Vargas SJ, Krege JH. Teriparatide reduces the fracture risk associated with increasing number and severity of osteoporotic fractures. *J Clin Endocrinol Metab* 2005; **90**: 1583–7.

26 Jiang Y, Zhao JJ, Mitlak BH *et al.* Recombinant human parathyroid hormone (1-34) [teriparatide] improves both cortical and cancellous bone structure. *J Bone Miner Res* 2003; **18**: 1932–41.

27 Zanchetta JR, Bogado CE, Ferretti JL *et al.* Effects of teriparatide [recombinant human parathyroid hormone (1-34)] on cortical bone in postmenopausal women with osteoporosis. *J Bone Miner Res* 2003; **18**: 539–43.

28 Horwitz M, Stewart A, Greenspan SL. Sequential parathyroid hormone/alendronate therapy for osteoporosis – robbing Peter to pay Paul? *J Clin Endocrinol Metab* 2000; **85**: 2127–8.

29 Ettinger B, San Martin J, Crans G, Pavo I. Differential effects of teriparatide on BMD after treatment with raloxifene or alendronate. *J Bone Miner Res* 2004; **19**: 745–51.

30 Tonino RP, Meunier PJ, Emkey R *et al.* Skeletal benefits of alendronate: 7-year treatment of postmenopausal osteoporotic women. Phase III Osteoporosis Treatment Study Group. *J Clin Endocrinol Metab* 2000; **85**: 3109–15.

31 Lindsay R, Nieves J, Formica C *et al.* Randomised controlled study of effect of parathyroid hormone on vertebral-bone mass and fracture incidence among postmenopausal women on oestrogen with osteoporosis. *Lancet* 1997; **350**: 550–5.

32 Lane NE, Sanchez S, Modin GW *et al.* Parathyroid hormone treatment can reverse corticosteroid-induced osteoporosis. Results of a randomized controlled clinical trial. *J Clin Invest* 1998; **102**: 1627–33.

33 Rehman Q, Lang TF, Arnaud CD, Modin GW, Lane NE. Daily treatment with parathyroid hormone is associated with an increase in vertebral cross-sectional area in postmenopausal women with glucocorticoid-induced osteoporosis. *Osteoporos Int* 2003; **14**: 77–81.

34 Lukert BP, Raisz LG. Glucocorticoid-induced osteoporosis: pathogenesis and management. *Ann Intern Med* 1990; **112**: 352–64.

35 Vanderschueren D, Boonen S, Bouillon R. Osteoporosis and osteoporotic fractures in men: a clinical perspective. *Baillieres Best Pract Res Clin Endocrinol Metab* 2000; **14**: 299–315.

36 Ebeling PR. Idiopathic or hypogonadal osteoporosis in men: current and future treatment options. *Treat Endocrinol* 2004; **3**: 381–91.

37 Orwoll ES, Scheele WH, Paul S *et al.* The effect of teriparatide [human parathyroid hormone (1–34)] therapy on bone density in men with osteoporosis. *J Bone Miner Res* 2003; **18**: 9–17.

38 Kurland ES, Cosman F, McMahon DJ *et al.* Parathyroid hormone as a therapy for idiopathic osteoporosis in men: effects on bone mineral density and bone markers. *J Clin Endocrinol Metab* 2000; **85**: 3069–76.

39 Body JJ, Gaich GA, Scheele WH *et al.* A randomized double-blind trial to compare the efficacy of teriparatide [recombinant human parathyroid hormone (1–34)] with alendronate in postmenopausal women with osteoporosis. *J Clin Endocrinol Metab* 2002; **87**: 4528–35.

40 Black DM, Greenspan SL, Ensrud KE *et al.* The effects of parathyroid hormone and alendronate alone or in combination in postmenopausal osteoporosis. *N Engl J Med* 2003; **349**: 1207–15.

41 Finkelstein JS, Hayes A, Hunzelman JL *et al.* The effects of parathyroid hormone, alendronate, or both in men with osteoporosis. *N Engl J Med* 2003; **349**: 1216–26.

42 Finkelstein JS, Klibanski A, Schaefer EH *et al.* Parathyroid hormone for the prevention of bone loss induced by estrogen deficiency. *N Engl J Med* 1994; **331**: 1618–23.

43 Fujita T, Inoue T, Morii H *et al.* Effect of an intermittent weekly dose of human parathyroid hormone (1-34) on osteoporosis: a randomized double-masked prospective study using three dose levels. *Osteoporos Int* 1999; **9**: 296–306.

44 Tashjian AH, Chabner BA. Commentary on clinical safety of recombinant human parathyroid hormone 1-34 in the treatment of osteoporosis in men and postmenopausal women. *J Bone Miner Res* 2002; **17**: 1151–61.

45 National Institute for Health and Clinical Excellence (NICE) guidelines: Technology Appraisal 87 – Bisphosphonates (alendronate, etidronate, risedronate), selective oestrogen receptor modulators (raloxifene) and parathyroid hormone (teriparatide) for the secondary prevention of osteoporotic fragility fractures in postmenopausal women. January 2005. *www.nice.org.uk*

Acknowledgements

Figure 2 is adapted from Neer *et al.*, 2001.[22]
Figure 3 is adapted from Gallagher *et al.*, 2005.[25]
Figure 4 is adapted from Ettinger *et al.*, 2004.[29]
Figure 5 is adapted from Lindsay *et al.*, 1997.[31]
Figure 6 is adapted from Orwoll *et al.*, 2003.[37]
Figure 7 is adapted from Finkelstein *et al.*, 2003.[41]

PATIENT NOTES
Dr Pam Brown

Drug treatment for osteoporosis

Although the diagnosis of osteoporosis can be alarming for the patient and their families, it is very reassuring that there are several very effective drugs currently available for both the prevention and treatment of the disease, and all of these (with the exception of teriparatide [Forsteo®]), can be prescribed by GPs working in primary care. These drugs are:

- calcium and vitamin D
- bisphosphonates (e.g. alendronate [Fosamax®], risedronate [Actonel®] and cyclical etidronate (Didronel® PMO).
- raloxifene (Evista®)
- strontium ranelate (Protelos®)
- teriparatide (Forsteo®)

In-depth reviews of the clinical evidence underlying the use of most of these drugs can be found in the preceding sections of this edition of *BESTMEDICINE*. Here, we will summarise the benefits and side-effects of each, and the recent guidance from the National Institute for Health and Clinical Excellence (NICE [see Reader's Guide for more information]) on how these drugs should be used.

How does drug treatment work?

As discussed in the Disease Overview and the earlier Patient Notes chapter, bone tissue is continuously being broken down (resorbed) by bone-eating cells (osteoclasts) and built up again by bone-building cells (osteoblasts). In people with osteoporosis, the osteoclasts are eating away bone faster than the osteoblasts can build it up again, resulting in a net loss of bone. The currently available treatments work by either slowing down the rate of bone resorption or speeding up the bone-building process. The bisphosphonates, raloxifene and hormone replacement therapy (HRT) all slow down bone resorption, whilst teriparatide works mainly by increasing bone formation. Strontium ranelate is the first of a new class of drug – the dual action bone agents (DABAs) – which work by decreasing bone resorption and increasing bone formation.

Calcium and vitamin D

Most vitamin D is made by the action of sunlight on the skin, and this is then converted into its active form by the liver and kidneys. Most housebound elderly people are vitamin D deficient

> *Currently available treatments work by either slowing down the rate of bone resorption or speeding up the bone-building process.*

because they eat a poor diet and do not get enough sunlight. Dietary sources of vitamin D include fish, margarines and some dairy products. Vitamin D is important for calcium absorption from the diet. Vitamin D deficiency can result in muscle weakness and increased body sway, leading to a greater risk of falling, thereby further increasing the risk of hip fractures.

Calcium and vitamin D are used in two ways. First, in frail, elderly, housebound people, calcium and vitamin D can help to reduce hip fractures by up to one-third. Vitamin D (given at a dose of 800 IU/day) and calcium (800–1200 mg/day) are both required, and are usually divided into two doses and taken with food to improve absorption. Second, calcium and vitamin D are also recommended as 'adjuvant' (additional) therapy for everyone who requires a bone-sparing treatment to prevent or treat osteoporosis, since most people participating in the clinical trials of these drugs also received calcium and vitamin D. The NICE technology appraisal also recommended that all patients should receive calcium and vitamin D unless they are known to be receiving an adequate amount from their diet. If you have chosen to buy calcium and vitamin D tablets, make sure that you buy a product with high enough doses and take them regularly.

The NICE technology appraisal recommended that all patients should receive calcium and vitamin D.

Bisphosphonates

The NICE Technology Appraisal published in January 2005 provides guidance on the use of the bisphosphonates (i.e. alendronate, etidronate, risedronate), the selective oestrogen receptor modulators (raloxifene) and parathyroid hormone (teriparatide) in postmenopausal women who have already suffered one or more fractures. Guidance on the prevention of osteoporosis in those who have not yet had a fracture and on the recently introduced strontium ranelate is expected later in 2005 or in early 2006.

The recommendations made in the NICE guidance for women with a fragility fracture are summarised below.

- Women 75 years and over should be started on bone-sparing therapy and do not require a dual energy X-ray absorptiometry (DXA) scan.
- Women aged 65–74 should receive treatment if their DXA scan confirms osteoporosis (i.e. a T-score of less than –2.5 SD).
- Women under the age of 65 years should only be treated if their DXA T-score is –3 SD or below, or if they have a T-score of below –2.5 SD and one or more additional age-independent risk factors, including a body mass index (BMI) below 19 kg/m^2, maternal hip fracture that occurred before the age of 75 years, untreated premature menopause, medical disorders associated with bone loss (including inflammatory bowel disease, rheumatoid arthritis, hyperthyroidism, coeliac disease) or conditions associated with prolonged immobility.

- Bisphosphonates should be used as first-line treatment in all of these women.
- Women who have an unsatisfactory response (i.e. another fracture despite adhering fully to therapy for 1 year, and evidence of decline in bone density below pre-treatment levels) should be considered for treatment with raloxifene.
- Women who are unable to tolerate bisphosphonate therapy (ulcers or strictures in the oesophagus, diarrhoea or abdominal pain severe enough to result in treatment discontinuation) should also be considered for raloxifene.

Whilst we await further guidance, doctors will continue to make decisions about which treatments to choose and which patients to treat, including those who have osteoporosis but have not yet had a fracture. As discussed previously, strontium ranelate has not yet been covered by the NICE guidance and so can be used first line if it is preferred to a bisphosphonate.

Although cyclical etidronate, alendronate and risedronate have all been shown to significantly increase bone density at both the hip and spine, and to decrease fractures at the spine, randomised controlled trials have only confirmed that alendronate and risedronate decrease hip fractures. All the bisphosphonates need to be taken exactly as directed to ensure that they are absorbed and also to minimise side-effects. Etidronate is taken daily for 14 days at the midpoint of a four-hour fast, followed by 76 days of calcium supplements. Alendronate and risedronate are available as once-daily or once-weekly tablets and must be taken on an empty stomach, first thing in the morning, swallowed whole with a full glass of water and at least 30 minutes before food, drink or other oral medications. The patient needs to remain upright after dosing to ensure that the tablet passes straight into their stomach.

Raloxifene

Raloxifene is a selective oestrogen receptor modulator (SERM), which means that it has oestrogen-like effects on some tissues, for example bone. Under NICE guidance, raloxifene is an alternative treatment for osteoporosis in women if bisphosphonates are contraindicated, not tolerated or not effective. Raloxifene can also be used in women who are unable to remain upright after therapy, and in women who have not yet had their first osteoporotic fracture as preventive therapy. Although raloxifene improves bone density at both the hip and spine, it does not reduce the risk of hip fractures and so is usually used in younger postmenopausal women. It increases the risk of blood clots in the legs and lungs slightly, and increases hot flushes, but also significantly decreases the risk of one type of breast cancer.

Raloxifene is usually used in younger postmenopausal women.

Strontium ranelate increases bone density and decreases fractures at all sites including the hip and spine.

Strontium ranelate

Strontium ranelate has only recently become available in the UK. It is a daily oral treatment, available in a 2 gram sachet of tasteless granules that are mixed with water and taken alone, preferably at bedtime, and at least 2 hours after food to ensure good absorption. It increases bone density and decreases fractures at all sites including the hip and spine. A small risk of blood clots in the legs and lungs has been shown in clinical trials, but it is not yet clear why this occurs. The incidence of heartburn and more serious upper gastrointestinal side-effects were shown to be comparable with placebo. Some patients may experience diarrhoea in the early stages of treatment but this appears to settle with time. As strontium ranelate therapy increases the bone density by a disproportionate amount, a special formula must be used to calculate the actual improvements on DXA scans.

Teriparatide

Teriparatide is given as an 18-month course of daily injections. The treatment has to be prescribed by a hospital specialist, but patients are taught how to give the injections at home. Since this is a new treatment and is expensive, NICE has laid down strict regulations for which patients can be given teriparatide:

- women aged 65 years and older who have had an unsatisfactory response to bisphosphonates (see above) or who are intolerant to them AND
- have an extremely low bone density (T-score approximately −4 SD or less) OR
- have a very low bone density (T-score approximately −3 SD or below) AND
  - multiple fractures (more than two) AND
  - one or more age-independent risk factors (BMI <19kg/m^2, maternal hip fracture before the age of 75 years, untreated premature menopause, conditions associated with prolonged immobility).

Teriparatide is not suitable for people who have high calcium levels, severe kidney failure, other types of bone disease (e.g. osteomalacia), or previous radiotherapy to their skeleton.

HRT

Although HRT improves bone density and reduces the risk of fractures, it is no longer recommended for long-term use to prevent or treat osteoporosis. This is due to the increased risk of breast cancer, coronary heart disease, stroke and dementia that has been demonstrated in randomised controlled studies. Short-term use for 3 or 4 years around the time of the menopause is probably safe to treat menopausal symptoms in most women.

8. Improving practice

Dr Pam Brown, BSc, MB ChB, DFFP, MBA, Dip Ther, Dip Sports Ex Med.
General Practitioner, Uplands, Swansea
Tutor, Diploma in Primary Care Rheumatology, University of Bath
Member Scientific Advisory Group, National Osteoporosis Society

Summary

Osteoporosis is a very common disease which exerts a significant burden of morbidity on the patient. As a consequence, the management of osteoporosis consumes significant healthcare resources, with an estimated annual cost of around £1.7 billion. A sizeable component of this cost relates to the management of osteoporotic fractures, which in many cases can be prevented with the implementation of appropriate systems of care that seek to identify individuals at high risk of fracture and thus who would benefit most from intervention. High-risk individuals can be identified in the community by a selective case-finding strategy in which risk is assessed either opportunistically when a patient presents in the surgery or by actively interrogating computer-based practice records. By targeting appropriate bone-sparing pharmacological interventions to these high-risk patients, we can go a long way to minimising the burden of the condition and also ensure that we use such interventions in a cost-effective fashion.

☞ *Remember that the author of the Improving Practice is addressing her healthcare professional colleagues rather than the 'lay' reader. This provides a fascinating insight into many of the challenges faced by doctors in the day-to-day practice of medicine (see Reader's Guide).*

The burden of osteoporosis in primary care

Osteoporosis is defined as a progressive systemic skeletal disease characterised by low bone mass and microarchitectural deterioration of bone tissue, with a consequent increase in bone fragility and susceptibility to fractures. It is a very common disease, with one woman in three over the age of 50 years affected. Between one-in-eight and one-in-twelve men are also affected. The prevalence increases amongst Caucasian women from 15% in those aged 50 years to more than 70% at age 80.

Osteoporosis is important clinically because of the fractures that it causes. In the UK every year it is estimated that there are more than 310,000 osteoporotic fractures, comprising 70,000 hip fractures, 70,000

In the UK every year it is estimated that there are more than 310,000 osteoporotic fractures.

Colles fractures, 120,000 vertebral fractures and 50,000 other fractures due to osteoporosis. Caucasian women at the time of menopause have a 30–40% lifetime risk of fracture, with a 14% risk of hip fracture.

Fractures result in pain, disability, loss of independence, hospitalisation and mortality, yet many osteoporotic fractures are preventable if people at high risk are treated appropriately. The number of fractures continues to increase year on year, out of proportion to the shifting demographics of the elderly population. Osteoporotic hip fractures occupy more than 20% of orthopaedic beds each year, and result in more than 14,000 deaths each year in the UK. Estimated costs are around £1.7 billion annually. The burden of fractures and costs for a typical primary care organisation (PCO) are shown in Table 1.

As well as the annual incident fractures, there is a burden of disease from the pool of previously diagnosed and undiagnosed osteoporotic fractures and people with osteoporosis, all of whom are also at very high risk of future fracture.

> GPs and the primary care team are in the best position to be able to identify and treat patients who have had a previous fracture to reduce the burden of further fractures.

Although around 80% of women are able to walk independently prior to a hip fracture, at 1 year post-fracture 20% will have died as a direct result, only 15–20% will be able to walk unaided and less than 10% can climb stairs unaided even though 60% were able to do this prior to the fracture.

We now know that those who have had a previous low trauma or fragility fracture are much more likely to have another, with as many as one-in-five patients who have had a vertebral fracture refracturing within 1 year. Where there is no fracture liaison service in secondary care, GPs and the primary care team are in the best position to be able to identify and treat these patients to reduce the burden of further fractures. The numbers likely to be at highest risk within an average practice are small enough to be manageable (Figure 1), yet tackling this group can have a dramatic impact on future fracture rates.

Practical strategies and identifying patients

The goals of osteoporosis management are to prevent initial and subsequent fractures. It is usually most appropriate to begin by tackling

Table 1. Fracture incidence and costs of fractures for a typical Primary Care Organisation (PCO).

Fracture type	Number of patients per PCO (100,000)	Hospital costs per fracture (£)	Total costs per fracture (£)	Total costs per PCO (£)
Hip	120	5,300	21,500	2,580,000
Wrist	120	500	500	60,000
Vertebral (diagnosed)	200 (40)	500	500	20,000
Other	100	1,400	1,400	140,600
Total cost				2,800,600

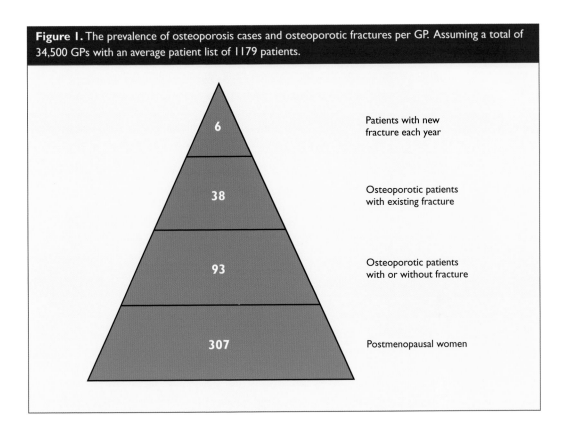

Figure 1. The prevalence of osteoporosis cases and osteoporotic fractures per GP. Assuming a total of 34,500 GPs with an average patient list of 1179 patients.

6 — Patients with new fracture each year

38 — Osteoporotic patients with existing fracture

93 — Osteoporotic patients with or without fracture

307 — Postmenopausal women

secondary prevention by targeting those who have already had a fracture. Two practical ways to identify this group are discussed later in this article. Once successful, the practice or PCO can then move on to primary prevention, which is, of course, more resource intensive.

The key strategies that can be used here are similar to those that can be used for other chronic diseases such as coronary heart disease (CHD) or diabetes – namely population strategies and individual or selective case-finding strategies. These are outlined in Table 2.

Population strategies

A 10% increase in bone mineral density (BMD) across the population would translate into a halving of osteoporotic fractures. However, the lifestyle advice involved (i.e. increasing dietary calcium, weight-bearing

Table 2. Practical strategies for managing osteoporosis.

Population strategies	• Improve bone mineral density across the whole population • Population screening
High-risk strategies (selective case-finding)	• Opportunistic identification of high-risk individuals • 'Search and rescue' strategies for high-risk groups

exercise and smoking cessation) is time consuming to deliver, and most people are unwilling or unable to make long-term lifestyle changes. In addition, there is little evidence from randomised controlled trials that this approach will actually decrease fractures in reality. Therefore, this approach should not be relied upon as the sole method for fracture prevention. Since this lifestyle advice is similar to that provided to reduce the risk of CHD, stroke and diabetes, it is important to remind patients of the likely benefits such lifestyle changes will have on their skeletons.

The second population strategy involves screening all perimenopausal women with dual-energy X-ray absorptiometry (DXA) scans at the time of the menopause, and then encouraging those found to be at high risk to take bone-sparing therapy. This strategy was piloted in Hull and Aberdeen but was not found to be cost-effective. DXA is expensive as a screening tool and has low sensitivity for identifying women who will fracture. Moreover, being aware that they were at risk of osteoporosis did not markedly influence women to take bone-sparing therapy.

Therefore, the recommended strategy that will be discussed in the remainder of this section is an individual and selective case-finding approach. This involves identifying those patients who are most at risk of osteoporosis and fragility fractures, and ensuring that they receive optimal advice and treatment to prevent first or subsequent fractures.

In a primary care setting, this approach would involve risk factor assessment, such as previous fracture or steroid use, to identify those at increased risk, either opportunistically when they present in surgery, or by searching the practice computer records for those with documented risk factors. Both methods can help to identify the prevalence pool of high-risk patients within the practice.

In secondary care, a separate method of selective case finding – the Fracture Liaison Service – operates in an increasing number of centres across the UK. Based on the premise that those who have already had one low-trauma fracture are at greatly increased risk of subsequent fractures, the Fracture Liaison Services assesses those with incident fractures, and identifies those who need further treatment with bone-sparing agents to reduce the risk of future fractures. Recommendations are then made for continuing drug therapy in primary care.

Goals of clinical management

Osteoporosis is important because of the fractures that it causes, and therefore the goals of management are to prevent first and subsequent fractures. Apart from vertebral fractures which result from normal activities of daily living, other osteoporotic fractures are usually caused by a combination of increased bone fragility and a fall. Therefore, to be most effective, one must identify and manage both the osteoporosis and the falls.

The overarching strategies to achieve this have been discussed earlier in this section. Here we will focus on the practical aspects of how to provide an osteoporosis service in the primary care setting.

To be most effective, one must identify and manage both the osteoporosis and the falls.

The main goals of osteoporosis prevention and management in primary care are to:

- maximise peak bone mass
- identify patients at highest risk of fracture
- use investigations cost-effectively
- exclude secondary osteoporosis
- provide lifestyle advice to all those at risk
- provide appropriate drug treatment to those at highest risk and encourage concordance
- identify and manage those at increased risk of falls.

Each of these goals will be discussed in detail in the following sections.

Maximise peak bone mass

The risk of osteoporosis and fracture in later life depends on three factors: the peak bone mass achieved in the teens and twenties, the age at which bone loss begins and the rate at which bone loss continues thereafter. It is therefore vital to ensure that children and teenagers optimise their peak bone mass by healthy eating, exercise and avoidance of smoking, anorexia and amenorrhoea. Supplementation with calcium can result in 1–5% increases in BMD, whilst consumption of milk and other dairy produce that also contain protein may be even more effective. The benefits derived from such an approach may be greatest in the pre-pubertal period and during early supplementation. Modest exercise is also beneficial, but excessive exercise that results in amenorrhoea is detrimental.

> It is vital to ensure that children and teenagers optimise their peak bone mass by healthy eating, exercise and avoidance of smoking, anorexia and amenorrhoea.

Identify patients at highest risk of fracture

High-risk groups for osteoporotic fracture include:

- a history of previous fragility fracture
- oral steroid use
- housebound, frail elderly individuals
- BMD T-score less than –2.5 on a DXA scan
- a maternal history of hip fracture
- premature menopause/hysterectomy (before 45 years of age)
- prolonged amenorrhoea not due to pregnancy
- Cummings Hip Fracture Risk score of five or more
- body mass index below 19 kg/m^2
- fallers.

Although osteoporosis can only be accurately diagnosed by axial DXA, several other factors can help to identify those at high risk of fracture. The World Health Organization (WHO) is currently preparing a model which will allow prediction of a 10-year fracture risk, similar to CHD risk scores. This will allow treatment to be targeted to those at highest fracture risk.

Peripheral DXA (pDXA) and quantitative ultrasound scans (QUS) can also be helpful in identifying those at high fracture risk. The National Osteoporosis Society (NOS) provides guidance on the use and limitations of these investigations – this can be downloaded from the Health Professionals' section of the website at *www.nos.org.uk*. Neither pDXA nor QUS can be used to monitor therapy, and QUS cannot be used to diagnose osteoporosis. When using pDXA, the NOS recommend using a triage approach with device-specific upper and lower thresholds chosen to have 90% sensitivity and specificity for identifying patients with osteoporosis at the hip or spine. If the pDXA measurement is below the lower threshold, treatment is recommended. If the measurement is above the upper threshold and no fractures are present, then no treatment is needed. Where the measurement is between the upper and lower thresholds, axial DXA is recommended. Thus, around 40% will need axial DXA.

Two commonly used scoring systems, the Cummings Hip Fracture Risk score and the Black Fracture Index are summarised in Tables 3 and 4. Patients with five or more hip fracture risk factors are 25-times more likely to suffer a hip fracture than those with two or less risk factors. These scoring systems can therefore help identify the highest-risk, frail elderly population. The Fracture Index provides an estimate of 5-year risk of osteoporotic fractures and can be calculated with or without DXA scores. Women with scores of six and higher, and four and above, with and without DXA respectively, need further assessment.

> The Cummings Hip Fracture Risk score and the Black Fracture Index can help identify the highest-risk, frail elderly population.

Table 3. Hip fracture risk factors used in determining the Cummings Risk Factor score.

- Age greater than 80 years
- Fracture since the age of 50 years
- Maternal hip fracture
- Poor or very poor health
- Anticonvulsant treatment
- Long-acting benzodiazepine treatment
- Weight below that at age 25 years
- Height above 168 cm at age 25 years
- Consumption of more than two cups of coffee per day
- On their feet for less than 4 hours per day
- No walking for exercise
- Unable to rise from chair without using arms
- Previous hyperparathyroidism
- Lowest quartile depth perception
- Lowest quartile contrast sensitivity

Table 4. Fracture index questions and scoring. BMD, bone mineral density.

	Score
1. Current age	
Under 65	0
65–69	1
70–74	2
75–79	3
80–84	4
85 or older	5
2. Fracture after the age of 50	1
3. Maternal hip fracture after the age of 50	1
4. Weight 57 kg or less	1
5. Current smoker	1
6. Uses arms to rise from chair	2
7. Hip BMD result if available	
T-score ≥–1	0
T-score between –1 and –2	2
T-score between –2 and –2.5	3
T-score <–2.5	4

Use investigations to confirm the diagnosis when appropriate

Axial DXA of the hip and lumbar spine is the 'gold standard' investigation for diagnosing osteoporosis, and the definition of osteoporosis is based on finding a T-score of –2.5 or less on axial DXA. However, DXA should be used only if it will change the patient's management. Guidelines from the National Institute for Health and Clinical Excellence (NICE) were published in early 2005 and recommend that women aged 75 years and over who have already had an osteoporotic fragility fracture do not require a DXA scan prior to starting bone-sparing therapy. Further guidance on women who have not yet had a fracture will be published later in 2005.

DXA has a high specificity but low sensitivity, which means that those with low BMD are at high risk of fracture, but around 50% of those who go on to fracture will have had a relatively normal BMD. Thus, DXA results should be viewed along with other risk factors in deciding which patients need therapy to prevent or treat osteoporosis.

> DXA results should be viewed along with other risk factors in deciding which patients need therapy to prevent or treat osteoporosis.

Exclude secondary osteoporosis

Our patients will not thank us if we treat their osteoporotic fracture but fail to identify an underlying condition that has caused it, or if we fail to identify that their vertebral fracture was due to bony secondaries rather than osteoporosis. We need to have a particularly high index of suspicion in patients who have had previous cancer, are elderly or who have evidence of systemic features such as weight loss or night pain. Investigations should be tailored to the particular patient, but may include:

- full blood count (FBC), erythrocyte sedimentation rate (ESR)
- myeloma screen (protein electrophoresis, Bence-Jones protein in urine)
- thyroid profile
- bone profile – calcium, alkaline phosphatase
- cortisol levels.

Provide lifestyle advice to all at risk

Lifestyle advice regarding healthy diet, exercise and smoking cessation to reduce the risks of CHD, stroke and diabetes, is provided routinely in primary care, but we rarely remember to stress the benefits that these interventions provide to the skeleton. These lifestyle messages need to be communicated from the 'cradle to the grave' to maximise peak bone mass, maintain bone mass and reduce bone loss later in life.

Population-based studies have demonstrated improved BMD and possibly reduced hip fracture rates amongst elderly people who eat a diet rich in fruit and vegetables, which are high in potassium, magnesium and vitamin K. High caffeine intake, particularly if combined with low calcium intake, may result in lower BMD and increased hip fracture rates. Adolescents and elderly patients are most at risk of vitamin D deficiency with 10–16% of teenagers having vitamin D-deficient diets and 37% of institutionalised elderly patients having low blood vitamin D levels.

One to two alcoholic drinks a day may improve BMD. In contrast, consumption of more than 14 units a week is associated with increased fracture risk. Postmenopausal smokers have an increased cumulative hip fracture risk up to the age of 85 years (19% in smokers compared with 12% in non-smokers).

High-impact weight-bearing exercise, such as jumping or jogging and slow-lifting of heavy weights (70–85% of personal maximum), can increase BMD in adults by 1–5%, but the benefits reverse once exercise stops. The FICSIT (Frailty and Injuries: Co-operative Studies of Intervention Techniques) meta-analysis demonstrated a significant reduction in falls with individually tailored exercise programmes, including a 50% reduction in falls after a Tai Chi programme.

Drug treatment for those at highest risk

Specific details about pharmacotherapy are beyond the scope of this article but can be found elsewhere in this edition of *BESTMEDICINE*. Here we will concentrate on the practical aspects of deciding who needs treatment and how to improve concordance with drug therapy.

Many GPs may be concerned by the impact that they believe tackling osteoporosis will have on their prescribing figures. However, this

> Lifestyle messages need to be communicated from the 'cradle to the grave' to maximise peak bone mass, maintain bone mass and reduce bone loss later in life.

need not be a concern. As is illustrated in Figure 1, the numbers of patients at the highest risk in each practice, who may require bisphosphonate or other drug therapy, are smaller than GPs might anticipate. Also, some practices may have patients who are currently treated with bisphosphonates but who are at a relatively low risk of future fracture. As with other medical interventions, targeting treatment to those at higher risk of fracture allows drugs to be used more cost-effectively.

Specific patient groups who may benefit from bone-sparing pharmacological intervention include those:

- aged 75 years and over who have had one or more fragility fractures
- aged 65–74 years who have had a fragility fracture and an axial DXA T-score of –2.5 or below
- aged under 65 years who have had a fragility fracture and an axial DXA T-score of –3.0 or below, or a T-score of –2.5 or below plus one or more additional age-independent risk factor: BMI <19 kg/m^2; family history of maternal hip fracture before 75 years of age; untreated premature menopause; certain medical disorders independently associated with bone loss (chronic inflammatory bowel disease, rheumatoid arthritis, hyperthyroidism or coeliac disease); conditions associated with prolonged immobility
- with a pDXA T-score below the device-specific lower threshold, especially if other risk factors and/or fractures are present
- aged over 65 years and commencing oral steroids for treatment courses of 3 months or more
- aged under 65 years commencing oral steroids where DXA T-score is –1.5 or less (start bone-sparing therapy immediately if a delay is likely before DXA available) for treatment courses of 3 months or more
- in nursing or residential homes (high-dose calcium and vitamin D) to prevent hip fractures.

Advice is usually available from local osteoporosis specialists or GPs with a special interest in osteoporosis to help guide treatment decisions in more complex cases, and in many parts of the UK the DXA scan report will include recommendations for treatment.

Whether drug treatment is initiated in primary or secondary care, patients need to be reviewed in primary care, ideally 3–4 months after starting treatment, to ensure they are continuing to take their medication, and, in the case of bisphosphonates, are taking medication in the correct way so that it is likely to be effective.

Monitoring with axial DXA after 18 months to 2 years of treatment will allow confirmation of a treatment effect, but this may not be appropriate in all patients.

Identify and manage those at increased risk of falling

Standard 6 of the National Service Framework (NSF) for Older People confirms that practices have a responsibility to identify fallers and those at risk of falling, and also those with osteoporosis or at high risk of fragility fractures or refracture, and to take appropriate action to manage these patients.

The risk of falling and the likelihood of resulting injuries increases steadily after the age of 60 years, with fall rates about three-times higher in nursing and residential homes than they are in the community. About 35–40% of mobile elderly patients will fall each year, and 5% will be hospitalised as a result. Several risk factors for falls have been identified and incorporated into fall-assessment risk tools. The simplest tool employs only three risk factors: hip weakness, unstable balance and taking four or more medications. Those with no risk factors have a 12% annual falls risk, compared with 100% for those with all three risk factors.

In practice, all older people or their carers should be asked once a year about falls. Those who have fallen should be assessed with the 'get up and go test', where the patient is asked to stand up from a chair without using their arms, to walk several paces and turn round and return to the chair. Those presenting after a fall, those reporting multiple falls, and those with gait or balance difficulties when tested, need referral for formal falls assessment.

There is evidence that multifactorial interventions can decrease risk of future falls when targeted at high-risk people. These include:

- medication assessment
- intervention for postural hypotension
- environmental hazard modification
- gait training and advice on the use of walking sticks and zimmer frames
- exercise programmes including balance training and Tai Chi
- treatment of comorbid cardiovascular problems.

Hip protectors may decrease the risk of hip fractures in fallers although not all studies confirm this. They are only likely to be acceptable to those in nursing or residential homes, and even in this group compliance and hygiene are a problem.

Improving osteoporosis management

Unfortunately, there are no quality points for osteoporosis within the new General Medical Services (GMS) contract currently, and therefore, if we are to make a significant impact on osteoporosis and fractures in Primary Care, it is likely that initiatives and incentives at the level of PCOs such as Primary Care Trusts (PCTs) and Local Health Boards (LHBs) will be needed to encourage widespread action. The National Osteoporosis Society has produced guidance for PCOs in England, Wales and Scotland to simplify the implementation of seamless primary and secondary care services. These can be accessed on the Health Professionals' section of the National Osteoporosis Society website at *www.nos.org.uk*.

A variety of other guidelines are available which can help primary care teams manage osteoporosis effectively. Two of the most useful are

> Those who have fallen should be assessed with the 'get up and go test', where the patient is asked to stand up from a chair without using their arms, to walk several paces and turn round and return to the chair.

the general osteoporosis guidelines produced by the Scottish Intercollegiate Guidelines Network (SIGN) (*www.sign.ac.uk*) and the Glucocorticoid Induced Osteoporosis Guidelines published in November 2002, by the Royal College of Physicians, the Bone and Tooth Society and the National Osteoporosis Society (*www.rcplondon.ac.uk*).

The impact of information technology and clinical audit

To meet the requirements of the NSF for Older People, it is important that all fallers and those with fractures should be identified and recorded in primary care. It is particularly important for the over 75s (or possibly even for the over 65s) that falls and osteoporosis risk assessments are carried out.

Datasets containing the necessary Read codes have been produced by Dr Mike Harvey and Dr Jonathan Bayly – members of the Scientific Advisory Group of the National Osteoporosis Society – and these are available on the Health Professionals' section of the National Osteoporosis Society website at *www.nos.org.uk*.

The NSF for Older People recommends clinical audit of the groups shown in Table 5. The fallers should be included in the practice Falls Register and those with previous fractures or diagnosed osteoporosis on a DXA scan can be included in an Osteoporosis Register. It is then very straightforward for practices to audit whether these patients have received appropriate assessments and management.

This will improve levels of care for osteoporosis patients and help reduce fracture risk from falls. Primary care teams need to work together with colleagues in secondary care who will be putting in place Fracture Liaison Programmes and working to improve rehabilitation after fractures, as per the recommendations of the *Blue Book* produced by the British Orthopaedic Association in 2003. Together this should provide a seamless service to identify and manage patients with incident and prevalent fractures.

Table 5. Clinical audit in osteoporosis, as recommended by the criteria of the National Service Framework (NSF) for Older People.

- Number of fallers in the last year
- Number with more than two falls or one fall and poor gait/balance as determined by the 'get up and go test' who need formal falls assessment
- Number of fallers who have received a falls assessment
- Number of fragility fractures in the last year by type
- Number of housebound/in residential accommodation who have received falls assessment
- Number of fallers who are prescribed high strength calcium and vitamin D
- Number on steroids who have received osteoporosis assessment

Conclusions

Osteoporosis is preventable and treatable, yet every year in the UK alone it is responsible for more than 310,000 fragility fractures, which in turn result in pain, disability and deaths, with a huge financial cost. Targeting interventions, whether lifestyle or drug therapies, at those with the highest risk of future fracture, will ensure that we make an impact on fracture rates whilst making the most cost-effective use of our resources, in terms of both people and pounds.

Key points

- Osteoporosis is a very common disease affecting up to one woman in two over 50 years but also affecting up to one-in-five men.

- Osteoporotic fractures result in pain, disability, loss of independence, hospitalisation and mortality, but can be prevented with appropriate systems of care which focus on high-risk individuals.

- The primary aim of management within primary care is to prevent initial and subsequent fractures, although primary prevention of initial fractures is more resource intensive than prevention of second fractures.

- The recommended strategy to identify patients at risk of osteoporotic fractures is an individual, selective case-finding approach, via risk factor assessment either opportunistically or by actively searching computer records.

- In addition to fracture prevention, it is essential to identify and manage patients at an increased risk of falls.

- Other goals of osteoporosis prevention and management include maximisation of peak bone mass via lifestyle intervention and the use of bone-sparing medication where most appropriate.

- No quality points are available for effective osteoporosis management in the new GMS contract, and thus other initiatives are required to encourage widespread action.

PATIENT NOTES

Dr Pam Brown

Improving the care of patients with osteoporosis

The preceding section of this edition of *BESTMEDICINE* discusses some of the practical aspects of delivering an osteoporosis service in primary care, including the importance of the patient's role. GPs need to identify those who may be at risk of osteoporosis or future fractures, use investigations to exclude any other underlying health problems and to confirm the need for treatment, then ensure that people continue to take their treatment correctly for long enough to benefit from it.

Although the drug treatment of osteoporosis is straightforward, most GPs have had little training in how to manage this disease and therefore many find it difficult to decide who needs treatment. Many parts of the UK still do not have access to the dual-energy X-ray absorptiometry (DXA) scanners required to diagnose the disease and to assess future fracture risk. In addition, practice teams are very busy managing other chronic diseases such as coronary heart disease, diabetes, asthma, chronic lung disease and cancer, which are all high priorities and targeted in the new General Medical Services (GMS) contract. These factors mean that most people with osteoporosis in the UK are still not receiving optimal treatment to prevent future fractures. The National Osteoporosis Society (NOS) has worked tirelessly to remedy this situation for nearly two decades, and treatment rates are slowly improving. It is hoped that the inclusion of osteoporosis in the National Service Framework (NSF) for Older People, and the National Institute for Health and Clinical Excellence (NICE) guidelines to be published in 2005 and 2006 will increase treatment rates further. However, it is vitally important that patients work closely with their doctor and/or nurse to help them manage the future risk of fracture, and be very assertive to ensure that the right care is given.

> *Most people with osteoporosis in the UK are still not receiving optimal treatment to prevent future fractures.*

Who should receive treatment for osteoporosis?

High-risk groups

All current guidelines encourage targeting treatment to people with the highest risk of future fracture. These include people who:

- have already had one or more fragility fractures
- will take oral steroids for at least 3 months
- are housebound, frail elderly.

Other groups may also be at increased risk, and the World Health Organisation (WHO) is developing a 10-year fracture risk score, similar to the 10-year risk score that is widely used for heart disease. This will incorporate risk factors such as smoking, lack of exercise or low bone density to calculate risk. Whilst we await this development, two risk factor scores are available to clinicians (Cummings hip fracture risk score and the Black Fracture risk score) and these are described in more detail in the preceding section of this book.

Other factors that may increase an individual's risk of future fracture include:

- increasing age
- a bone mineral density T-score of less than –2.5 on a DXA scan
- a maternal history of hip fracture occurring under the age of 75 years
- smoking
- premature menopause/hysterectomy (before the age of 45 years)
- prolonged amenorrhoea (absence of periods) not due to pregnancy
- being underweight (a body mass index [BMI] below 19 kg/m^2)
- falls.

Glucocorticoid-induced osteoporosis

It is important that everyone who is taking oral steroids also receive high-dose calcium and vitamin D supplements.

The Royal College of Physicians, the Bone and Tooth Society and the NOS combined their expertise to provide updated guidelines on the prevention and management of glucocorticoid-induced (steroid-induced) osteoporosis in 2002. These guidelines stress the high risk of osteoporosis and fracture in people who take oral steroids, and that bone loss is greatest during the first few months of treatment. Therefore, it is important that everyone who is taking oral steroids also receive high-dose calcium and vitamin D supplements. Prophylaxis with bone-sparing drug treatment is recommended for all high-risk individuals such as those with previous fragility fractures and those aged 65 years and over. Those under the age of 65 years should have a DXA scan to assess their risk, and be offered bone-sparing treatment if their T score is –1.5 SD or less (a higher level than would warrant treatment for other types of osteoporosis). Bisphosphonates are usually the drugs of choice in this situation, as they have been shown to be effective for the prevention and treatment of glucocorticoid-induced osteoporosis, whilst the data for some of the other treatments are inconsistent.

Falls

The risk of falling and the likelihood of resulting injuries increase steadily after the age of 60 years, and fall rates are three-times higher in nursing and residential homes than they are in the community. About 35–40% of elderly individuals living in the community will fall each year, and 5% will become hospitalised as a result of the fall. Several fall risk factors have been identified and incorporated into falls assessment risk tools. The simplest tool uses only three risk factors – hip weakness, unstable balance and taking four or more medications. Those with no risk factors had a 12% annual risk of a fall, compared with 100% for those with all three risk factors.

All older people should be asked once a year about falls. Those who have fallen should be assessed with the 'get up and go' test (where the patient is asked to stand up from a chair without using their arms, walk several paces, turn round and return to the chair). Those presenting after a fall, those reporting multiple falls, and those with gait or balance difficulties when tested, need referral for formal falls assessment. Multifactorial interventions can decrease the risk of future falls and these are described in the preceding section of this book.

Hip protectors are lightweight protective discs in pockets in underpants, designed to dissipate the force around the hip when someone falls. Some studies (but not all) have shown that they decrease the risk of hip fractures in fallers, but they are only acceptable to those in nursing or residential homes, and even in this group compliance is a problem.

Strategies for managing osteoporosis

Doctors use different strategies to identify people at risk of osteoporosis and fractures. For example, computer searches can identify all postmenopausal women who have had a fracture, and these women can then be seen and offered appropriate investigations and treatment to prevent further fractures. Alternatively, people at risk can be identified opportunistically when they attend surgery for another reason. The 'search and rescue' strategy is more cost-effective for the highest risk groups listed above, as these are all easily identified by computer searches. However, the important message is that if you think you are at risk, you should discuss this with your doctor or practice nurse who can use the appropriate tools to quantify your risk.

Further investigations

As we have seen in earlier sections of this book, X-rays are used to diagnose fractures and DXA scans are needed to diagnose osteoporosis in those under 75 years of age. Some other underlying conditions can cause osteoporosis or fractures,

If you think you are at risk, you should discuss this with your doctor or practice nurse.

particularly spinal fractures, so doctors will also usually conduct a range of blood tests before starting treatment. These will check that the liver and kidneys are working properly and that the level of calcium in the blood is normal.

Persistence and adherence with therapy

One of the major problems with all drug treatments, but particularly in the area of osteoporosis, is that many patients either do not take their treatment correctly or stop it prematurely without discussing this with their doctor so that alternative treatment can be prescribed. Follow-up appointments with either the GP or practice nurse can improve persistence with therapy, but this can be very time-consuming for both the patient and the practice team. If you do not feel able to continue with your therapy for whatever reason, it is very important to discuss this with your doctor so that alternatives can be considered.

Conclusion

Osteoporosis is preventable and treatable, yet every year in the UK it is responsible for more than 310,000 fragility fractures that result in pain, disability and even deaths, all at huge financial cost. Targeting lifestyle interventions and drug therapies at those at highest risk of future fracture will ensure that we make an impact on fracture rates whilst making the most cost-effective use of resources.

Since you are reading this book, it is likely that you will either have osteoporosis, or care for someone who has the disease. Being well informed about the disease will maximise your chances of getting appropriate treatment, taking your medication properly and reducing your future fracture risk. Investing in your health is always justified!

Many patients either do not take their treatment correctly or stop it prematurely without discussing this with their doctor.

Glossary

1,25-dihydroxyvitamin D – The biologically active form of vitamin D. Vitamin D is necessary for the body to absorb calcium. If a person is deficient in vitamin D, the body will take calcium from the bones. Vitamin D is produced by the action of sunlight on the skin and is obtained from certain foods, such as dairy products, egg yolk, liver and fish.

17β-estradiol – The main and most potent oestrogen hormone produced by the ovaries. It is necessary for normal female sexual development and for proper functioning of the female reproductive system. It also has an effect on the bones, slowing bone resorption (breakdown).

Absorption – The movement and uptake of a drug into cells or across tissues (such as the skin, intestine and kidney).

Achalasia – A rare disease where the muscle at the end of the oesophagus does not relax sufficiently to enable it to open and allow food to pass into the stomach. Symptoms include difficulty in swallowing and chest pain.

Active gastrointestinal bleeding – Bleeding from the gastrointestinal (GI) tract that becomes more severe. Signs of GI bleeding include the vomiting of blood and the passage of blood from the anus. Possible causes of GI bleeding include an ulcer, cancer, Crohn's disease (an inflammatory disease of the GI tract), irritable bowel syndrome (abdominal pains, diarrhoea and constipation) and haemorrhoids (swollen veins that bleed easily).

Acute – A relatively short course of drug treatment lasting days or weeks rather than months. Can also refer to the duration of a disease or condition.

Adjunctive therapy – Treatment used in conjunction with the primary therapy in order to enhance the therapeutic outcome.

Adverse event – An unwanted reaction to a medical treatment.

Aetiology – The specific causes or origins of a disease, usually a result of both genetic and environmental factors.

Agonistic effects – Effects elicited by a drug or substance that has affinity for, and stimulates physiological activity at, cellular receptors which are normally stimulated by naturally occurring substances, thereby triggering a biochemical response.

Albumin – A protein produced by the liver. The most common protein in blood.

Alkaline phosphatase – An enzyme that catalyses the cleavage of inorganic phosphate from phosphate esters, in particular, it is present in osteoblasts where it plays a role in bone mineralization. When these cells are destroyed, the enzyme leaks into the blood and levels of the enzyme increase. Total serum alkaline phosphatase levels can be used as a marker of bone formation, however, bone-specific alkaline phosphatase is a more specific marker of bone formation.

Aluminium – A silvery, metallic element which appears to have no beneficial effects in the body, and a small percentage of people are allergic to it. It has also been linked to Alzheimer's disease (dementia). Some antacids (drugs used to treat heartburn) contain aluminium.

Ambulatory – Able to walk around freely.

Amelioration – Improvement or moderation in the severity of a disease or the intensity of its symptoms.

Amenorrhoea – The absence of menstrual periods in women of reproductive age. Possible causes include pregnancy, anorexia nervosa, excessive exercise, emotional stress and hormonal disorders.

Amino acids – Small molecules that link together in chains to form proteins. In other words, they are the building blocks of proteins. There are 20 different types of amino acid.

Amino-terminal fragment – A broken-off piece of a protein consisting of the end of the protein with a free amino (NH_3) group. This distinguishes it from the other end of the protein which will always contain a free carboxyl (COOH) group.

Ampicillin – A type of antibiotic. It is used to treat bacterial infections.

Anabolic – Pertaining to anabolism, the build-up or synthesis of molecules within the body. The build-up of proteins in the body leading to the development of muscle is an example of anabolism.

Angiotensin-converting enzyme (ACE) – An enzyme that converts angiotensin I to angiotensin II, a substance which influences blood pressure and kidney function.

Anion-exchange resins – Insoluble polymers that contain negatively charged (anionic) groups capable of undergoing exchange reactions. Used to separate substances according to their ionic charge.

Anorexia – Loss of appetite, leading to significant weight loss.

Antacids – Drugs that neutralise acid in the stomach and are used to treat heartburn. Examples include aluminium hydroxide and magnesium hydroxide.

Antagonists – Substances (e.g. drugs) that block the action of other substances by binding to specific cell receptors without eliciting a biological response (see Reader's Guide).

Anticonvulsants – Drugs used to prevent convulsions (involuntary and violent muscle contractions) by preventing abnormal electrical activity in the brain. Convulsions are commonly associated with epilepsy and as a result, these drugs are often referred to as antiepileptics. Examples include sodium valproate, carbamazepine, diazepam and phenytoin.

Antiosteoporotic agent – An agent that either slows bone loss or stimulates bone formation and is therefore effective against osteoporosis.

Antiresorptive agent – An agent that slows down or prevents bone loss (resorption).

Apoptosis – The death of cells through a programmed sequence of events. This is a normal and essential process that occurs throughout the body and is a means by which the body gets rid of damaged or unwanted cells.

Appendicular bones – The bones relating to the limbs, in particular those of the shoulders, arms, pelvis and legs.

Areal bone mineral density – The amount of bone tissue in a given area measured in grams per square centimetre (g/cm^2). It is used to indicate bone strength and is more commonly simplified to bone mineral density (BMD).

Aromatase – An enzyme that catalyses (speeds up) the conversion of androgens (male hormones) into oestrogens (female hormones). The enzyme is found in the ovaries and other tissues that produce oestrogen, such as the liver, adrenal glands, placenta and testes.

Arthralgia – Pain in the joints.

Asthenia – A lack of energy and strength (weakness).

Asthma – A chronic (long-lasting or recurring) inflammatory disorder of the airways, characterised by coughing, wheezing and difficulty in breathing.

Asymptomatic – No symptoms.

Atomic number – The total number of protons (positively charged particles) in the nucleus (centre) of an atom of a chemical element.

Atraumatic – Not related to a sudden injury.

Axial cross-sectional moment of inertia – The force required to spin a cross-sectional area (a section of the object cut at right angles to its length) of an object around its axis (central line) measured in kilograms per square metre (kg/m^2). It provides an indication of the strength of the object. Applied to bone, it would indicate how strong the bone was and whether it was at an increased risk of fracture.

Axial DXA – Dual-energy X-ray absorptiometry (DXA) of bones in the axial skeleton, usually those in the lower spine, is a technique for measuring the density of those bones. It involves passing low-dose X-rays through the bones. The X-rays that emerge are detected and analysed using a computer, and this enables the density of the bones to be calculated.

Axial skeleton – The bones that make up the skull, spine, ribs and breastbone.

β-blockers – Drugs that block the β-adrenoceptors in the sympathetic nervous system, thus inhibiting the effects of the neurotransmitter, noradrenaline. This can reduce blood pressure and heart rate, and stabilise the heart beat. β-blockers are commonly used to treat hypertension, cardiac arrhythmias and angina pectoris.

Basic side chain – A group of atoms or molecules that is alkaline (has more hydroxide [OH⁻] than hydrogen [H⁺] groups) and is attached to a more complex molecule.

Baseline – The starting point to which all subsequent measurements are compared. Used as a means of assessing improvement or deterioration during the course of a clinical trial.

Bence-Jones protein – A protein found in the urine of many patients with myeloma (cancer of the blood-making cells in the bone marrow). The protein is a fragment of a large immunoglobulin molecule (a protein that helps to protect the body against invading organisms) secreted by myeloma cells.

Benzodiazepines – A family of drugs that dampen the activity of the nervous system, they are used to treat a variety of conditions including seizures, epilepsy, anxiety, agitation and insomnia. They have a sedative (sleep-inducing) effect, and may also cause breathing and behavioural problems.

Benzothiopene – A non-steroidal chemical from which the antiosteoporotic drug, raloxifene, is derived.

Biliary excretion – Refers to a compound being removed from the body via the bile ducts and gall bladder. From there, the compound passes into the small intestine and out of the body through the anus. The bile ducts are a system of ducts that carry the fluid bile from the liver (where it is produced) to the gallbladder (where it is stored), and from the gallbladder to the small intestine.

Bioavailability – The amount of a drug that enters the bloodstream and hence reaches the tissues and organs of the body. Usually expressed as a percentage of the dose given.

Biochemical markers – Biological or chemical substances that act as an indicator of disease. For example, blood levels of the protein, prostate specific antigen, are used as an indicator of prostate cancer.

Biopsies – Samples of tissue that are removed surgically from the body and then examined under the microscope (e.g. for the presence of cancer cells).

Bisphosphonates – A group of non-hormone drugs used in the treatment of osteoporosis. These drugs slow bone resorption (breakdown), thus helping to maintain bone density and reduce the risk of fracture. Examples of bisphosphonates include alendronate and risedronate.

Body mass index (BMI) – A measure of body fat which takes into account both weight and height. Used to determine whether a person is over- or underweight. Calculated by dividing weight (in kilograms) by the square of height (in metres) [i.e. $BMI = kg/m^2$].

Bone apatite – A form of calcium phosphate that is present in bone.

Bone geometry – The size, shape and location of the bones.

Bone mineral density (BMD) – The amount of bone tissue in a certain area of bone, measured as a surrogate for bone strength. BMD is sometimes referred to as areal BMD and is measured in grams per square centimetre (g/cm^2), commonly using dual-energy X-ray absorptiometry (DXA). A low BMD is associated with a greater risk of fracture.

Bone mineralisation – The incorporation of hydroxyapatite, a form of calcium phosphate, into bone. This gives the bone its hardness and rigidity.

Bone proliferative lesions – Areas of abnormal bone tissue that grow. Examples include bone tumours and bone spurs (outgrowths of bone).

Bone turnover – The process of bone renewal; the balance between bone breakdown and the formation of new bone.

Bone-specific alkaline phosphatase (BSAP) – An enzyme present in bone cells that plays an important role in bone mineralisation (the incorporation of calcium phosphate into bone). When the cells that produce this enzyme are destroyed, the enzyme leaks into the blood. Serum levels of BSAP are commonly measured as a marker of bone formation in clinical trials of drugs for osteoporosis.

Broadband attenuation – The reduction in magnitude of an energy source as it travels through a material due to absorption by the material. The reduction in magnitude of ultrasound waves as they travel through bone can be measured to provide an indication of the risk of bone fracture.

C-terminal propeptide of type I procollagen (PICP) – The carboxyl end (COOH) of type 1 procollagen, which is the precursor molecule for type 1 collagen (the main protein in bones and tendons). Type 1 procollagen is split by enzymes into type 1 collagen and two propeptides (the N- and C-terminal propeptides). Serum levels of the C-terminal propeptide are used as a marker of bone formation.

Calcium – A mineral that is necessary for many bodily functions, including the maintenance of healthy bones, muscle contraction, the beating of the heart and the conduction of nervous impulses in the nervous system. Calcium is needed for bone growth, and a lack of calcium in the diet contributes to the development of osteoporosis.

Calcium carbonate – A form of calcium used as a dietary supplement.

Calcium-channel blocker – Drugs that block the calcium channels in cell membranes, thus preventing calcium ions (Ca^{2+}) from flowing into cells. Prevents the smooth muscle cells in the walls of blood vessels from contracting, thereby keeping the blood vessels dilated and reducing blood pressure. Calcium-channel blockers are effective in the treatment of hypertension.

Cancellous bone – Denoting bone that has a lattice-like or spongy structure.

Candidate genes – Genes (segments of DNA on the chromosomes) that may be related to a particular disease or condition.

Candidate loci – Specific locations on the chromosomes that may be related to a particular disease or condition.

Carbon – A non-metallic element present in all organic molecules, such as proteins, fats and carbohydrates. These molecules form the basis of all living organisms. Pure carbon exists in nature as coal, diamond and graphite (pencil lead).

Carcinogenicity – The ability of a substance to cause cancer.

Calcitriol – The biologically active form of vitamin D. Also known as 1,25-dihydroxyvitamin D.

Cardiac glycosides – Chemicals found in certain plants (e.g. digitoxin found in foxgloves) that consist of a sugar and a non-sugar joined together. Such chemicals are often poisonous to animals, but are useful in treating heart failure in humans because they stimulate the heart to beat and strengthen the force of contraction of the heart muscle.

Cation-sensing receptor – A protein on the surface of a cell or inside a cell, that senses and responds to cations which are molecules or atoms with a positive charge. For example, calcium receptor proteins in the cells of the parathyroid gland and kidney enable these organs to sense and respond to changes in blood levels of calcium.

Central oxygen atom – An atom of oxygen at the centre of a molecule.

Cerebrovascular – Pertaining to the blood vessels that supply blood to the brain.

Chemical analogues – Chemical compounds with a similar structure to another chemical, but differing from it in some respect. Such analogues may have a similar or opposite effect in the body.

Cholesterol biosynthesis – The production of cholesterol. Cholesterol is an important component of cells, and also acts as a precursor for steroid hormones and bile acids. Some of the cholesterol in the body is produced in the liver, and some is absorbed from food in the digestive tract. High blood levels of cholesterol increase the risk of heart disease.

Chromosomal loci – The unique positions that given genes occupy on the chromosomes.

Chronic – A prolonged course of drug treatment lasting months rather than weeks. Can also refer to the duration of a disease or condition.

Chronic Obstructive Pulmonary Disease (COPD) – A potentially fatal, slowly progressive disease of the airways that is characterised by airflow obstruction that is not fully reversible. This is in contrast to asthma, in which the airflow obstruction is reversible. Tobacco smoking is a major cause of COPD, and leads to chronic inflammation of the small airways and lung tissue, and the destruction of lung tissue by certain enzymes. The main symptoms of COPD include chronic cough and/or wheezing, a tight chest, shortness of breath, difficulty in breathing, increased sputum production and frequent clearing of the throat. There is no cure, and treatment is aimed at controlling symptoms and preventing further progression of the disease through the use of bronchodilators.

Cirrhosis – A disease in which the liver accumulates scar tissue and fat and consequently, is unable to function properly. The most common causes of cirrhosis are infection (hepatitis) and long-term alcohol abuse.

Cleave – Split or break.

Clinical sequelae – Complications of a disease or illness that produce symptoms. For example, the complications of a cold may include clinical sequelae such as infection of the ear, sinusitis (infection of the sinuses) and bronchitis (infection of the tubes leading to the lungs).

Clinical vertebral fracture – A split or break in one of the vertebrae (the bones that make up the spinal column) that causes symptoms, such as pain.

Coadministration – The simultaneous administration of more than one type of medication.

Cognition – Mental ability; thought processes.

Colecalciferol – Another name for vitamin D_3, which is one of a group of related substances known as vitamin D. Vitamin D_3 is the form of vitamin D that is produced by the action of sunlight on the skin.

Colestyramine – A drug used to treat hypercholesterolaemia (abnormally high blood cholesterol levels). It acts by binding to bile salts (molecules which break down fats in the digestive tract) and promoting their excretion preventing their role in absorbing cholesterol. Cholesterol is thus metabolised instead (converted to bile salts) and blood cholesterol levels are reduced. The drug is also used to treat diarrhoea caused by the abnormal digestion of fat, such as occurs in Crohn's disease (an inflammatory disorder of the digestive tract).

Collagen synthesis – The production of collagen, which is the main protein in bone, tendons, ligaments, cartilage, skin and connective (supporting) tissue. It provides strength and resilience to these tissues. There are twelve different types of collagen in the body (types I-XII).

Collagen – A fibrous protein found in connective tissue (e.g. bone, cartilage and tendons).

Collagen type-1 α1 – One of the chains of amino acids that makes up collagen type 1. Collagen type 1 is the most abundant type of collagen in the body, being found in bones and tendons. It consists of three coiled chains of amino acids, two of which are the same and are known as α1 chains, and one of which is known as the α2 chain.

Colles fractures – A break in the radius (one of the bones in the lower arm) just above the wrist. It is generally caused by a fall onto an outstretched hand such that the wrist and hand are pushed backwards (in contrast to a Smith's fracture which is a fracture angled toward the palm). The fracture is usually associated with severe pain and swelling and is the most common type of fracture in people over the age of 40 years.

Comorbid – A coexisting medical condition.

Connectivity density – A measure of how connected or how continuous the meshwork is in a given volume of spongy (trabecular) bone. The fewer the gaps the greater the connectivity density. It provides an indication of how compact the bone is.

Continuous conjugated equine oestrogens – Treatment every day of the month (as opposed to a certain number of days each month) with a mixture of several different oestrogens derived from the urine of pregnant horses. These oestrogens are used in menopausal and postmenopausal women to replace the oestrogen that is no longer produced.

Contraindication – Specific circumstances under which a drug should not be prescribed, for example, certain drugs should not be given simultaneously.

Cortical bone – The hard, outer layer of bone. This type of bone consists of columns of bone cells.

Cortical steal hypothesis – A situation in which a drug induces an increase in trabecular bone mass concurrently with a reduction in cortical bone mass.

Corticosteroids – Hormones produced by the adrenal glands. These compounds can be used to treat a variety of inflammatory conditions, including asthma, rheumatoid arthritis, eczema and hay fever. They can also be used to prevent the rejection of a transplanted organ.

Cranial-caudal ends – Refers to the two ends of the spinal column. The cranial end is close to the head whilst the caudal end is at the bottom and is known as the coccyx or tailbone.

Creatinine clearance – The rate at which creatinine (a protein produced by muscle from the breakdown of creatine) is cleared from the blood by the kidneys. It is measured as the amount excreted in the urine over a certain amount of time, and provides an indication of how well the kidneys are functioning.

Cross-linked C-terminal telopeptides of type I collagen (CTX) – Short proteins (peptides) attached to the carboxyl end (COOH) of the triple helix (three coiled protein chains) that comprises a molecule of type 1 collagen. These telopeptides are highly interactive, and can cross-link (join together) with each other. When type 1 collagen is broken down, the telopeptides are released into the bloodstream. Blood levels of these peptides can therefore be used as an indicator of the extent of bone resorption (breakdown).

Cross-linked N-telopeptides of type I collagen (NTX) – Short proteins (peptides) attached to the amino end (NH_3) of the triple helix (three coiled protein chains) that comprises a molecule of type 1 collagen. These telopeptides are highly interactive, and can cross-link (join together) with each other. When type 1 collagen is broken down, the telopeptides are released into the bloodstream. Blood levels of these peptides can therefore be used as an indicator of the extent of bone resorption (breakdown).

Crossover study – A clinical trial in which every subject receives each treatment being tested, in a random order. In this type of trial, subjects act as their own control.

C-terminal telopeptide – A short protein (peptide) attached to the carboxyl end (COOH) of a larger protein molecule.

Cummings Hip Fracture Risk score – A score obtained by comparing the bone mineral density in the hip of a patient with osteoporosis with that in a young population of the same gender. The score gives an indication of the person's risk of hip fracture.

Cyclic adenosine-3', 5'-monophosphate (cAMP) – A small, ring-shaped molecule that is present in many of the body's cells and acts as a chemical messenger within the cells.

Cyclically – Occurring or being given in cycles, which are recurring sequences of events. For example, some forms of hormone replacement therapy are given only on certain days of each month.

Cytoskeletal function – The role of the cytoskeleton or how well it is working. The cytoskeleton is a network of protein fibres in each cell that gives the cell shape and support. In other words, it is the framework of each cell.

D receptor – A protein present in cells of the intestines, bones, kidney, skin, and endocrine and immune systems that is activated by vitamin D. It mediates the biological effects of vitamin D by stimulating gene transcription (the copying of a sequence of DNA into messenger RNA, which serves as a blueprint for the synthesis of a particular protein) in the cell nucleus.

Deep vein thrombophlebitis – The blockage of a vein lying deep in the leg by a blood clot, leading to inflammation of the vein.

Deoxypyridinoline – A substance produced from the breakdown of collagen type 1, the protein present in bone. When this happens, deoxypyridinoline (sometimes abbreviated to free DPD, or fDPD) is released into the blood stream and excreted via the kidneys. Urinary levels of the compound can therefore be used as an indicator of bone resorption (breakdown).

Digestive enzymes – Complex proteins in the digestive tract that break down food. There are three classes of digestive enzymes: proteolytic enzymes that help to break down proteins; lipases that help to break down fat; amylases that help to break down carbohydrates.

Differentiated cells – Cells that have developed into a specialised type of cell with a specific function (e.g. muscle cell, liver cell, bone cell).

Distal – Refers to a part of the body that is remote from the centre of the body, as opposed to proximal (denoting nearness). For example, the fingers are distal to the arm.

Distal forearm – The part of the forearm (the part of the arm between the elbow and wrist) that is furthest away from the centre of the body. In other words, the part nearest the wrist rather than the part nearest the elbow.

Distal metaphysic of the femur – The metaphysic of the femur furthest from the centre of the body – the one near the knee, as opposed to the one near the hips. The metaphysic (or metaphysis) is the segment of a long bone located between the end part (epiphysis) and the shaft (diaphysis). It consists mostly of cancellous bone within a thin cortical shell.

Diuretics – A group of drugs that remove excess water from the body by increasing the production of urine. Diuretics are used to treat many conditions associated with water retention, including heart failure, certain kidney and liver disorders, high blood pressure, glaucoma and premenstrual syndrome.

Double blind – A clinical trial in which neither the doctor nor the patient are aware of the treatment allocation.

Double dummy – The use of two different types of placebo in a clinical trial so that participants do not know which treatment they are receiving. If the mode of administration of the two active treatments is different, participants will be able to deduce which treatment they are receiving.

Downregulate – Reduce; lower; decrease.

Drug interactions – In which the action of one drug interferes with that of another, with potentially hazardous consequences. Interactions are particularly common when the patient is taking more than one form of medication for the treatment of multiple disease states or conditions.

Dual-energy X-ray absorptiometry (DXA) scanning – A technique used to measure the density of bone, bone mineral content and body fat content. It is particularly useful for the diagnosis of osteoporosis and assessing the response to treatment for this condition. A scanner machine beams X-rays from two different sources at the part of the body being examined. Any X-rays not absorbed are picked up by a detector, which produces an image of the bone.

Dual-photon absorptiometry (DPA) – A technique for measuring the density (thickness) of bones. It involves passing a beam consisting of two different types of electromagnetic radiation through the bones. The radiation that is not absorbed is detected and analysed using a computer, and this enables the density of the bones to be calculated. The introduction of dual X-ray absorptiometry (DXA) has made DPA largely obsolete.

Duodenal erosion – A break in the inner lining (mucosa) of the duodenum (the first part of the small intestine that connects to the stomach).

Duodenitis – Inflammation of the duodenum (the first part of the small intestine that connects to the stomach).

Duration dependent – Being dependent on the length of time for which something (e.g. a disease) has lasted.

Dyspepsia – Also known as indigestion. A feeling of pain or discomfort in the upper middle part of the stomach. Other symptoms include bloating of the stomach, nausea, vomiting, belching and heartburn.

Dysphagia – Difficulty in swallowing.

Efficacy – The effectiveness of a drug against the disease or condition it was designed to treat.

Electrolyte – A substance that dissolves in water to form ions which are able to conduct electricity. Examples of electrolytes are sodium and potassium salts. These dissolve in water to produce sodium and potassium ions, respectively.

Elimination profile – The way in which a substance (e.g. a drug or hormone) is removed from the body.

Endogenous inorganic compound – A chemical substance that is produced or found naturally in the body but is of mineral (as opposed to plant or animal) origin and does not contain carbon or hydrogen.

Endometrial cancer – Cancer of the endometrium.

Endometrial cavity fluid – The presence of fluid in the cavity of the uterus or womb.

Endometrium – The inner lining of the uterus or womb.

Endpoint – A recognised stage in the disease process, used to compare the outcome in the different treatment arms of clinical trials. Endpoints can mark improvement or deterioration of the patient and signify the end of the trial.

Enterohepatic recycling – The recycling of certain lipids (fats) in the body. In this process, fats are absorbed from the digestive tract, carried to the liver, excreted via bile into the digestive tract, reabsorbed, carried to the liver, and so on. It is an efficient process for the conservation of bile salts (organic molecules that help to break down fats in the digestive tract) and certain hormones.

Epidemiology – The incidence or distribution of a disease within a population.

Erythrocyte sedimentation rate (ESR) – A blood test that measures how quickly red blood cells fall to the bottom of a test tube. The test is used as an indicator of swelling and inflammation in the body, the sedimentation rate being increased in inflammation, infection, cancer, rheumatic disease and diseases of the blood and bone marrow.

Estradiol (or 17β-estradiol) – The main and most potent oestrogen hormone produced by the ovaries in women. It is necessary for normal female sexual development and for proper functioning of the female reproductive system. It also has an effect on the bones, slowing bone resorption (breakdown).

Excretion – The elimination of a drug or substance from the body as a waste product, for example, in the urine or faeces.

Extracellular calcium-sensing receptor – A protein on the surface of a cell that senses and responds to calcium ions. Calcium-sensing receptors on the cells of the parathyroid gland and kidney enable these organs to sense and respond to changes in blood levels of calcium.

Extraskeletal uptake – The uptake of a substance by tissues other than those in the skeleton.

Farnesyl diphosphate synthase – An enzyme in the liver that is involved in the synthesis of farnesyl diphosphate. This compound is necessary for the synthesis of steroids, such as cholesterol and the sex hormones.

Femoral neck – The neck of the thigh bone. The neck is the area under the head of the thigh bone that joins the head to the shaft (main body) of the bone.

Femur – The thigh bone, which is the bone in the upper leg (the part of the leg between the hip and knee).

First-pass glucuronidation – A biochemical process that occurs with some drugs when they are administered orally (via the mouth), whereby some of the drug is metabolised in the intestines or in the liver before it is circulated around the body in the bloodstream. As a result, only a proportion of the drug reaches its site of action.

Fischer 344 rats – A particular strain of rat that is used in medical research.

Fluoride treatment – The use of compounds containing fluorine, such as sodium fluoride, to strengthen teeth and bones. Fluoride treatment is used worldwide to prevent tooth decay: fluoride is added to toothpaste, mouth washes and tap water, and can also be applied directly to the surface of the teeth. However, fluoride treatment is not recommended for osteoporosis because studies have shown that such treatment has no beneficial effect on the bones. In fact, some studies have shown that such treatment actually increases the risk of bone fracture.

Fracture index – A questionnaire for predicting the risk of bone fracture in postmenopausal women. The questionnaire takes into account seven variables, including age, bone mineral density, weight, smoking status and fracture status. It provides an overall score, which gives an indication of the risk of bone fracture.

Full blood count (FBC) – A collection of blood tests that measure a number of different features of the blood, including the amount of haemoglobin, the number, percentage and volume of red and white blood cells, and the number of platelets.

Full length parathyroid hormone – A whole molecule of parathyroid hormone consisting of a chain of 84 amino acids. This form of the hormone is split into smaller molecules in the liver. These fragments of the hormone circulate in the blood along with the 'full-length' molecules.

Gastric erosions – Breaks in the inner lining (mucosa) of the stomach.

Gastritis – Inflammation of the inner lining (mucosa) of the stomach.

Gastrointestinal tract – The part of the digestive system consisting of the mouth, oesophagus, stomach, small intestine, large intestine and rectum.

Genetic predisposition – An individuals' susceptibility to developing a disease or condition as a result of their genetic make-up.

Genotoxic – Capable of causing damage to the genetic material (DNA) in cells.

Geriatric Depression Scale (GDS) – A questionnaire designed to determine the severity of depression in elderly people. It is also useful for monitoring the effects of antidepressant therapy. The questionnaire comprises 15 questions to which a yes or no answer is required.

Glucocorticoid-induced osteoporosis – Osteoporosis (thinning of the bones) caused by the use of glucocorticoids, which are synthetic steroid (fat-like) hormones used to treat allergic and inflammatory conditions (e.g. asthma and rheumatoid arthritis). Glucocorticoids have direct and indirect effects on bone tissue, ultimately leading to bone loss.

Glucocorticoids – Also known as glucocorticosteroids, these are the steroid (fat-like) hormones produced by the adrenal glands that regulate energy metabolism and play a role in immune and inflammatory responses. Cortisol is the most important glucocorticosteroid produced by the adrenal glands. Synthetic glucocorticosteroids are used to suppress allergic and inflammatory diseases (such as asthma) and the rejection of transplanted organs.

Glucocorticosteroids – See Glucocorticoids.

Glycaemic – Pertaining to blood glucose (sugar) levels.

Gout – Inflammation of the joints due to the accumulation of uric acid crystals. The condition most commonly affects the joint of the big toe. It is caused by a defect in uric acid metabolism in the body, leading to high levels of uric acid in the blood.

Growth plates – The areas of growing tissue at the ends of the long bones (the bones in the arms, legs, hands and feet) in children and adolescents. Each long bone has at least two growth plates: one at each end. The growth plates determine the length and shape of the mature bone. When growth is complete, the growth plates close and are replaced by solid bone.

H1 antagonists – Agents that bind to histamine H1 receptors and block binding and activity of histamine at these receptors. In this way, H1 antagonists block the symptoms normally associated with allergic reactions, such as sneezing, itching and contraction of the smooth muscle in the walls of the respiratory system. The most well known H1 antagonists are antihistamines.

H2 antagonists – Agents that bind to histamine H2 receptors and block binding and activity of histamine at these receptors. In this way, H2 antagonists block acid secretion in the stomach. Such agents are used in the treatment of gastric and duodenal ulcers (sores in the lining of the stomach and duodenum, respectively), as decreased acid production in the stomach helps the ulcers to heal.

Haematology – The study of blood and blood formation.

Haematopoietic progenitor cells – Precursor cells in the bone marrow that develop into mature blood cells.

Half-life – The time taken for half of the amount of an agent (e.g. drug) to be removed from the blood.

Hepatic – Pertaining to the liver.

Hepatic blood flow – The flow of blood in the liver.

Heterocyclic ring – A ring of atoms consisting of more than one type of atom.

Heterogeneous – Diverse; composed of different elements or substances.

High specificity – Describes a substance that binds specifically to a certain target molecule, such as a receptor, in preference to any other possible target molecule.

Histomorphometric indices – Pointers indicating the health of the bones that are obtained by studying bone tissue under a microscope and measuring certain parameters.

Homeostasis – The process by which a living organism maintains a constant internal environment despite external changes. Examples of homeostatic processes include the regulation of blood pressure, body temperature and blood sugar levels.

Hormone replacement therapy (HRT) – Use of the female hormones oestrogen and/or progestin (a synthetic form of progesterone) in menopausal women to replace the hormones that are no longer produced in the body after the menopause. Such treatment slows bone resorption (breakdown) and therefore helps to maintain bone density and reduce the risk of fracture.

Hydrolysis – The breakdown of a molecule through the addition of a water molecule.

Hydroxyapatite crystals – A form of calcium phosphate (the substance in bone that makes it hard) in which the molecules of calcium phosphate are arranged in a repeating, orderly fashion.

Hydroxyapatite – A form of calcium phosphate found in bone. It is the substance that makes bones hard.

Hypercalcaemia – Abnormally high levels of calcium in the blood. Possible causes of hypercalcaemia include cancer, the overproduction of parathyroid hormone (which helps to regulate blood calcium levels) and excessive intake of vitamin D. Hypercalcaemia causes nausea, vomiting, lethargy, depression, thirst and excessive urination. If left untreated, it may lead to an irregular heartbeat, kidney failure, coma and ultimately death.

Hypercalciuria – The presence of abnormally high levels of calcium in the urine. This is most commonly caused by excessive bone resorption (breakdown), such as occurs in hyperparathyroidism (the overproduction of parathyroid hormone) or osteoporosis.

Hyperparathyroidism – Overactivity of the parathyroid glands – pea-sized glands located beside the thyroid gland in the neck. This leads to the overproduction of parathyroid hormone (which controls the level of calcium in the body), and hence high blood calcium levels (hypercalcaemia). Hyperparathyroidism is most commonly caused by a benign (non-cancerous) tumour in the parathyroid glands.

Hyperthyroidism – The overproduction of thyroid hormones by the thyroid gland which leads to overactivity of the body's metabolism, resulting in hyperactivity, insomnia, anxiety, increased appetite, diarrhoea and weight loss.

Hypocalcaemia – Abnormally low levels of calcium in the blood. The condition can lead to softening of the bones due to the removal of calcium. Severe hypocalcaemia causes painful muscle spasms.

Hypoglycaemic – Having abnormally low blood levels of glucose (sugar). The condition occurs most commonly in people with insulin-dependent diabetes if they inject too much insulin, miss a meal, don't eat enough carbohydrate (sugar) or exercise too much. Symptoms of hypoglycaemia include sweating, weakness, hunger, dizziness, headache, confusion, aggressive behaviour and uncoordinated movement. Severe hypoglycaemia can cause coma.

Hypogonadism – Reduced secretion of sex hormones from the testes (in men) or ovaries (in women). This may be caused by abnormal functioning of the sex organs (primary hypogonadism) or abnormal functioning of the centres in the brain that control them (central hypogonadism). In children, hypogonadism results in a lack of sexual development. In adults, it causes sexual dysfunction and loss of body hair.

Hysterectomy – Surgical removal of the uterus or womb.

Idiopathic – A disease or condition of unknown cause.

Iliac crest – The curved edge at the side of the hip bone. It contains bone marrow and is usually the site from which bone marrow is taken in order to diagnose diseases of the blood.

Inactivating genetic mutation – A change (mutation) in a person's genetic material (DNA) that causes a particular gene (a region of DNA) to be inactivated.

Incident fracture – A new fracture.

Indometacin – A non-steroidal anti-inflammatory drug (NSAID) that reduces fever, pain and inflammation. It is used to relieve the pain, tenderness and inflammation caused by gout, arthritis and other inflammatory conditions. It is similar to ibuprofen, and works by reducing the production of prostaglandins (chemicals that cause pain and inflammation) in the body.

Inorganic pyrophosphate – A form of phosphorus in the body that is found in abnormal calcium deposits in soft tissues, such as the cartilage that covers the ends of bones. In this case, the abnormal deposits of calcium and phosphorus can give rise to joint inflammation, causing a condition similar to gout known as pseudogout.

Insoluble complexes – A complex is a group of molecules or atoms that is joined together by weak chemical bonds that can be easily broken. An insoluble complex is a complex that does not dissolve in blood or other body fluids and tends to form a solid mass.

Intertrochanter – Between the two trochanters, which are two bumps of bone near the top of the femur (thigh bone) to which muscles attach.

Intestinal reabsorption – The selective reuptake by the intestines of useful substances (e.g. bile salts and certain hormones) that have been excreted from the body into the intestines via bile (a fluid produced by the liver that helps to break down fats in the intestines).

In vitro – 'In glass'. Used with reference to experiments performed outside the living system in a laboratory setting.

In vivo – Used with reference to experiments performed within the living cell or organism.

Ionising radiation – Energy in the form of X-rays (electromagnetic radiation produced by a special machine), gamma rays (electromagnetic radiation produced by the decay of radioactive substances) or particles from atoms (e.g. protons, neutrons or electrons). These forms of energy can knock electrons (small, negatively charged particles that orbit the nucleus of an atom) out of atoms, creating ions (particles with an electrical charge), hence the term ionising radiation.

Isoprenoid lipids – A group of fat-like substances whose structure is based on isoprene, a molecule consisting of five carbon atoms and eight hydrogen atoms.

Lateral spine – Refers to the sides of the spine as opposed to the front or back.

Lipids – Fats and fat-like substances which are insoluble in water yet dissolve freely in non-polar solvents (e.g. alcohol). All lipids contain aliphatic hydrocarbons.

Logistic regression relationship – A statistical technique that is used to analyse data where there are two possible outcomes: yes or no. The technique is used to predict whether a certain variable (e.g. temperature) will affect the outcome.

Low density lipoprotein cholesterol (LDL-C) – Cholesterol that is carried in the blood by the lipid–protein complex, low density lipoprotein (LDL). LDL-cholesterol is known as 'bad' cholesterol because high levels increase the risk of heart disease.

Low-energy trauma – A physical injury or wound (e.g. fracture) caused by a mild external force, such as bumping into something.

Lumbar spine – The part of the spine between the lowest pair of ribs and the top of the pelvis. The lumbar spine consists of five bones (vertebrae).

Macular – Pertaining to maculae, which are pale or coloured markings on or in an organ or, more commonly, on the skin. Macular may also pertain to the macula retinae, the central area of the retina.

Magnesium hydroxides – Substances commonly used as laxatives (substances that encourage defecation) or to neutralise acid in the stomach. The most well known example is probably milk of magnesia, which is a milky white, liquid suspension of magnesium hydroxide.

Markov model – A statistical model that is commonly used to analyse systems that may exist in different states. The model measures the probability of the system being in a given state at a given time point, the amount of time the system spends in a given state and the expected number of transitions between different states.

Marrow fibrosis – The growth of fibrous tissue (scar tissue) in the bone marrow.

Marrow star volume – The average volume of the bone marrow, as seen unobscured from a point within the bone marrow. It is a relatively new parameter that provides a measure of the porosity (the amount of space in a material) of trabecular (spongy) bone and can be estimated using bone marrow samples.

Mean annual slopes – The mean change in a parameter (e.g. bone mineral density) over 1 year compared with baseline, expressed as a percentage.

Mechanism of action – The manner in which a drug exerts its therapeutic effects.

Medroxyprogesterone acetate – A form of the hormone progesterone, which is a female sex hormone produced in the ovaries that prepares the uterus to receive a fertilised egg, controls menstruation and maintains pregnancy. It is used to treat abnormal uterine bleeding, to stimulate menstrual cycles and to treat symptoms of the menopause.

Memory Assessment Clinics (MAC) battery – A series of tests designed to assess short-term, verbal and visual memory.

Meta-analysis – A set of statistical procedures designed to amalgamate the results from a number of different clinical studies. Meta-analyses provide a more accurate representation of a particular clinical situation than is provided by individual clinical studies.

Metabolism – The process by which a drug is broken down within the body.

Metabolites – The products of metabolism.

Mevalonate pathway – A series of biochemical reactions resulting in the production of cholesterol and isoprenoid lipids, such as farnesyl diphosphate. These compounds are necessary for the synthesis of steroid hormones.

Microarchitectural deterioration – Thinning of the meshwork of bone tissue in trabecular (spongy) bone and the loss of connections in the meshwork.

Micronised 17β-estradiol – Very small particles of 17β-estradiol, which is the main and most potent oestrogen hormone in women. See also Estradiol.

Mineral apposition rate – How quickly hydroxyapatite (calcium phosphate) is incorporated into the bones.

Mineralisation – The incorporation of minerals into a material. For example, the incorporation of hydroxyapatite (calcium phosphate) into bones.

Mineralised – Having undergone mineralisation, which is the incorporation of minerals into a material. For example, having incorporated hydroxyapatite (calcium phosphate) into bones.

Monotherapy – Treatment with a single drug.

Morbidity – A diseased condition or state or the incidence of a disease within a population.

Morphology – The shape and structure of an organism or any of its parts.

Morphometric – Pertaining to morphometry, which is the measurement of the shape and structure of an object (e.g. length, volume, surface area, curvature, the number of subunits, etc.).

Mortality – The death rate of a population. The ratio of the total number of deaths to the total population.

Multicentre – A clinical trial conducted across a number of treatment centres, either abroad or in the same country.

Multifactorial – A disease or state arising from more than one causative element.

Multinucleated cells – Cells which contain many nuclei. Osteoclasts (the cells in bone that break down and remove old bone) are one example.

Multiphasic pattern – A pathway or cycle of events that has multiple stages or phases.

Murine – Pertaining to mice.

Musculoskeletal – Pertaining to the muscles and bones.

Mutagenic – Having the potential to cause a mutation (change) in the genetic material (DNA) of a cell.

Myeloma screen – To test for the presence of cancer of the cells of the bone marrow.

Negatively correlated – Describes the relationship between two parameters, such that one parameter increases as the other decreases.

Neonatal – Referring to the first 4 weeks of a newborn baby's life.

Non-calcified tissues – Tissues of the body that, unlike bone, do not normally contain deposits of calcium. This includes most of the tissues in the body.

Norethisterone acetate – A synthetic form of the hormone progesterone, which is a female sex hormone produced in the ovaries that prepares the uterus to receive a fertilised egg, controls menstruation and maintains pregnancy. It is used to treat abnormal uterine bleeding, to stimulate menstrual cycles and to treat symptoms of the menopause.

N-terminal – Refers to the end of the protein with a free amino group (NH_3).

N-terminal propeptide of type I procollagen (PINP) – The amino end (NH_3) of type 1 procollagen, which is the precursor molecule for type 1 collagen (the main protein in bones and tendons). Type 1 procollagen is split by enzymes into type 1 collagen and two propeptides (the N- and C-terminal propeptides). Serum levels of the N-terminal propeptide are used as a marker of bone formation.

Oesophageal – Pertaining to the oesophagus, which is the muscular tube that carries food from the throat to the stomach.

Oesophageal disease – An abnormal condition of the oesophagus.

Oestrogen agonist – A substance that mimics or promotes the effects of oestrogen hormones by stimulating oestrogen receptors.

Oestrogen deficiency – A lack of oestrogen where oestrogen is a group of hormones normally produced by the ovaries in women. These hormones are necessary for normal female sexual development and for proper functioning of the female reproductive system. They also have an effect on the bones, slowing bone resorption (breakdown). The ovaries stop producing oestrogen hormones at the time of the menopause.

Oestrogen receptor – A protein present in certain cells that binds to oestrogens and mediates the biological effects of this group of hormones.

Oestrogen receptor-negative – Refers to cells containing no oestrogen receptors.

Oestrogen receptor-positive – Refers to cells containing oestrogen receptors.

Open label – A clinical trial in which all participants (i.e. the doctor and the patient) are aware of the treatment allocation.

Oral anticoagulants – Drugs that are taken in tablet form to stop or slow clotting of the blood. They work by inhibiting vitamin K, which is necessary for the synthesis of blood clotting factors. They are used to treat conditions where the patient is at risk of thrombosis (the development of blood clots). The most well known example is warfarin.

Orthogonal – Pertaining to right angles. It is commonly taken to mean movement in two or three axes at right angles to each other.

Orthopaedic management – The prevention or correction of injuries or diseases of the skeletal system and associated muscles, joints and ligaments.

Osteoblast precursor replication – The production of many identical copies of the cells in the bone marrow that eventually develop into oesteoblasts.

Osteoblast progenitor cells – Cells in the bone marrow that develop into oesteoblasts.

Osteoblasts – Cells present in bone that form new bone tissue.

Osteocalcin – A protein produced by bone cells or osteoblasts that plays a role in bone formation. Serum levels of osteocalcin provide an indication of bone turnover.

Osteoclasts – Cells present in bone that break down and remove old bone, a process known as resorption.

Osteolytic cancer metastases – Cancerous growths in the bones that arise from a tumour elsewhere in the body (cells from this tumour spread to the bones via the blood and lymphatic systems) and cause the breakdown of bone.

Osteomalacia – Softening, weakening and demineralisation (loss of calcium phosphate) of the bones due to a deficiency of vitamin D, the latter being necessary for the body to absorb calcium from the diet. The main symptoms are pain in the bones, muscle weakness, muscle spasms and bones that break easily.

Osteopenia – A condition where the bone is less dense than normal, but insufficiently so to be classed as osteoporotic.

Ovariectomised – Having had the ovaries removed.

***p*-value** – In statistical analysis, a measure of the probability that a given result occurred by chance. If the *p*-value is less than or equal to 0.05 then the result is usually considered to be statistically significant, and not due to chance.

Paget's disease of the bone – A disease characterised by abnormally fast breakdown of bone and the growth of new bone that is softer and more porous than normal bone. These soft bones tend to bend and break more easily than normal. They may also grow larger than normal. The disease can affect any bone in the body, but most commonly affects the bones of the skull, hips, pelvis, legs and back.

Parathyroid hormone – An 84 amino acid peptide hormone produced by the parathyroid glands (four small glands in the front of the neck). It helps to regulate blood levels of calcium by increasing the levels when they become low by stimulating osteoclast bone resorption.

Pathological – Pertaining to disease or to pathology, which is the study of disease, its causes, mechanisms and effects on the body.

Pathophysiology – The functional changes that accompany a particular syndrome or disease.

P-C-P structure – Having a chemical structure that contains a carbon atom linked to two phosphorus atoms. Bisphosphonates (a group of non-hormone drugs used in the treatment of osteoporosis) have a central backbone consisting of this grouping of atoms.

Perimenopausal – Around the time of the menopause, which is the time of a woman's life when the ovaries stop producing oestrogens and menstruation ceases.

Periosteal – Pertaining to the periosteum, which is the membrane of fibrous tissue that covers the surface of all bones apart from the ends of bones at joints.

Peripheral DXA (pDXA) – Refers specifically to dual-energy X-ray absorptiometry (DXA) of bones in the peripheral skeleton (the bones of the shoulders, arms, pelvis and legs), usually those of the thigh and wrist rather than those of the trunk (i.e. vertebral).

Peripheral oedema – The abnormal accumulation of fluid in the peripheral (away from the central core of the body) tissues or cavities of the body, such as the legs.

Peripheral quantitative computed tomography – A technique for measuring the density of bones in peripheral areas of the body, usually the wrist. A beam of X-rays is passed through the wrist, and the absorption of X-rays by the wrist bones is analysed using a computer. The data is then used to calculate the bone mineral density.

pH – A measure of the concentration of hydrogen ions (hydrogen atoms with a single positive charge due to the loss of one negatively charged electron) in a solution. The greater the concentration of hydrogen ions, the lower the pH. A pH of less than 7 indicates an acidic solution (high concentration of hydrogen ions), a pH of 7 indicates a neutral solution and a pH of more than 7 indicates an alkaline solution.

Pharmacodynamics – The physiological and biological effects of a drug, including its mechanism of action – the process by which it exerts its therapeutic effects.

Pharmacokinetics – The activity of the drug within the body over a period of time.

Pharmacology – The branch of science that deals with the origin, nature, chemistry, effects and uses of drugs.

Pharmacotherapy – The treatment of a disorder with drugs.

Phosphorus-carbo-phosphorus bond – Containing a carbon atom linked to two phosphorus atoms. Bisphosphonates (a group of non-hormone drugs used in the treatment of osteoporosis) have a central backbone consisting of this grouping of atoms.

Physiotherapy – The treatment of injuries and other disorders using physical methods, such as exercises, massage, heat treatment, ice packs and water. Such treatment is used to reduce joint stiffness and to restore muscle strength after a fracture has healed. It is also used to treat pain, inflammation and muscle spasms, and to retrain joints and muscles after a stroke or nerve injury.

Placebo – An inert substance with no specific pharmacological activity.

Placebo controlled – A clinical trial in which a proportion of patients are given placebo in place of the active drug.

Planar triphenylethylenes – A group of compounds that contain three phenyl rings (a ring of six carbon atoms with five attached hydrogen atoms). The compounds are flat (planar) and rigid in their structure.

Plasma – The acellular fluid in which blood cells are suspended. In the laboratory, it is isolated by the immediate centrifugation (high-speed spinning) of fresh whole blood before clotting has occurred.

Plasma concentrations – The amount of a substance (e.g. a drug) in a given volume of plasma (the fluid component of blood).

Plasma protein binding – The binding of substances that circulate in the blood (e.g. a drug or hormone) to proteins present in the fluid component of blood (plasma), such as albumin.

Pluripotent precursor cells – Cells that have the ability to develop into a number of different cell types.

Polar cross-sectional moment of inertia – The ability of an object to resist being twisted. In bones, this parameter provides an indication of how rigid they are.

Polygenic control – Controlled by a number of genes.

Polymorphism – Existing in a number of different forms.

Polymyalgia rheumatica – An uncommon disease of the elderly characterised by pain and stiffness in the muscles of the hips, thighs, shoulders and neck, especially first thing in the morning. The condition affects twice as many women as men, and is uncommon before the age of 50 years.

Polyvalent cations – Atoms with a double or more positive electrical charge due to the loss of two or more negatively charged electrons. Examples of polyvalent cations include calcium and magnesium ions, which both carry a double positive charge.

Pooled analysis – The amalgamation and processing of data derived from multiple clinical trials.

Porosity – The extent to which a material (e.g. bone) is permeated with pores and cavities through which fluid or air can move.

Posteroanterior spine – From the back to the front of the spine.

***Post hoc* analysis** – Analysis of the data from a completed clinical study to see if any results were obtained that were not specified at the start of the study (i.e. coincidental results).

Postural hypotension – A sudden fall in blood pressure after standing or sitting up quickly. Symptoms include dizziness, lightheadedness, blurred vision and, sometimes, fainting.

Prevalent fracture – A previous or past fracture.

Procollagen I carboxy-terminal – The end of the precursor molecule for collagen type 1 (the main protein in bones and tendons) containing a carboxyl group of atoms (COOH). See also C-terminal propeptide of type 1 procollagen (P1CP).

Progestin – A synthetic form of the hormone progesterone, which is a female sex hormone produced in the ovaries that prepares the uterus to receive a fertilised egg, controls menstruation and maintains pregnancy. It is used to treat abnormal uterine bleeding, to stimulate menstrual cycles and to treat symptoms of the menopause.

Prophylaxis – Preventative treatment. Steps taken to prevent a disease before it occurs.

Protein electrophoresis – A technique for separating the different proteins in a protein mixture. An electric current is passed through a fine gel containing the protein mixture, and each type of protein travels through the gel at a different rate, depending on its electrical charge and size.

Protein isoprenylation – The addition of hydrophobic (does not dissolve in water) molecules to a protein to help the protein attach to the cell membrane.

Protein matrix – The framework or mesh of protein in bone. All other bone material (e.g. osteoblasts, osteoclasts and hydroxyapatite) is embedded in this framework.

Proton pump system – A system for transporting protons (hydrogen ions) from the inside to the outside of a cell across the cell membrane in order to maintain an electrical charge across the cell membrane. The proton pump is a protein (H^+/K^+-ATPase) embedded in the cell membrane. It exchanges hydrogen ions for potassium ions, transporting hydrogen ions out of the cell. It uses energy to do this.

Proximal femur – The part of the femur (thigh bone) closest to the centre of the body. In other words, the top part near the hips as opposed to the lower part near the knee.

Proximal tibia – The part of the tibia (the larger of the two long bones in the lower leg) closest to the centre of the body. In other words, the top part near the knee as opposed to the lower part near the ankle.

Pulmonary embolism – Blockade of the pulmonary artery by a blood clot. This causes shortness of breath, difficulty in breathing and, if left untreated, death.

Pulsatile administration – Given in short bursts or pulses.

Qualitative – Pertaining to the quality of a variable as opposed to the amount. For example, a person's gender, the extent of a disease or the amino acids that make up a particular protein.

Quantitative – Pertaining to the amount of a variable as opposed to the quality. For example, a person's height or the amount of each amino acid in a protein.

Quantitative computed tomography (QCT) – An established technique for measurement of bone mineral density in the axial spine or peripheral skeleton. A beam of X-rays is passed through the part of the body being examined, and the absorption of X-rays by the bone is analysed using a computer. The data is then used to determine in three dimensions the true volumetric density (mg/cm^3) of trabecular or cortical bone.

Quantitative morphometric methods – Techniques that enable the numerical measurement of the shape and structure of an object. For example, quantitative computed tomography (QCT), dual-energy X-ray absorptiometry (DXA) and quantitative ultrasound (QUS) enable the density of bones to be measured.

Quantitative ultrasound (QUS) – The use of high-frequency sound waves (ultrasound) to measure a variable, such as the density of bones. High-frequency sound waves are aimed at the bone being investigated, and the resulting echoes are detected and analysed using a computer. The data is then used to calculate the bone mineral density.

Quinolone antibiotics – A group of antibiotics derived from the substance nalidixic acid. These antibiotics are effective against a wide range of bacteria and are used to treat a variety of bacterial infections. Examples include ciprofloxacin, levofloxacin and moxifloxacin.

R2 side chain – A chain of atoms attached to the central carbon atom in a bisphosphonate drug (drugs used to treat osteoporosis). This central carbon atom is also bonded to another chain of atoms (the R1 side chain) and two phosphorus atoms.

Radial shaft – The main trunk of the radius, which is one of the bones in the lower arm extending from the elbow to the wrist.

Radiographically defined – Clearly characterised by radiography, which is the use of X-rays to form an image of the body on a photographic film.

Radiolabelled – Tagged with a radioactive substance. Commonly used to visualise biological processes *in vivo*.

Random non-fasting glucose value – The amount of sugar in the blood measured in a sample of blood taken at any time of the day and not after the patient has fasted (not eaten).

Ranelic acid – An organic compound that is combined with the element strontium to produce strontium ranelate, a drug used in the treatment of osteoporosis.

Receptor-ligand complex – A molecule bound to a receptor (a protein on the surface of a cell or within a cell that acts as a binding site for a particular molecule and mediates the biological effects of that molecule) through weak chemical bonds.

Recombinant – A biologically active substance formed *in vitro* by the joining together of segments from different sources.

Regression analysis – A statistical technique that is used to analyse data where there are two possible outcomes: yes or no. The technique is used to predict whether a certain variable (e.g. temperature) will affect the outcome.

Remodelling balance – The balance between bone formation and bone resorption (breakdown). If the rate of bone formation is faster than the rate of bone resorption, the bone remodelling balance will be positive. If the rate of bone resorption is faster than the rate of bone formation, the bone remodelling balance will be negative.

Renal – Pertaining to the kidneys.

Renal synthesis – The production of a substance by the kidneys.

Resorption – The breakdown of a substance and the absorption of the breakdown products into the tissues of the body. Commonly used to describe the breakdown of bone in the bone remodeling process.

Retinal vein thrombosis – Blockage, by a blood clot, of the small veins that drain blood from the retina of the eye.

Revascularisations – Improving blood supply to a tissue or organ, usually by joining together functional (patent) blood vessels.

Rheumatoid arthritis – A chronic (long-lasting or recurring) inflammatory disease of the joints in the body caused by the body's immune system attacking the joint tissues. It is characterised by painful, swollen, stiff joints that ultimately lose their ability to work properly.

Ruffled border – An area of the cell membrane of osteoclasts (the cells that break down bone) that has many inward folds. The part of the osteoclast cell membrane lying against the bone develops these inward folds, which then play a role in the process of bone resorption.

Run-in period – A period of time before a clinical trial starts when no treatment is given. This time is used to increase the efficiency of the trial by screening out patients who are unlikely to comply with treatment, by ensuring that patients are in a stable condition and by providing baseline observations.

Sacrum – A triangle of bone at the base of the spine consisting of five fused vertebrae. It connects the spine to the pelvis.

Safety and tolerability – The side-effects associated with a particular drug and the likelihood that patients will tolerate a drug treatment regimen.

Selective oestrogen receptor modulators (SERMs) – Drugs used to treat osteoporosis. They act on the bones in a similar way to oestrogen, slowing bone resorption (breakdown). This helps to maintain bone density and reduce the risk of fracture. The only SERM currently available for the treatment of osteoporosis is raloxifene.

Serum – The clear, straw-coloured, fluid component of blood, after the clotting agents (e.g. fibrinogen and prothrombin) have been removed.

Serum intact N-terminal propeptide – See N-terminal propeptide of type 1 procollagen (P1NP).

Sham-operated – Having undergone a fake or simulated operation. A sham operation is designed to resemble a real operation, and is used as a type of placebo (inactive treatment) in studies that are testing a particular type of operation.

Single blind – A clinical trial in which only the patient is unaware of the treatment allocation.

Single-energy X-ray absorptiometry (SXA) – A technique for measuring the density of bones. It involves passing low-dose X-rays through the bones. The X-rays that emerge are detected and analysed using a computer, and this enables the density of the bones to be calculated.

Single photon absorptiometry (SPA) – A technique for measuring the density of bones. It involves passing a beam of one type of electromagnetic radiation through the bones. The radiation that is not absorbed is detected and analysed using a computer, and this enables the density of the bones to be calculated. The introduction of dual X-ray absorptiometry (DXA) has made SPA largely obsolete.

Skeletal mass – The amount of matter in the skeleton, measured in the same units as weight (e.g. kilograms). Although mass is different from weight, the two terms are often used interchangeably.

Small signalling molecules (GTPases) – Small molecules that play a role in relaying messages within a cell. One such example is the family of enzymes (proteins) known as GTPases.

Socioeconomic impact – Social and economic factors that characterise the influence of a disease. Incorporates the financial cost incurred by the healthcare provider, patient and/or their employer.

Stable non-radioactive strontium – A form of the chemical element strontium that does not spontaneously emit radiation (energy in the form of particles or rays).

Statistical significance – A measure of the probability that a given result derived from a clinical trial – be it an improvement or a decline in the health of the patient – is due to a specific effect of drug treatment, rather than a chance occurrence.

Steady state – A condition whereby all the components of a system remain at a constant concentration and do not fluctuate. For example, the steady-state concentration of a drug in the blood is the concentration at which drug levels are constant.

Steroid – A lipid (fat-like) molecule with a basic skeleton consisting of four interconnected carbon rings. Examples of steroids include the sex hormones, the corticosteroid hormones produced by the adrenal glands, vitamin D and cholesterol.

Subcutaneous injection – Use of a syringe and needle to push fluids or drugs into the body just beneath the skin.

Subcutaneous nodules – Small lumps just beneath the skin.

Surrogate markers – Laboratory or physical parameters that are used as a substitute for a direct biological measurement, such as how a patient feels, or how effective a particular treatment is.

Synergy – An interaction between two or more agents (e.g. drugs) such that the effect produced is greater than the effects of the agents on their own.

Systemic – Pertaining to or affecting the entire body. Systemic treatment is treatment that reaches and affects cells throughout the body.

Tai Chi – A traditional form of Chinese exercise combining mental concentration, slow breathing and slow, gentle movements. The idea is to promote the flow of internal energy (chi) to give health benefits, such as improved co-ordination and well-being, stress relief and a stronger immune system.

Target cells – The cells in the body upon which a particular molecule or chemical acts.

Tertiary nitrogen atom – A nitrogen atom that is attached by chemical bonds to three carbon atoms.

Tertile – One-third of a particular population.

Testosterone – Male sex hormone (androgen) secreted by cells of the testis and responsible for triggering the development of sperm and other secondary sexual characteristics.

Tetracycline – An antibiotic that is effective against a wide range of bacteria.

Third distal radius – A particular region of the radius, which is one of the bones in the lower arm extending from the elbow to the wrist. The distal radius is the part of the radius furthest from the elbow and this region itself is further divided into three regions. The third distal radius is the third of the distal radius that is closest to the elbow.

Thoracic spine region – The part of the spine consisting of twelve thoracic vertebrae. These are located in the chest region between the cervical (neck) vertebrae and the lumbar (lower back) vertebrae.

Thromboembolic disease – The blockage of a blood vessel by a fragment of a blood clot that has broken off and been carried around in the circulating blood.

Thyroid C cells – One of the two types of cell found in the thyroid gland. Also known as the parafollicular cells, the C cells secrete the hormone calcitonin, which plays a role in the regulation of blood calcium levels.

Thyroid profile – The measurement of blood levels of the thyroid hormones tri-iodothyronine (T_3) and thyroxine (T_4), and thyroid stimulating hormone (TSH), which is a hormone produced by the pituitary gland that stimulates the thyroid gland to secrete T_3 and T_4.

Tibial metaphysic – A layer of cartilage (a type of connective tissue) between the ends of the tibia (the shin bone) and its main shaft.

Torsional loading – An uneven load that causes twisting of an object.

Trabecular architecture – The structure of the soft, spongy, mesh-like inner layer of bone.

Trabecular bone – The soft, spongy, mesh-like, inner layer of bone. The spaces in this type of bone contain bone marrow, where red and white blood cells are made.

Transforming growth factor (TGF)-β3 – One of a family of small proteins that regulates growth and differentiation in a variety of cells. TGF-β3 is thought to play a role in the growth and development of osteoblasts (bone forming cells), the production of collagen (the main protein in bone) and wound repair.

Trauma – Physical injury or a wound caused by an external force or violence.

Trochanter – One of two bumps of bone near the top of the femur (thigh bone) to which muscles attach.

T-score – A number that shows how dense a person's bones are in comparison to a young adult of the same gender. It is essentially bone mineral density quoted as the number of standard deviations from the mean bone mineral density in a young adult of the same gender. A score above –1 is considered normal. A score between –1 and –2.5 is classified as osteopenia (bones less dense than normal) and a score below –2.5 is defined as osteoporosis.

Tubular reabsorption – The reuptake by the kidneys of useful substances (e.g. sodium, water, glucose, amino acids, small proteins) that have been filtered out of the blood into the nephrons (the functional units of the kidneys) ready for excretion. These substances then pass back into the blood circulation.

Tunnelling resorption – A pattern of bone loss observed in certain disorders, such as hyperparathyroidism (abnormally high levels of parathyroid hormone). Cortical bone (the hard, outer layer of bone) is lost in such a way that a pattern of tunnels or grooves is observed in the bone.

Type 1 collagen – The main protein found in bones and tendons. There are twelve different types of collagen in the body (types 1–12), and type 1 is the most abundant.

Type 1 diabetes – A disease in which the body is unable to regulate the amount of glucose (sugar) in the blood because it does not produce enough insulin (the hormone produced by the pancreas that reduces blood glucose levels when they are high). The disease is caused by the destruction of the cells in the pancreas that normally produce insulin. It usually develops in childhood or adolescence but may appear at any age. This form of diabetes is also known as insulin-dependent diabetes.

Type 2 diabetes – A disease in which the body is unable to regulate the amount of glucose (sugar) in the blood because it does not respond to insulin (the hormone produced by the pancreas that reduces blood glucose levels when they are high) or the amount of insulin produced is too low. Type 2 diabetes usually develops later in life, and is also known as late-onset diabetes or non-insulin dependent diabetes mellitus. In most cases, insulin injections are unnecessary and the disease can be controlled by appropriate diet, weight loss and oral medication.

Ulcerative colitis – A disease characterised by inflammation and ulceration of the inner lining of the colon and rectum (the lower sections of the digestive tract). Symptoms include bloody diarrhoea, abdominal discomfort, loss of appetite and weight loss.

Ulna proximal – The part of the ulna (one of the two long bones in the lower arm) that is closest to the centre of the body. In other words, the part nearest the elbow as opposed to the part nearest the wrist.

Ultra distal – A particular region of a long bone. The distal region of a long bone is the part of the bone furthest from the centre of the body (i.e. the lower end of the bone), and this region itself is further divided into three regions. The ultra distal region is the third of the distal region that is furthest from the centre of the body (i.e. the lowest third of the distal region).

Upper gastrointestinal mucosa – The soft, pink lining of the upper digestive tract, which consists of the oesophagus, stomach and first part of the small intestine. The main functions of the mucosa are to give protection and support to the underlying structures, to absorb nutrients and to secrete mucus, enzymes and salts.

Upper-gastrointestinal endoscopy – Examination of the upper digestive tract (the oesophagus, stomach and first part of the small intestine) using a thin, flexible, lighted tube.

Upregulation – An increase in the number of receptors for a certain chemical on the cell surface. This leads to an increase in the response that normally occurs when the relevant chemical binds to the receptor.

Urea nitrogen – The nitrogen found in urea (a chemical produced by the breakdown of proteins). This is different from the nitrogen found in blood proteins and serum levels of urea nitrogen provide a marker of kidney and liver function.

Uric acid – A substance found in blood and urine that is a waste product of protein breakdown. High blood levels of uric acid may lead to deposits of uric acid in the joints, a painful condition called gout.

Urinary C-telopeptide – See Cross-linked C-terminal telopeptides of type 1 collagen (CTX).

Urinary hydroxyproline excretion – The removal of hydroxyproline from the body via the kidneys and urine. Hydroxyproline is an amino acid (the building blocks of proteins) found only in collagen (the main protein in bone). Blood and urinary levels of this amino acid can be used as a marker of bone resorption (breakdown).

Urolithiasis – Another name for kidney stones, which are hard deposits of substances normally found in urine, such as calcium, magnesium, phosphate and uric acid. Kidney stones may form in the kidneys or ureters (the narrow tubes that carry urine from the kidneys to the bladder) and can vary in size from a grain of sand to a golf ball.

Vasculitis – Inflammation of the blood vessels.

Vasomotor – Pertaining to the nerves and muscles that control narrowing and widening of the blood vessels.

Vasomotor events – Symptoms caused by widening or narrowing of the blood vessels, such as fainting, hot flushes and night sweats.

Venous thromboembolism – The blockage of a vein lying deep in the legs or pelvis by a blood clot. This may be accompanied by a pulmonary embolism, which is the blockage of the arteries in the lungs leading to difficulty in breathing and, possibly, respiratory failure. A pulmonary embolism is caused by the breaking off of a fragment of a blood clot in the deep veins of the leg, which then travels in the bloodstream to the lungs and lodges in the arteries supplying blood to the lungs.

Vertebral cancellous bone – The soft, spongy, mesh-like, inner layer of bone (also known as trabecular bone) in the vertebrae, which are the bones that make up the spinal column.

Vertebral fracture – A split or break in one of the vertebrae, which are the bones that make up the spinal column.

Vitamin D synthesis – The production of vitamin D in the body due to the action of sunlight on the skin. Vitamin D can also be obtained from certain foods, such as dairy products, egg yolk, liver and fish. Vitamin D is necessary for the body to absorb calcium. If a person is deficient in vitamin D, the body will take calcium from the bones.

Vitamin K – A vitamin that is essential for the normal clotting of blood, for the absorption of calcium and proper bone growth, for normal functioning of the liver and for the storage of sugar in the body. It is produced by bacteria that live in the human gastrointestinal tract, and is also found in leafy green vegetables, tomatoes and egg yolk.

Volumetric bone mineral density – The amount of bone tissue in a given volume of bone, measured in grams per cubic centimetre (g/cm^3).

Walter Reed Performance Assessment Battery (PAB) – A series of computerised psychological tests that are used to determine the effects of various factors on mental ability.

Wash-out – A period of time during a clinical trial when the participants do not receive any treatment so that the variables being evaluated (e.g. blood pressure) can return to their normal values.

Useful contacts

The organisations listed below represent an accurate cross-section of what we believe to be reliable and up-to-date sources of information on osteoporosis and its management.

National Osteoporosis Society

Camerton
Bath
BA2 0PJ
Osteoporosis helpline: 0845 450 0230
Email: *nurses@nos.org.uk*
Website: *www.nos.org.uk*
**UK patient support group
and registered charity**

International Osteoporosis Foundation

73 cours Albert-Thomas
69447 Lyon Cedex 03
France
Email: *info@osteofound.org*
Website: *www.osteofound.org*
Independent professional organisation

International Bone and Mineral Society

Email: *info@ibmsonline.org*
Website: *www.ibmsonline.org*
Independent professional organisation

The British Pain Society

21 Portland Place
London W1B 1PY
United Kingdom
Tel: 02076 31 8870
Email: *info@britishpainsociety.org*
Website: *www.britishpainsociety.org*
Registered charity

The Bone and Tooth Society

Website: *www.batsoc.org.uk*
Independent professional organisation and registered charity

Best Treatments UK

Website: *www.besttreatments.co.uk/btuk/home.html*
Produced by the British Medical Association

BBC health website

www.bbc.co.uk/health

NHS Direct

Website: *www.nhsdirect.nhs.uk*

Index

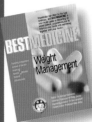
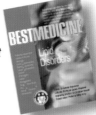
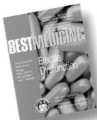
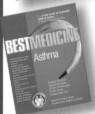
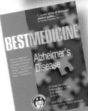
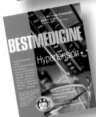
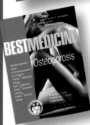
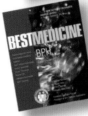
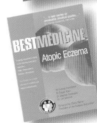
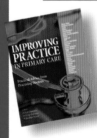
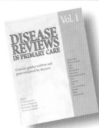
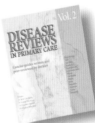
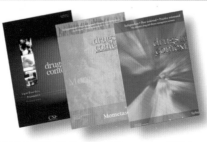